Strength Training

SECOND EDITION

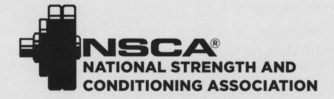

NSCA®
NATIONAL STRENGTH AND
CONDITIONING ASSOCIATION

Lee E. Brown

Editor

HUMAN KINETICS

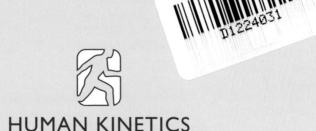

Library of Congress Cataloging-in-Publication Data

Names: Brown, Lee E., 1956- editor. | National Strength & Conditioning
    Association (U.S.)
Title: Strength training / National Strength and Conditioning Association ;
    Lee E. Brown, editor.
Description: Second edition. | Champaign, IL : Human Kinetics, [2017] |
    Includes bibliographical references and index.
Identifiers: LCCN 2016043063 | ISBN 9781492522089 (print) | ISBN 9781492542803 (ebook)
Subjects: LCSH: Physical education and training. | Muscle strength. |
    Physical fitness--Physiological aspects.
Classification: LCC GV711.5 .S775 2017 | DDC 613.7--dc23 LC record available at https://lccn.loc.
gov/2016043063

ISBN: 978-1-4925-2208-9 (print)

The web addresses cited in this text were current as of August 2016, unless otherwise noted.

Acquisitions Editor: Justin Klug; **Senior Managing Editor:** Amy Stahl; **Copyeditor:** Mandy Eastin-Allen; **Indexer:** Alisha Jeddeloh; **Permissions Manager:** Dalene Reeder; **Senior Graphic Designer:** Nancy Rasmus; **Cover Designer:** Keith Blomberg; **Photograph (cover):** © Human Kinetics; **Photographs (interior):** Neil Bernstein, unless otherwise noted; **Photo Asset Manager:** Laura Fitch; **Visual Production Assistant:** Joyce Brumfield; **Photo Production Manager:** Jason Allen; **Senior Art Manager:** Kelly Hendren; **Illustrations:** © Human Kinetics, unless otherwise noted; **Printer:** Versa Press

We thank the National Strength and Conditioning Association in Colorado Springs, Colorado, and The Fitness Center in Champaign, Illinois, for assistance in providing a location for a photo shoot for this book.

Printed in the United States of America   10   9   8   7   6   5   4   3   2   1

The paper in this book is certified under a sustainable forestry program.

Human Kinetics
Website: www.HumanKinetics.com

United States: Human Kinetics
P.O. Box 5076
Champaign, IL 61825-5076
800-747-4457
e-mail: info@hkusa.com

Canada: Human Kinetics
475 Devonshire Road Unit 100
Windsor, ON N8Y 2L5
800-465-7301 (in Canada only)
e-mail: info@hkcanada.com

Europe: Human Kinetics
107 Bradford Road
Stanningley
Leeds LS28 6AT, United Kingdom
+44 (0) 113 255 5665
e-mail: hk@hkeurope.com

Australia: Human Kinetics
57A Price Avenue
Lower Mitcham, South Australia 5062
08 8372 0999
e-mail: info@hkaustralia.com

New Zealand: Human Kinetics
P.O. Box 80
Mitcham Shopping Centre, South
Australia 5062
0800 222 062
e-mail: info@hknewzealand.com

E6705

Strength Training

SECOND EDITION

Contents

PART III Exercise Technique

PART IV Sample Programs

Preface

We are pleased you have chosen this book for your strength training needs. Our purpose is to provide you with information on strength training that is supported by the latest scientific research. Each chapter is written by an expert in the field. This entire book fills a need for a science-based examination of strength training for those who want to know the best way to build strength. The information herein is supported by the National Strength and Conditioning Association, a worldwide authority on strength and conditioning.

We have organized the book in a way that will facilitate your progress in understanding and building a complete strength training program. In part I, you will benefit from a detailed explanation of the scientific foundation of strength. You will find a description of muscle anatomy as well as information on how you can maximize your training program by identifying training variables. Part II provides information on assessing your strength and power and interpreting the results of such tests. It also covers ways to prevent injury while strength training so that you can correctly design your workout schedule. The heart of this book is part III, which presents comprehensive exercise techniques through pictures and instructions for all major muscles in the upper body, lower body, and core. Part III concludes with a section on explosive power training movements. In part IV, sample programs are provided for beginners through advanced strength trainers as well as for youths and seniors.

We hope you will find the unique features of this book, including the detailed photos of the start and midpoint of each exercise and the sample training programs, helpful in your search for strength training knowledge to help you attain your fitness goals.

PART I

The Origin of Strength

This part of the book focuses on the science of strength and its foundation. First you need to understand how muscles work and develop in order to plan your strength training program. Chapters 1 through 4 introduce you to many fundamental aspects of muscle physiology, various forms of program design, and proper nutrition for enhancing muscle growth.

Chapter 1, "Muscle Anatomy 101," discusses the various types of muscles and their function as well as muscular contraction and recruitment. This information will allow you to choose exercises targeted for specific body parts as well as to understand the benefits of different types of movements such as pushing and pulling exercises.

Chapter 2, "How Muscle Grows," lays the physiological foundation of the muscular adaptation process. This information is important when you are designing your strength training program because it will guide you in choosing the correct exercises and rest intervals according to your training needs.

Chapter 3, "Types of Muscle Training," introduces the program variables included in a resistance training regimen. It also presents various types of training programs and modalities so you can choose the right workout for you. Finally, it makes recommendations for your training program as they relate to your purpose for exercising.

Chapter 4, "Nutrition for Muscle Growth," describes your body's metabolism, how it works, and how you can maximize your efforts to enhance your strength. It further illustrates how food and water interact in your body to provide fuel for maximum muscle development.

Muscle Anatomy 101

William J. Kraemer and Jakob L. Vingren

When trying to prescribe various types of strength training protocols, it is important to understand the body's fundamental structures that help mediate the body's different functions. Thus, understanding the basic anatomy of the body is fundamental to knowing how the body works. The general architecture of skeletal muscles as a whole—as well as the specific composition of individual muscles—determines how each muscle functions. Many of the training principles described throughout this book are based on this knowledge; thus, learning some basic anatomy will help you better understand these training principles and how to use them in strength training.

About 40 percent of the body's tissues are made up of skeletal muscle (based on mass). Skeletal muscles are the muscles that are attached to bones and produce movement across joints. We start at the smallest anatomical level of the muscle—the proteins that make up each muscle fiber—and gradually expand on each structure to show how they all come together to make an intact, functioning muscle. We include an overview of the muscle anatomy of the human body along with the functions of the major muscle groups.

This chapter also covers how a muscle is stimulated by the nervous system. As you will see, this is important in strength training because only those muscles that are stimulated by exercise will be trained and, thus, developed. In addition, we explain the principles of how different resistance loads stimulate different amounts of muscle due to the activation of different types of muscle fibers in the muscle. Finally, we cover different types of muscle action and how these actions, along with the structures of the muscle, affect force and power production.

Muscle Organization

Skeletal muscle consists of many noncontractile proteins that provide the optimal structural alignment of the contractile proteins, actin and myosin, which are vital for muscle function. As noted in figure 1.1, a variety of noncontractile proteins provide a latticework that structurally holds in place the contractile proteins,

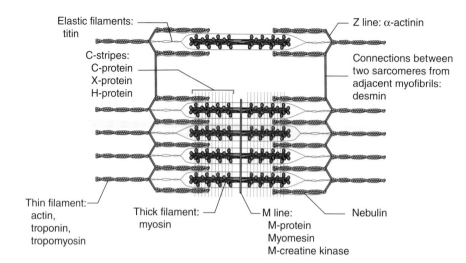

FIGURE 1.1 The sarcomere is made up of a latticework of noncontractile proteins that hold the two contractile proteins, actin and myosin, in place for optimal interactions during muscle force production.

thereby allowing strict spatial orientations for optimal interactions and muscle force and power production.

The smallest contractile unit in the muscle is called a *sarcomere*. The sarcomere is made up of various noncontractile proteins (e.g., titin, nebulin, Z proteins, and so on; see figure 1.1 for the array of noncontractile proteins) as well as the two contractile proteins, actin and myosin, which produce the various muscle actions and associated force and power output. Myofibrils make up a single muscle fiber, also called a *muscle cell*. The muscle fibers are grouped together into bundles, and these bundles of muscle fibers make up the intact muscle. Figure 1.2 shows different types of connective tissue, called *fascia*, that surround the bundles of muscle fibers and the muscle itself.

The noncontractile proteins and connective tissue found in muscle are what create the elastic component in muscle. Just as a rubber band stretches and then recoils, so too can the connective tissue stretch and recoil, adding greater force to the shortening of the muscle. This is part of the stretch–shortening cycle of the muscle, which consists of an eccentric elongation followed by a rapid concentric shortening of the muscle. The noncontractile proteins in the muscle and the connective tissue wrapping the muscle all contribute to the elastic component of the muscle, which can contribute an additional 15 to 30 percent to power production when brought into play using the stretch–shortening cycle (Kraemer et al. 2016). The reason that plyometric training, such as bounding exercises or depth jumps, is so effective in improving muscular power is that it trains this elastic component in muscle (i.e., the stretch–shortening cycle).

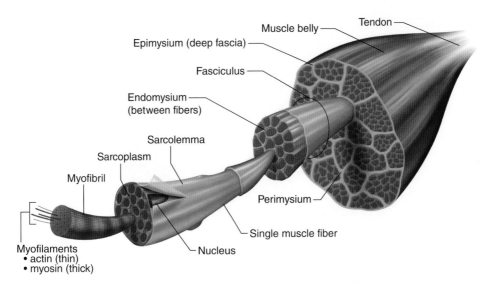

FIGURE 1.2 Tendons attach the muscles to the bones, allowing muscles to cause movement. The intact whole muscle is made up of bundles of muscle fibers, each with a connective tissue sheath surrounding it. A muscle fiber is made up of myofibrils, which contain many different contractile proteins. The key contractile proteins in the myofibrils of the muscle are actin and myosin.

Sarcomere

The sarcomere is the basic contractile unit of skeletal muscle, and all force produced in human movement starts with the fundamental interactions of actin and myosin within this small element of the muscle. A sarcomere runs from one Z line to the next Z line and is the smallest functional unit in the muscle that can shorten. Each sarcomere contains several distinct light and dark areas. These areas give skeletal muscle a striped or striated appearance when examined under a special microscope (figure 1.3); because of this, skeletal muscle is also called *striated muscle*. These light and dark areas reflect the arrangement of the actin and myosin filaments. The light areas represent the H zone, which contains no actin and only a small amount of myosin. The I bands are at the ends of the sarcomere and contain only actin filaments. The dark areas, which represent the A bands, contain both actin and myosin filaments in an overlapping region. Sarcomeres are attached to each other longitudinally at the Z line to form a myofibril. Many myofibrils stacked parallel to each other make up a muscle fiber (refer back to figure 1.2).

Contraction essentially shortens the sarcomere—the myosin protein is stationary, and cross bridges coming from the myosin filaments pull the actin filaments together from opposing directions, causing the actin to move over the myosin. Amazingly, this process, called the *sliding filament theory*, was first described

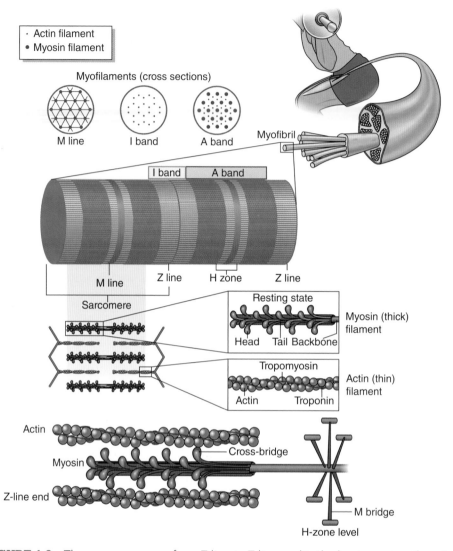

FIGURE 1.3   The sarcomere runs from Z line to Z line and is the basic contractile unit of the muscle. The interactions of the actin and myosin create force production that causes the muscle to contract.

independently in 1954 by two research teams, one consisting of Andrew F. Huxley and Rolf Niedergerke from the University of Cambridge and the other consisting of Hugh Huxley and Jean Hanson from the Massachusetts Institute of Technology. They eloquently showed that force actually is produced by muscle through the interactions of the actin and myosin filaments—an incredible discovery in the 20th century. This is discussed in greater detail later in the chapter.

Muscle Fibers

Skeletal muscle is made up of thousands of muscle fibers ranging in length from about 1.9 to 3.5 inches (3-9 cm); in shorter muscles, such as the biceps, some fibers run all the way from the origin to the insertion. Connective tissue binds the muscle fibers and blood vessels in place, and nerves run through this tissue. Muscle fibers are unique in that they are individual cells with multiple nuclei that contain the DNA material of the cell. This provides the muscle fiber with greater potential for both repair and hypertrophy via protein synthesis because each nucleus regulates only a small section of the cell.

Muscle fibers come in two basic types: Type I (also called *slow-twitch fibers*) and Type II (also called *fast-twitch fibers*). In addition, each of these types has various subtypes that we do not discuss in this chapter (for a complete review, see Fleck and Kraemer 2014; Kraemer et al. 2016). Type I fibers have a high oxidative capacity (i.e., high aerobic capability) and are made for endurance, with lower contractile force capabilities. Type II fibers, on the other hand, have a high glycolytic capacity and are made for strength and power, with high contractile force capabilities. The percentage of Type I and Type II muscle fibers in the body varies for each person and in each muscle; for example, postural muscles such as the abdominals have a high percentage of Type I muscle fibers. These percentages reflect the role of the muscle in human movement. Genetics dictate the percentage of Type I or Type II fibers in a muscle. Interestingly, training contributes only to the gain potential of a given muscle fiber for a specific characteristic (e.g., oxidative potential, fiber size, enzyme content, and so on). We now know that an individual cannot alter the percentage of Type I or Type II muscle fibers he or she possesses. Nor can an individual significantly increase the number of muscle fibers, despite the long debate on hypertrophy (increase in muscle fiber size) versus hyperplasia (increase in muscle fiber number) that raged in the 1970s and 1980s. Thus, because an athlete cannot change his or her muscle fiber type, the terms *aerobic athlete* and *strength power athlete* have surfaced over the past decade. As noted before, different muscles in the body have different percentages of Type I and Type II muscle fibers. Additionally, no significant differences in fiber type have been observed between men and women when appropriate comparisons are made between the sexes (e.g., elite distance runners for both sexes). However, if one compares similar populations of men and women, men generally have a higher number of muscle fibers (especially in the upper-body musculature) and larger muscle fibers.

As noted earlier, different athletes have different fiber type profiles that explain, in part, their unique abilities in a given event or sport. For example, elite endurance athletes have higher percentages of Type I muscle fibers in their lower-body musculature (i.e., thigh and leg muscles), whereas elite weightlifters and powerlifters have higher percentages of Type II muscle fibers, except for muscles dedicated to postural control where everybody has Type I muscle fibers.

This difference in muscle fiber composition is due to the genetic predispositions of these athletes, who are able to excel at their respective sport in part because of the fiber types they were born with. Although training may cause a small change in fiber type composition (or what is called fiber transitions within a subtype), the major reason for improved performance is the increase in the fiber size of the muscle fibers all contributing to the increase in the actual muscle and the improved metabolic pathways. Again, a person cannot change his or her inherent fiber type through training; that is, a person cannot change Type I muscle fibers to Type II muscle fibers. However, fiber subtype transitions (e.g., Type IIX to Type IIA) occurs with training when motor units are trained in the exercise. Regardless of whether the athlete trains for strength or endurance, the fiber subtype change appears to go strictly in the direction of increasing the oxidative capacity of the fibers. For example, Type IIX fibers (fast-twitch glycolytic) are converted to Type IIA fibers (fast-twitch oxidative glycolytic) through either resistance or endurance training. It may seem counterintuitive that resistance training will make muscle fibers more oxidative; however, the resistance training per se may not be making the fibers more oxidative as much as restoring the fibers from an untrained state to a more conditioned and functional state. The magnitude of this transformation, however, will not be sufficient to create the fiber type compositions seen in elite athletes unless the genetic predisposition is already present in the individual.

Figure 1.4 shows how these different fibers are classified under a microscope using staining or coloring of the muscle fibers to differentiate between Type I and Type II fibers. Depending on the fiber type makeup, each person has different genetically determined strength, power, and endurance capabilities. Because Type I fibers cannot be converted to Type II fibers (and vice versa) through training, a person cannot develop a training program to change the overall fiber type composition. However, as discussed later in this chapter, altering training loads and movement speeds changes the involvement of the muscle fiber types affecting force production capabilities.

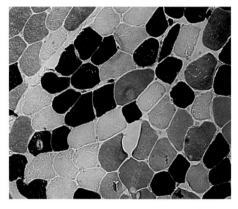

FIGURE 1.4 Muscles can be artificially stained in the laboratory to produce different-colored fibers in order to classify what percentage of Type I and Type II muscle fibers exist in the muscle. In this picture, Type I muscle fibers are black and Type II muscle fibers are light gray (Type IIA) and dark gray (Type IIX).

Reprinted, from J. Wilmore and D. Costill, 2004, *Physiology of sport and exercise*, 2nd ed. (Champaign, IL: Human Kinetics), 39. By permission of D. Costill.

Motor Units

The activation or recruitment of muscle tissue is a key factor in any exercise program, especially resistance training. The greater the activation of muscle tissue, the greater the force exerted. Muscle fibers are recruited when the nervous system activates muscle tissue via the activation of motor units. How motor units are recruited is reflected in the size principle (discussed later in this chapter), which is vital to understanding resistance exercise and training—or all exercise training programs, for that matter.

Muscle activation or recruitment starts with the motor unit. A motor unit is inclusive of the alpha motoneuron and all the muscle fibers it stimulates or activates to produce force. A motor unit comprises either all Type I (slow twitch) or all Type II (fast twitch) muscle fibers; no motor units contain mixed muscle fiber types.

The muscle fibers in a motor unit are not all located adjacent to each other but rather are spread out in the muscle in microbundles of about 3 to 15 fibers. Thus, adjacent muscle fibers do not necessarily belong to the same motor unit. Because of how the fibers of a motor unit are spread out within a muscle, fibers are activated throughout the whole muscle when a motor unit is activated. If fibers of a motor unit were all adjacent to each other, activating that motor unit would appear to stimulate only one segment of the muscle. When a muscle moves, those motor units that are not activated (and their associated muscle fibers) do not generate force; rather, they move passively through the range of motion as the muscle moves to follow the activated motor units.

Muscles of the Body

The body contains more than 600 skeletal muscles varying in size, shape, and use (figure 1.5, *a* and *b*). The major purpose of skeletal muscles is to provide force to move the joints of the body in the different directions or planes in which they are designed to move. Many joints, such as knee and finger joints, are hinge joints that can be moved in only one plane—they can extend and flex. Other joints, such as the hip and shoulder joints, are ball-and-socket joints that can move in all planes—extend, flex, adduct, and abduct—as well as rotate. Each joint generally has one or more muscles for each of the movements it can perform. These muscles or muscle groups are usually paired so they have opposite functions to each other; if one causes flexion of the joint, the other causes extension. This arrangement is required because muscles can produce only an active shortening and not a lengthening of themselves. Thus, two muscles or muscle groups with opposite functions are required for each dimension or plane in which a joint can move.

The muscles that are the primary movers of a joint in one direction are called the *agonists* for that movement, and muscles that assist in that movement are called *synergists*. Muscles that can oppose a movement are called *antagonists* to that movement. For example, during an arm curl the biceps brachii and the brachialis are the agonists, the brachioradialis is a synergist, and the triceps brachii is an antagonist to the movement.

A muscle usually is connected to the bones it acts on via two kinds of attachment sites. One site is called the *origin* of the muscle. The origin can be either

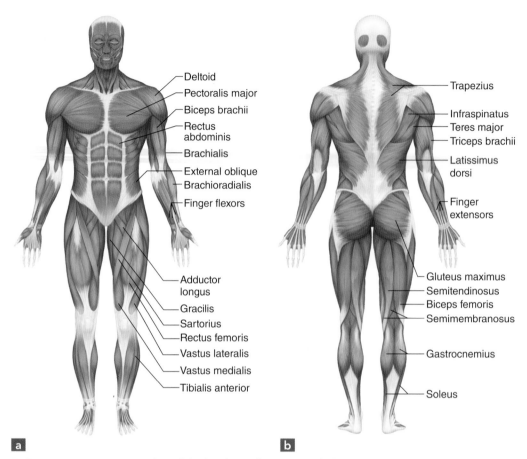

FIGURE 1.5 Major muscles of the body: (*a*) front view, (*b*) back view.

a small, distinct site on a bone or a large area covering most of the length of the bone. The origin is generally on the bone closest to the core of the body. The other attachment site for the muscle is called the *insertion*. This end of the muscle usually is connected to a tendon that spans the joint on which the muscle functions. A muscle can have more than one origin or insertion; in such cases, the muscle is divided into segments called *heads*. This allows the muscle to fine tune its function (when heads function on the same joint but at slightly different angles) or to span more than one joint while still affecting these joints independently of each other. The triceps brachii, for instance, has three heads that all function across the elbow joint, whereas only two of its heads function across the shoulder joint.

Figure 1.5, *a* and *b*, and tables 1.1 and 1.2 present the major muscles of the human body that are involved in resistance exercise. Note that some muscles consist of several heads, or segments, that attach on different sites on the body and that some muscles span more than one joint. These features give the muscles

TABLE 1.1 Major Muscles in the Body and Their Origin, Insertion, and Function

Muscle name	Origin	Insertion	Function
Abductors (tensor fasciae latae, gluteus medius, gluteus minimus)	Ilium	Femur	Moves hip sideways away from body
Adductors (adductor longus, adductor brevis, adductor magnus)	Pubis	Femur	Moves leg back and across body sideways
Biceps brachii	Scapula	Radius and ulna	Flexes elbow and moves forearm
Brachialis	Humerus and septum	Coronoid process and ulna	Flexes elbow
Brachioradialis	Humerus and septum	Radius	Flexes and rotates elbow
Deltoids	Clavicle, deltoid tuberosity, acromion, and scapula	Deltoid tuberosity (humerus)	Raises and rotates arm in all directions
Erector spinae	Sacrum and ilium	Upper thoracic vertebrae	Extends spine and trunk backward
Gastrocnemius (calf muscle)	Femur, lower leg, and back	Calcaneum (by Achilles tendon)	Raises heel when leg is straight
Gluteus maximus	Ilium	Femur	Moves hips forward
Hamstrings (made of 3 muscles): 1. Biceps femoris 2. Semitendinosus 3. Semimembranosus	1. Ischium 2. Ischium 3. Ischium	1. Fibula and femur 2. Tibia 3. Tibia	1. Bends knee 2. Bends knee 3. Bends knee
Iliopsoas	Ilium, sacrum, and thoracic and lumbar vertebrae	Femur	Moves hips backward
Latissimus dorsi	Lower thoracic and lumbar vertebrae and sacrum	Humerus	Moves shoulders and arms back to body
Pectoralis major and minor	Sternum	Humerus	Moves humerus (arm) to chest
Quadriceps (made of 4 muscles): 1. Rectus femoris 2. Vastus lateralis 3. Vastus medialis 4. Vastus intermedius	1. Ilium 2. Femur 3. Femur 4. Femur	1. Tibia (patella tendon) 2. Tibia (patella tendon) 3. Tibia (patella tendon) 4. Tibia (patella tendon)	1. Extends leg out 2. Extends knee 3. Extends knee 4. Extends knee

> *continued*

TABLE 1.1 > *continued*

Muscle name	Origin	Insertion	Function
Rectus abdominis	Costal cartilages and medial inferior costal	Margin and xiphoid	Brings trunk forward and aids expiration
Rhomboids	Upper thoracic vertebrae	Scapula	Pulls back scapula (shoulder blade)
Soleus (calf muscles)	Tibia and fibula	Calcaneum (by Achilles tendon)	Raises heel when leg is bent
Tibialis anterior	Tibia	First metatarsal (big toe)	Raises front of foot
Trapezius	Starts at base of skull; ends at last thoracic vertebra	Scapula and clavicle elevation	Elevates and lowers pectoral girdle; moves scapula toward spine
Triceps brachii	Scapula and humerus	Olecranon process (elbow)	Extends forearm

TABLE 1.2   Major Resistance Exercises and the Muscles Involved

Exercise	Muscles used
Barbell bench press	Pectoralis major, anterior deltoid, triceps brachii
Barbell incline bench press	Pectoralis major, anterior deltoid, triceps brachii
Dumbbell biceps curl	Biceps brachii
Machine seated triceps push-down	Triceps brachii
Standing military press	Deltoids, triceps brachii
Lat pull-down	Latissimus dorsi, biceps brachii
Cable seated row	Latissimus dorsi, trapezius, posterior deltoid, biceps brachii
Barbell shrug	Upper trapezius, levator scapulae
Bent-knee sit-up	Rectus abdominis
Back squat	Gluteals, hamstrings, quadriceps
Leg extension	Quadriceps
Seated leg curl	Hamstrings
Leg press	Gluteals, quadriceps, hamstrings
Calf raise	Gastrocnemius, soleus
Back extension	Erector spinae, gluteals, hamstrings

The muscles are listed in order of their involvement in the exercise. Only the agonists and major synergists to each exercise are listed.

added function. The quadriceps, for example, does not only extend the knee: One of its heads (medial) also keeps the kneecap (patella) in place during leg extensions, and another head (long) is involved in movements of the hip.

Muscle Actions

The Huxley sliding filament theory (for a complete review see Huxley 2004; see also Kraemer et al. 2016) attempts to explain how the muscle fibers produce force. This production of force starts at the level of the sarcomere through the interactions of the two major contractile proteins (i.e., actin and myosin; see figure 1.3).

As discussed early in the chapter, in the relaxed state, the muscle has a striated appearance. When muscle is in the contracted (fully shortened) state there are still striations of the muscle tissue, but they have a different pattern. This change in the striation pattern occurs because of the sliding of the actin over the myosin protein filaments. The actins are anchored to the Z line at each end of the sarcomere. Upon muscle contraction, the A bands maintain their length but the I bands shorten, pulling the Z lines closer together. This causes the H zone to diminish as actin filaments slide into it and give it a darker appearance. The I bands become shorter as the Z lines move closer to the ends of the myosin filaments. When the sarcomere relaxes and returns to its original length, the H zone and I bands return to their original size and appearance (figure 1.6, *a* through *d*).

The neural signals involved in muscle contraction converge in the zoma—the body of the alpha motor neuron located in the spinal cord. This neuron can be stimulated (or inhibited) from the central nervous system and from sensory and reflex neurons. If the sum of the stimuli is sufficient to create an electric signal that is sufficiently large enough to meet the stimulatory electrical threshold for the motor unit (i.e., depolarization) in the zoma, this signal (i.e., action potential) then propagates along the axon of the efferent motor neuron to the neuromuscular junction. Here the signal causes the release of a chemical neurotransmitter, acetylcholine (ACh), from the nerve ending. The ACh subsequently travels across the junction to the outer membrane of the muscle fiber (sarcolemma). When ACh reaches the sarcolemma, it attaches to ACh receptors, causing a depolarization of the sarcolemma; the signal has now reached the muscle fiber. The signal then spreads rapidly throughout the surface of the muscle fiber. This ionic current triggers the release of calcium ions ($Ca++$) from the sarcoplasmic reticulum into the interior fluid of the muscle fiber. The sarcoplasmic reticulum is a membranous structure that surrounds each muscle fiber and acts as a storage space for $Ca++$. The released $Ca++$ binds to the troponin molecule; this triggers a change in the arrangement of troponin and tropomyosin so that the active sites on the actin become exposed, allowing binding of the myosin cross bridges. This is referred to as the *excitation-coupling phase* of the contraction process (figure 1.7).

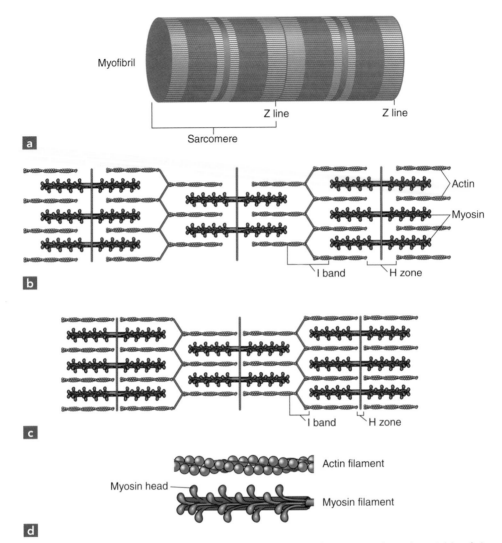

Myofibril

Z line   Z line

Sarcomere

a

Actin

Myosin

I band   H zone

b

I band   H zone

c

Myosin head

Actin filament

Myosin filament

d

FIGURE 1.6   As a muscle contracts, the Z lines move closer together, the width of the I bands decreases, and the width of the H zones decreases, but no change occurs in the width of the A band. Conversely, as a muscle is stretched, the width of the I bands and H zones increases, but still no change occurs in the width of the A band.

Since both of the Huxley research groups proposed the sliding filament theory more than 60 years ago, a great deal more has been discovered about how the protein filaments of muscle interact. At rest, the projections, or cross bridges, of the myosin filaments can touch the actin filaments, but they cannot interact to cause muscle shortening because the actin filaments have active sites to which the myosin cross bridges must bind in order to cause shortening. At rest, however, the active sites are covered by troponin and tropomyosin, two regulatory proteins that are associated with the actin filament (figure 1.8).

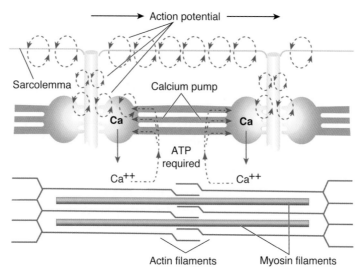

FIGURE 1.7   As the signal for contraction (action potential) spreads across the surface (sarcolemma) of the muscle fiber, the signal causes the release of Ca++ from the sarcoplasmic reticulum (SR). To pump Ca++ back into the SR after a contraction, adenosine triphosphate (ATP) is required.

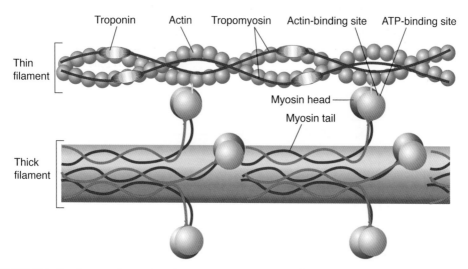

FIGURE 1.8   At rest, the active sites on actin are covered by troponin and tropomyosin. As Ca++ binds to troponin, the troponin and tropomyosin proteins move, thereby exposing the active sites on the actin filament and allowing the binding with the myosin heads to occur.

Once the myosin cross bridge attaches to an active site on actin, contraction (shortening) of the sarcomere can take place. The binding between the myosin cross bridge and actin results in the head of the myosin swiveling forward or collapsing, causing the actin to slide over the myosin, resulting in the sarcomere shortening. (The swivel movement of the head of the myosin is often referred to as the *power stroke*.) At this point, the movement stops, and the myosin cross bridge remains attached to the actin. For further shortening to occur, the cross bridge must first detach from the actin, swivel back, and then attach to another active site on the actin filament—a site that is closer to the Z line than the site to which it was previously attached.

Detachment from the actin is caused by the binding of an adenosine triphosphate (ATP) molecule to the cross bridge. The ATP molecule is then broken down to adenosine diphosphate, causing the cross bridge to swivel back (cock) into its original position. At this point, one cross bridge cycle has been completed (figure 1.9). If the active sites on the actin are still exposed, the cross bridge can bind to a new active site closer to the Z line, and the sarcomere can shorten further. The energy for this cocking of the myosin cross bridge, which is the only energy-requiring step in the cross bridge cycle, is provided by the breakdown of ATP by an enzyme called *myosin adenosine triphosphatase* that is located on the myosin cross bridge. Thus, as for many cellular activities, ATP is the only energy source used directly for muscle contractions. The process of breaking contact with one active site and binding to another is called *recharging*. This cyclical process (referred to as the *ratchet theory*) is repeated until the sarcomere has shortened as much as possible, no more ATP is available, or relaxation of the muscle takes place.

Relaxation of the muscle occurs when the impulse (or signal) from the motor neuron ends. Without a continuous stream of signals from the motor neuron,

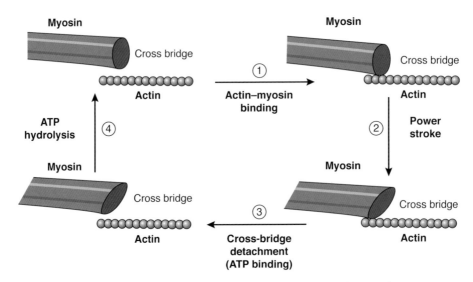

FIGURE 1.9 The cross bridge cycle. (1) The cross bridge attaches to the active site on the actin. (2) The power stroke moves actin over the myosin. (3) ATP attaches to the cross bridge, which then detaches from the active site on the actin. (4) ATP is broken down by adenosine triphosphatase in the cross bridge, and the cross bridge cocks back to its starting position. If a new active site on the actin is available, the cross bridge will attach to the site, and the cycle can continue. (For a more detailed schematic of myosin heads, see figure 1.8.)

◼◼◼◼ Whole-Muscle Design

The overall design of the muscle plays an important role in the muscle's function because it influences the force and velocity of contractions. In general, the more sarcomeres arranged in series (producing a longer muscle), the faster the velocity of the muscle contraction. This is because each sarcomere has a maximal contraction velocity; when sarcomeres are arranged in series, their contraction velocities become additive and the overall contraction velocity of the muscle increases. An additional benefit to sarcomeres being arranged in series is that they can achieve a fast overall velocity of contraction while staying close to their optimal length–tension relationship (the length of the sarcomere at which it produces maximal force). There exists an optimal number of cross bridges of myosin with actin that for a given length provides the highest range of force production. Outside this range, fewer interactions exist, or the actin-myosin filaments are too bunched up to provide any further force application arising from the sarcomere.

In contrast to velocity, the force of contraction increases as more sarcomeres are arranged parallel to each other (producing a wider muscle). Each sarcomere has a maximal force production capability; when sarcomeres are arranged parallel to each other, their force outputs become additive. In this manner, a large force can be produced without a large change in the length of the muscle, again potentially keeping the individual sarcomere close to its optimal length–tension relationship.

Another important aspect of whole-muscle design is pennation (figure 1.10). Pennation is the angle between the muscle fiber orientation and the direction in which the overall muscle force is directed during contraction. A greater angle of pennation allows for more sarcomeres in parallel to be packed into the space between the origin and insertion of a given muscle, thus increasing the potential force production of that muscle. Pennation does have a drawback: As the angle of pennation increases, the resultant force that a given muscle fiber relays to the tendon is reduced. However, the angle of pennation must be greater than approximately 30 degrees before the additional increase in force from packing in more muscle fibers is lost.

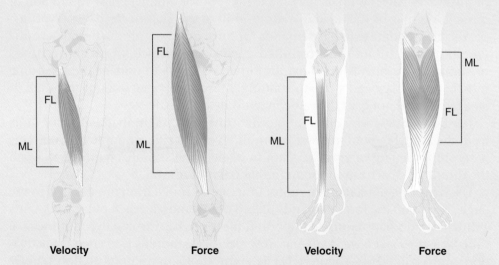

Velocity   Force   Velocity   Force

FIGURE 1.10 Pennation angle, muscle fiber length (FL), and muscle length (ML) for muscles with either high-force or high-velocity functions. Relatively long muscle fibers make the muscle well suited for high-velocity movements; relatively short fibers arranged in parallel make the muscle well suited for high-force movements.

the release of Ca++ stops, and the Ca++ already released is actively pumped back into storage within the sarcoplasmic reticulum. As for the cross bridge cycle, this pump mechanism requires energy from the breakdown of ATP to function. Thus, ATP is required for both contraction and relaxation of the muscle fiber. As Ca++ is removed, the troponin and tropomyosin assume their original position covering the active sites on the actin. The cross bridges of the myosin filament now have no place to attach to on the actin in order to pull it over the myosin. With relaxation, cross bridge activity of the muscle stops, and the muscle will remain in the shortened state unless pulled to a lengthened position by gravity or an outside force. Muscles are only able to actively shorten; there is no mechanism within the muscle that actively causes a lengthening of that muscle to occur.

The neurons of the higher-threshold motor units recover more quickly (i.e., become available for reactivation faster) than the neurons of the lower-threshold motor units after a contraction. This allows the higher-threshold motor units to be activated more quickly than the lower-threshold motor units in repeated actions. Therefore, although the high-threshold Type II motor units fatigue quickly, the ability of their neurons to recover quickly makes them ideal for repeated high-force, short-duration activities.

Motor Unit Recruitment: The Size Principle

Over his career, Dr. Elwood Henneman published eloquent scientific papers that contributed to what is called the *size principle*. The size of the motor units within a muscle varies, as does the number and type of muscle fibers in a motor unit within different muscles. Thus, sizing of motor units relates to the number of fibers, the type of fibers, the size of the muscle fibers, and so on. In the muscles of the eye, as few as 6 fibers may make up a motor unit, whereas 450 to 800 or more fibers may be included in a motor unit of the quadriceps. The size principle dictates that the external demands for force or power production determine the number of motor units recruited. Again, how muscle fibers are recruited or stimulated is one of the most important concepts to understand regarding muscle physiology and strength training. Motor units that are not recruited in an exercise will not gain the same magnitude of benefit.

The body uses several different mechanisms to recruit individual motor units from the available pool in order to produce very specific amounts of force. This is accomplished by varying the amount of electrical stimulus required to reach the threshold of activation for an individual motor unit.

The size principle states that motor units are recruited from the smallest to the largest based on the force demands placed on the muscle. Each muscle contains a different number of muscle fibers and motor units. The smaller motor units, called *low-threshold motor units* (i.e., low electrical stimulus is needed for activation), are recruited first (figure 1.11). Low-threshold motor units predominantly comprise Type I fibers. Then, motor units with progressively higher thresholds are recruited based on the increasing demands of the activity. The higher-threshold motor units predominantly comprise Type II fibers.

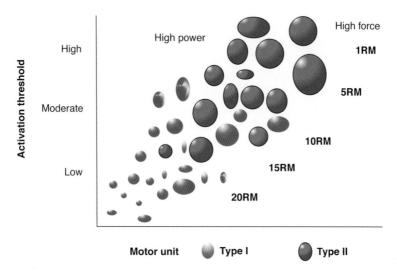

FIGURE 1.11 Recruitment of motor units (alpha motor neuron and the associated muscle fibers; depicted as circles) occurs based on size. Small motor units are recruited first, going up to larger motor units that produce high force and power. Some people and some muscles do not have many fast-twitch, or Type II, motor units. Also, if not stimulated with resistance exercise, motor units can be lost with age. The force requirement needed to stimulate motor units varies.

Heavier resistance, such as that used in lifts that a person can perform for only three to five repetitions maximum (RM), requires the recruitment of motor units with a higher threshold than those required for a lighter resistance (e.g., 12-15RM). However, according to the size principle, lifting heavier resistance starts with the recruitment of low-threshold motor units (Type I) and progressively recruits more and more motor units as the external force demands progressively increase until maximal force is reached. This process of recruiting progressively larger motor units is very rapid because only the motor units that are recruited benefit from the training. As noted previously, this principle has important implications for training programs. Therefore, to maximize strength gains from a resistance training program, high resistance (1-5RM) must also be used to stimulate adaptation in the largest motor units, which need to be trained in order to improve maximal strength.

The size of the motor units within a muscle varies. In keeping with the size principle, motor units with fewer fibers are recruited first. This selective activation of motor units and the difference in size of motor units allow for graded force production and thus more precise control of the amount of force that the whole muscle can generate. This in turn allows for more precise control of body movements. Motor unit recruitment progresses in an orderly fashion from lower-threshold motor units to higher-threshold motor units that require a greater neural stimulus to activate the motor unit. Recent findings show that exercising to failure with a resistance exercise does not increase the number of motor units recruited. Thus, if a person has a maximal strength of 220 pounds (100 kg) in a bench press, more motor units would be required to lift 187 pounds (85 kg) than to lift 88 pounds (40 kg) even if that person exercises to failure in the set. The size principle applies to both concentric and eccentric muscle actions attempting to meet the external demands of an exercise (e.g., lifting or lowering a weight).

Depletion of energy sources, which with endurance exercise takes more than a few hours, can also cause recruitment of higher-threshold motor units or more motor units higher in the recruitment order. Elite endurance athletes can maintain high speeds for long distances due to the additional recruitment of more oxidative Type I motor units, whereas elite sprinters would hit the wall when they had to use their Type II motor units (containing Type II muscle fibers), which produce greater amounts of force and are not very economical for energy. Thus, athletes with different genetic capabilities at the muscle level excel at different distances in running events. Although very fast for short distances, elite sprinters cannot keep up speed for long durations because the recruitment of Type II motor units is not efficient in maintaining the needed power output.

In any activity, especially strength training, the external resistance or power demands dictate the number of motor units used. The duration of most resistance exercise programs typically is not long enough to deplete glycogen from the lower-threshold motor units (thereby forcing upward recruitment to occur), even with sets of more than 100 repetitions to failure with light weights. Therefore, heavier loads are needed to train the entire motor unit pool and challenge the muscle to get bigger and stronger.

All-or-None Law

Another important concept is the all-or-none law, which states that when a specific motor unit reaches its threshold level for activation, all of the muscle fibers in that motor unit are activated fully. If the threshold is not reached, then none of the muscle fibers in that motor unit are activated. Although this holds true for individual motor units within a muscle, whole muscles, such as the biceps, are not governed by the all-or-none law.

The fact that motor units follow the all-or-none law is one reason why a muscle can vary the amount of force it produces. The more motor units stimulated within a muscle, the more force that muscle produces. In other words, if one motor unit in a muscle is activated, that muscle produces only a very small amount of force. If several motor units are activated, the muscle produces more force. If all of the motor units in a muscle are activated, maximal force is produced by the muscle. This method of varying the force produced by a muscle is called *multiple motor unit summation*.

Muscle Activation and Strength Training

Periodization of training (see chapter 3) is based on the principles stated previously—that different loads (light, moderate, or heavy) or power requirements

◀■■■ Protective Mechanisms:
Muscle Spindles and Golgi Tendon Organs

The muscle uses two neural mechanisms or reflexes to protect itself from acute damage. One protects against the muscle becoming overstretched, and the other protects the muscle from tearing itself from its tendon.

Muscle spindles—sets of specialized muscle fibers wrapped with sensory nerves—are located between the regular muscle fibers within the muscle. Because the muscle spindles are attached to the regular muscle fibers, they can sense when the muscle is being stretched rapidly. This signal is sent directly to the spinal cord, where it can trigger a signal in the muscle's motor neurons, causing the muscle to reflexively contract. In this manner, the muscle spindle monitors the lengthening of the muscle and helps prevent the muscle from being overstretched. This mechanism, however, protects the muscle during fast stretches only; if the muscle is stretched slowly, the muscle spindles will not be stimulated to send a signal to the spinal cord.

The Golgi tendon organs are not located in the muscle itself; however, they play an important role in protecting the muscle from being torn from its tendon. As the name suggests, the actual location of the Golgi tendon organ is in the tendon near the point at which the muscle fibers and tendon intersect. The Golgi tendon organ senses tension in the tendon and operates as a strain gauge. When the Golgi tendon organ is stimulated by high tension in the tendon, it sends a signal to the spinal cord to inhibit the contraction of the muscles to which the tendon is attached (agonists) and to excite the muscle on the opposite side of the joint (antagonist). Experts have speculated that this reflex can be diminished with training and that the inhibition of this reflex may play a role in the strength gains seen with resistance training.

recruit different types and numbers of motor units. On a light training day, you would allow some muscle fibers to rest by recruiting fewer of them than on a heavy training day. For example, if your maximal lift (1RM) for one dumbbell biceps curl is 100 pounds (45.4 kg), then 10 pounds (4.5 kg) of resistance represents only about 10 percent of your maximal strength in the biceps curl exercise. Performing 15 repetitions of the dumbbell biceps curl with 10 pounds would activate only a small number of your motor units in the biceps. Conversely, performing a biceps curl with 100 pounds would require all of the available motor units.

The size principle's order of recruitment ensures that low-threshold motor units are predominantly recruited to perform lower-intensity, long-duration (endurance) activities, whereas the higher-threshold motor units are used only to produce higher levels of force or power. This helps delay fatigue during submaximal muscle actions because the high activation threshold for the highly fatigable Type II motor units is not reached unless high levels of force or power are needed; instead, mainly the lower-threshold, fatigue-resistible Type I motor units are recruited. In conjunction, higher-threshold motor units will be recruited only when enough total work has been performed to dramatically reduce the glycogen stores in the lower-threshold motor units. However, this typically has not been observed with resistance exercise because the activity does not tend to reduce muscle glycogen stores significantly. When force production needs are low to moderate, motor units can be alternately recruited to meet the force demands (asynchronous recruitment). This means that a motor unit may be recruited during most of the first repetition of a set with a light weight and then not (or only minimally) recruited during the second repetition. This ability to rest motor units when submaximal force is needed also helps to delay fatigue. When velocities are very slow and loads are very light—as in super-slow training—this type of recruitment may predominate during the exercise, leaving many muscle fibers not stimulated and thus primarily promoting endurance.

Recruitment order is important from a practical standpoint for several reasons. First, in order to recruit Type II fibers and thus achieve a training effect in these fibers, the exercise must be characterized by heavy loading or demands for high power output. Second, the order of recruitment is fixed for many movements, including resistance exercise; if the body position changes, however, the order of recruitment can also change and different muscle fibers can be recruited (e.g., in a flat vs. an incline bench press). The magnitude of recruitment of different portions of the quadriceps also varies among different types of leg exercises (e.g., a leg press vs. a squat). Order and magnitude of recruitment may contribute to strength gains being specific to a particular exercise. The variation in recruitment order provides some evidence to support the belief held by many strength coaches that a particular muscle must be exercised using several different movement angles to develop completely.

Not every person has the same complement of motor units available; thus, not every person has the same strength potential. This, along with differences in the total number of muscle fibers available, allows for differences in force and power capabilities among individuals. These differences are determined largely by genetics; however, various forms of endurance and resistance training as well as detraining can slightly change fiber type composition. The effects of detraining are seen especially with the loss of Type II motor units during aging. Some people and some muscles, such as abdominal muscles, may have only low-threshold motor units predominantly comprising Type I muscle fibers, thus limiting their capability to produce power and force. The type, number, and size of muscle fibers in the motor unit dictate the functional abilities of that individual motor unit and, eventually, the functional abilities of the whole muscle.

Types of Muscle Actions

Muscles can perform a number of different types of actions, including concentric, eccentric, and isometric actions (figure 1.12).

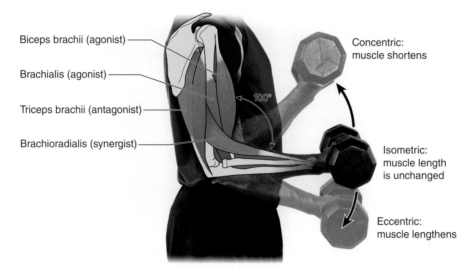

Biceps brachii (agonist)

Brachialis (agonist)

Triceps brachii (antagonist)

Brachioradialis (synergist)

100°

Concentric:
muscle shortens

Isometric:
muscle length
is unchanged

Eccentric:
muscle lengthens

FIGURE 1.12 Concentric, eccentric, and isometric muscle action. The arrow indicates the direction of the movement.

Reprinted, by permission, from R. McAtee, 2014, *Facilitated stretching*, 4th ed. (Champaign, IL: Human Kinetics), 7.

Normally, when a weight is lifted (i.e., the muscle produces more force than the resistance it is trying to move), the muscles involved are shortening while producing force. This is called a *concentric* muscle action. Because shortening occurs during a concentric muscle action, the use of the word *contraction* for this type of muscle action is appropriate.

When a weight is lowered in a controlled manner (i.e., the resistance is greater than the force that the muscle is producing), the muscles involved are lengthening while producing force. This is called an *eccentric* muscle action. Muscles can only pull or lengthen in a controlled manner; they cannot push against the bones to which they are attached. In most exercises, gravity pulls the weight back to the starting position. To control the weight as it returns to the starting position, the muscles must lengthen in a controlled manner or the weight will fall.

If no movement of a joint takes place due to the external load being too heavy but a muscle is activated and developing force (i.e., the force produced by the muscle equals the resistance), the action is called an *isometric* or *static* muscle action. This can occur when a weight is held stationary or the weight is too heavy to lift any higher. Some muscles, such as the postural muscles of the spine, primarily perform isometric muscle actions; they act to stabilize the upper body during most lifts.

The maximal force that a muscle can produce changes throughout the range of motion and is a function of the architecture of the muscle and the joint angle. This relationship is described by the strength curve for the muscle. The "sticking point" (i.e., a point where the external resistance is too great and stops the movement) of an exercise often is related to a low point on the strength curve.

The ascending curve is characterized by the ability to produce greater and greater force over the range of motion. This is the most common curve for exercise movements. Exercises such as the bench press, squat, shoulder press, and leg press follow this strength curve. Rubber band resistance also matches this curve best. Descending curves are less common but are seen in movements that are performed at unusual angles. The leg curl is one example of an exercise in which the most force that can be exerted occurs at the beginning of the range of motion. A bell curve represents exercises in which the highest force that can be produced over the range of motion occurs somewhere in the middle of the curve. The biceps curl is a great example of an exercise that follows this strength curve.

Let's briefly cover how some different types of resistance training use these muscle actions and strength curves. More information on each of these types of lifting can be found in chapter 6.

- **Free weights** such as barbells and dumbbells require the use of both concentric and eccentric muscle actions. This type of training is considered free-form exercise because the bar movement has no set path; rather, the user must control the movement. Thus, assistance and support provided by the prime mover or core muscles are vital when using this type of equipment.

- **Stack plate machines** allow fixed-form exercise because the movement pattern is, for the most part, dictated by the machine itself. Both concentric and eccentric muscle actions are part of the repetition. A person often can lift more weight when using these machines than when performing a free-weight exercise because less need for balance and stability exists. However, the stabilizing muscles get less training than they do during free-weight lifts because the machine is guiding the movement.

- **Rubber band resistance** is unique in that it produces more resistance as the rubber or elastic polymers stretch to their length limits. The return resistance follows a different pattern back to the starting position. This direction-dependent action of the rubber band is called *hysteresis*. The elastic resistance is directly related to an ascending strength curve in which the person can exert continually increasing force over the range of motion. If the band is not set up properly, little or no resistance often is observed during the first 10 degrees to 30 degrees of a range of motion.

- **Isokinetic movements** occur when the velocity of the movement of a joint is held constant. This muscle action can be either concentric or eccentric and usually is performed using a computerized device that controls the speed. The load is determined solely by how much force the person produces. Although no specific resistance is used, the force produced by the muscles involved can be measured. Isokinetic movements are most often used for research testing purposes and in rehabilitation settings.

- **Pneumatic resistance,** developed by the Keiser Corporation (Fresno, CA), eliminates the dependence on gravity and the momentum associated with iron weights, thus allowing an individual to train at any speed with consistent concentric and eccentric resistance. This resistance system trains both the force and the speed components of a movement, thereby providing the means to help athletes develop the explosive power needed for certain movements (e.g., upper-body movements and knee extensions) in competitive sport.

- **Hydraulic resistance** uses concentric muscle action only. The equipment consists of a piston that moves in and out of a fluid cylinder under pressure; thus, the athlete pushes out and pulls in when performing an exercise. No eccentric loading is available in this type of lifting, which has been popularized in many women's fitness clubs. The lack of eccentric loading in this type of resistance makes it less efficient: Double the reps are needed to gain the same effects as a normal concentric–eccentric repetition.

Length–Tension (Force) Curve

The length–tension (force) curve demonstrates that there is an optimal length at which muscle fibers can generate their maximal force (figure 1.13). The total amount of force developed depends on the total number of myosin cross bridges interacting with active sites on the actin. At the optimal length, potential exists for maximal cross bridge interaction and thus maximal force. Below this optimal length, less tension is developed during muscle fiber activation because an overlap of actin filaments occurs with excessive shortening. As a result, the actin filaments interfere with each other's ability to interact with the myosin cross bridges. The reduction in cross bridge interaction with the active sites on the actin results in a smaller potential for force and power development.

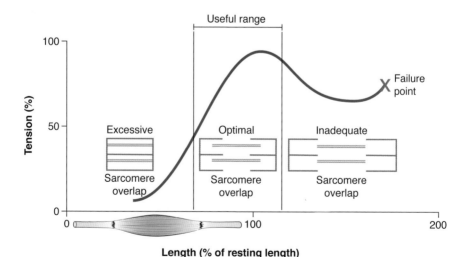

FIGURE 1.13 The relationship between the length of the sarcomere and the sarcomere's tension (force) production capability. Optimal force production capability is achieved when all myosin cross bridges are opposed by an active actin filament and no overlap of actin filaments exists.

At lengths greater than optimal, less and less overlap of the actin and myosin filaments occurs, resulting in fewer cross bridges attaching to the active sites on the actin. The cross bridges close to the center of the myosin filament will not have an actin site across from them to attach to. Thus, if the sarcomere's length is greater than optimal, less force and power can be developed.

The length–tension curve shows that the muscle's capacity for force development changes throughout a particular movement. In addition, the curve indicates that some prestretch of the muscle before the initiation of a contraction increases the amount of force generated. Too much prestretch, however, actually decreases the total amount of force developed. This is especially important during isometric muscle actions; for maximal force to be produced, the length of the muscle must correspond to the optimal point on the length–tension curve.

Force–Velocity Curve

As the velocity of movement increases, the force a muscle is able to produce concentrically (while shortening) decreases (figure 1.14). This is empirically true. If an athlete is asked to bench press the maximal amount of weight possible (1RM), the weight will move very slowly, but if the athlete is asked to bench press half of his or her 1RM, the weight will move at a faster velocity. Maximal velocity of shortening occurs when no resistance (weight) is being moved or lifted and is determined by the maximal rate at which cross bridges can attach to and detach from the active sites on the actin. The force–velocity curve is important when examining various forms of weight training such as isokinetic training, in which the velocity of the movement is controlled but the resistance is not. (See chapter 6 for other examples, including free weights and variable-resistance machines.)

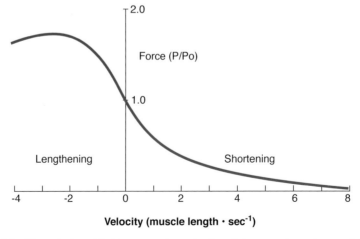

FIGURE 1.14 The relationship between the velocity of the muscle action and the muscle's force production capability. The faster the velocity of a concentric muscle action, the lower the force production capability. For an eccentric muscle action, the opposite is true: The faster the velocity, the higher the force production capability.

Increases in the velocity of movement actually increase the force that a muscle can develop during eccentric (lengthening) action. This increase is thought to be attributable to the elastic component of the muscle, although the explanation for such a response remains unclear. It is interesting to note that eccentric force at even low velocities is higher than the highest concentric force or isometric force. Development of such high force when performing maximal eccentric muscle actions has been related to muscle damage in untrained people. However, it has been demonstrated that muscle that is exposed to repeated eccentric actions can adapt by strengthening part of the connective tissue so that the damage per training session is reduced in subsequent training sessions. At the percentages of 1RM normally used for resistance training, eccentric force is not maximal. Thus, the eccentric portion of the repetition may not be optimal for strength gains. New methods and equipment that allow higher loads to be applied only during the eccentric phase of a lift are being developed (see chapter 3 for a discussion).

Summary

Understanding the basic structures of muscle allows a better understanding of the primary elements affected by a resistance training program. These muscle structures begin with the smallest organizational parts and build into a system allowing human movement. Progressive resistance training enhances the muscular system by making it stronger and more powerful, and it conditions the large tissue mass, which is important not only in sport but also in fighting the effects of aging. Health is in part also related to appropriate muscle fitness, and only with proper weight training can muscle become healthy and fit.

How Muscle Grows

William J. Kraemer

Muscle growth is complex, and many of the mechanisms that mediate it are still not completely understood. Furthermore, it is an integrated process in which the involvement of various mechanisms depends on the demands of repair and remodeling. Simply understanding the multiple signaling networks and genetic underpinnings is a daunting challenge at best. Thus, although our understanding of resistance exercise–induced muscle growth advances each year, is still evolving. Essentially, muscle growth is an adaptation to external work stimuli that activates motor units and results in some extent of damage. When discussing muscle hypertrophy, we think of the muscle's response to exercise—more specifically, strength or resistance exercise and training. Figure 2.1 provides a general overview of the process of muscle growth.

With the recruitment of motor units, muscle fibers are stimulated to produce force. With continued exposure to such training in a progressive manner, the response by the muscles is to adapt over time and get bigger in order to reduce the cross-sectional stress on the intact muscle. In essence, by getting stronger, the muscle is capable of producing more force per unit of cross-sectional area. This adaptation continues until the maximal growth potential of the muscle fibers is reached or until errors in training create an overtraining syndrome.

In addition to increasing muscle size, resistance training improves muscle strength and can improve athletic performance. For athletes, training the musculature creates stronger muscle and connective tissue components that are resistant to injury. An athlete with trained muscles also recovers from competition more rapidly.

Resistance training helps both men and women stay healthy and offset the natural aging process, which can lead to loss of muscle mass (sarcopenia) and bone mass (osteoporosis) and to subsequent disability. After age 35 an inactive individual can lose between 0.5 and 1 percent of muscle mass annually. Maintaining muscle mass or reducing its decline with resistance training can help prevent loss of function.

The author acknowledges the significant contributions of Barry A. Spiering to this chapter.

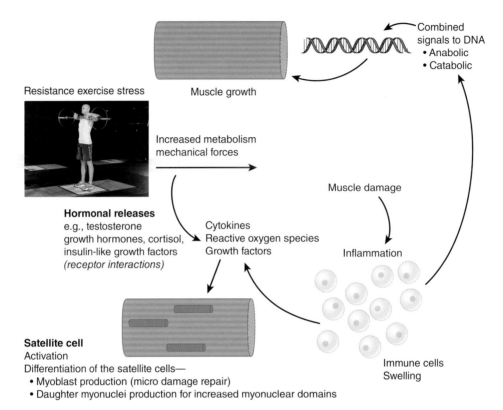

FIGURE 2.1 A general overview of the growth stimuli applied to skeletal muscle during resistance exercise stress. The growth of muscle tissue is caused by a multitude of integrated responses and stimuli from the physical demands of loading; such physical demands result in muscle tissue damage, leading to inflammation and subsequent release of cytokines and other chemical messengers from immune cells. Various products act as signals for growth and stimulation of hormones from endocrine glands to produce either myoblasts for microdamage repair or daughter myonuclei, allowing for greater protein accretion and growth of muscle fibers. In total, a host of factors contribute to stimulating growth processes in muscle.

Too often, people (frequently women) do not engage in progressive heavy resistance training because they are afraid it will make them too big. This unfounded fear can prevent them from obtaining the full benefits of a strength training program. Women have fewer muscle fibers than men, especially in the upper body, and the primary anabolic (muscle building) hormone, testosterone, is dramatically lower in women than in men. Every individual's body type is different, and some men and women (e.g., those of the mesomorph somato-type) are more genetically capable of developing muscle size because they have a greater number of muscle fibers. However, men and women rarely develop excessive hypertrophy except through the use of anabolic drugs.

Elite female athletes have shown that highly trained and developed muscu-latures do not make a woman less feminine. With a well-designed resistance training program, women typically see an increase in muscle size and a corresponding decrease in body fat, resulting in smaller dimensions and improved muscle definition. For men, the increase in muscle size depends on proper training and nutrition, and the upper limits of size are related to genetics and number of muscle fibers.

Many individuals seek to improve their strength because a close relationship exists between the size of a muscle and its strength. Adhering to a resistance training program of progressive overload stimulates the muscle to enhance its size by increasing the amount of proteins. Structurally, this adaptation results in an increase in both contractile and noncontractile proteins (see chapter 1), which therefore permits more actin–myosin cross bridges to be formed during muscle activation. Subsequently, this allows the muscle to produce greater force and an observed increase in strength. To fully appreciate the importance of strength training, one must grasp how the exercise stimulus affects the basic underlying mechanisms of muscle growth—that is, how muscle size increases.

In this chapter, we discuss muscle growth in a natural environment. The extreme muscle size seen in certain bodybuilders or individuals using anabolic drugs is beyond the typical results attained through a sport- or fitness-based, progressive heavy resistance training program and is outside the scope of this chapter.

Muscle Growth

In order for a muscle to get bigger it must increase in size. Historically, two primary mechanisms—hypertrophy and hyperplasia—have been proposed to explain how an increase in the size of an intact muscle might occur. *Hypertrophy* refers to an increase in the size of individual muscle fibers, whereas *hyperplasia* refers to an increase in the number of muscle fibers.

Research over the past 40 years has shown that the predominant mechanism for increasing muscle size is hypertrophy. Hyperplasia in humans may exist but is still very controversial as a major mechanism for increasing the intact size of a muscle (MacDougall et al. 1984; Alway et al. 1989; McCall et al. 1996). If hyperplasia does occur, it likely contributes very little (<5 percent) to absolute muscle growth, and anabolic drugs may play a role. Its existence may also be attributable to a mechanism called *neural sprouting*, where part of a muscle fiber without any neural connection that breaks away from the main fiber due to a clean breakage due to mechanical damage from exercise stress are attached to a neural sprout from another motor neuron and take on the characteristics of that motor unit, thereby increasing the number of fibers for that type of motor unit. However, we focus on skeletal muscle hypertrophy via an increase in muscle fiber size because this response has been demonstrated clearly in the research.

Two principles form the foundation of muscle growth. First, muscle must be stimulated to increase in size. However, that stimulus must be anabolic in nature. The anabolic stimulus appears to be related to the amount of resistance used in a lift and the associated neural activation in both men and women (Campos et al. 2002; Schuenke et al. 2013). Heavier resistance produces higher neural activation voltages in the recruitment of motor units. High voltage is needed for neural stimuli to activate high-threshold motor units; this high voltage also exposes lower-threshold motor units to the neural stimuli because recruitment always progresses from low- to high-threshold motor units. This was evidenced with biopsy training studies on the thigh muscle from Dr. Robert Staron's research groups (Campos et al. 2002; Schuenke et al. 2013). These studies showed that when using only light weights (20-28RM), no hypertrophy of the Type I muscle fibers was seen. However, when using heavier resistance (9-11RM and 3-5RM), increases in cross-sectional area of all muscle fiber types were observed with training. In this context, the most prolific stimulus for muscle growth is a well-designed resistance exercise program of sufficient volume and sufficiently high intensity.

Second, increasing muscle size requires energy and the building blocks for new protein growth, both of which come from a properly designed and well-balanced diet that incorporates adequate calories and needed nutrients. As discussed in greater detail in chapter 4, nutrient intake is vital for optimal muscle development. The body needs carbohydrate, protein, and fat to repair and remodel muscle. Thus, everyday dietary patterns (including the timing of nutrient intake around the workout), appropriate sleep, and a healthy lifestyle all contribute to the effectiveness of muscle repair and, therefore, muscle growth.

If either of these principles is ignored, muscle simply will not adapt optimally for the desired hypertrophy. Figure 2.2 shows the basic paradigm of muscle growth and illustrates that the foundation for muscle growth consists of a proper resistance training stimulus and sound nutritional intake.

Magnitude of Skeletal Muscle Growth

As discussed in chapter 1, human muscles generally can be classified as Type I or Type II. Type II fibers are often further subclassified into Type IIA or Type IIX; however, many "hybrid" fibers exist in between each of these fiber type classifications—for example, there are fiber types that exist between Type I and Type IIA, between Type IIA and Type IIX, and so forth. Therefore, fiber types should be considered to exist on a continuum, not just as finite classifications. This continuum ranges from Type IIX to Type IIA of which represents the fully trained Type II fiber profile and the Type IC to the Type I with the Type I being the fully trained fiber type profile. With training, one sees the movement of the enzymes and capabilities ending with Type I or Type IIA. Type II muscle fibers are high in the recruitment threshold and can exert greater force when recruited, whereas Type I fibers are made for repetitive recruitment and are found in the lower portions of the recruitment profile. For simplicity's sake, we discuss the major fiber types.

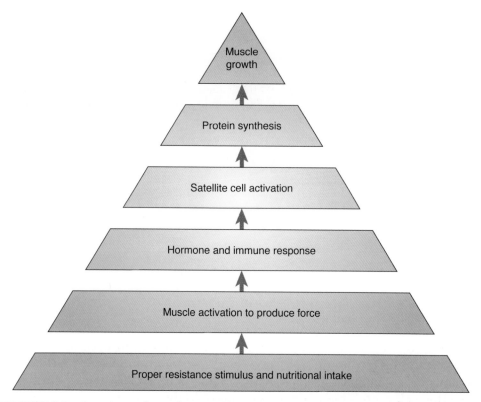

FIGURE 2.2 Paradigm of muscle growth. Muscle growth begins with a solid foundation consisting of a proper resistance training stimulus and adequate nutritional intake.

As noted before, the number of muscle fibers dictates the absolute growth of an intact muscle. The type of muscle fiber affects the rate of growth and other physiological functions (e.g., protein synthesis rates; Kraemer et al. 2016). Type I muscle fibers grow at a slower rate than Type II muscle fibers because the synthesis rates of Type II fibers are higher than those of Type I fibers for the contractile proteins. The greater the number of muscle fibers, the greater the potential for absolute muscle growth in response to a progressive heavy resistance training program (Fleck and Kraemer 2014). The growth of the individual muscle fibers upon their recruitment with resistance exercise loading contributes to the growth of the whole muscle. Thus, it is important that as many muscle fibers as possible are stimulated with a resistance exercise training program; again, this implicates the importance of load and intensity.

Body somatotyping takes into account the muscle mass of an individual. Three standard body types exist: ectomorph, endomorph, and mesomorph. However, most individuals are a combination of two (e.g., mesomorph–endomorph or endomorph–ectomorph), and body somatotypes run along a continuum in both men and women (see figure 2.3). The ectomorph is typified by a low number

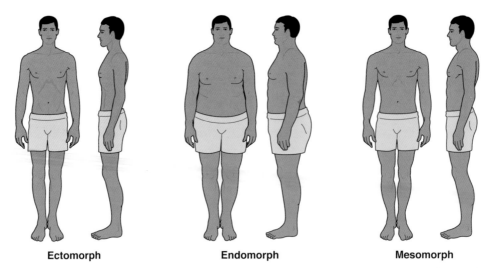

Ectomorph	Endomorph	Mesomorph

FIGURE 2.3.   Three basic body somatotypes: ectomorph, mesomorph, and endomorph. Body types are related to the potential for absolute changes in muscle growth due to the number of muscle fibers associated with each body type.

of muscle fibers and low fat mass; many elite endurance athletes are classified as ectomorphs. The mesomorph is typified by a high number of muscle fibers and lower body fat; many strength and power athletes are classified as this body type. The endomorph has a higher amount of body fat, which masks either an underlying mesomorph or, in some cases, ectomorph body type. Because resistance training and solid nutritional practices reduce body fat, a transformation to the underlying body type typically is observed. The existing research does not show that it is possible to increase muscle fiber number, so an individual cannot transform from an ectomorph to a pure mesomorph. However, muscular strength, power, and definition can be seen in trained endomorph body types. A properly designed progressive heavy resistance training program optimizes body somatotypes.

Neural Contributions to Muscle Growth

Neural adaptations help mediate growth-related processes. The early increase in strength is attributable mainly to improved neural function, primarily from the eccentric component of the resistance. (This again points to the importance of concentric–eccentric repetition with training.) Greater strength in turn increases the quality of the training stimulus, which also contributes to a greater anabolic stimulus for muscle hypertrophy.

A dramatic increase in strength occurs during the first few weeks of a strength training program. However, intact muscle and muscle fiber size change very little during this initial phase. The observed changes take place in the quality (e.g., increased packing density of the myofibrils) and type of protein (i.e., change in the myosin isoform X to A) in the growth of the muscle fibers. In general, resistance training stimulates a transition of Type II fibers: The fiber profile of the muscle shifts from Type IIX toward Type IIA. This is part of the adaptation of the muscle to a more metabolically active fiber (Staron et al. 1994). However, it is doubtful that muscle fibers transform from Type II to Type I, or vice versa, under normal training conditions. Thus, changes in the quality of muscle proteins occur with shifts in the myosin heavy chains toward the Type IIA fiber. Enzyme changes also occur that help mediate growth-related metabolism. Many of these changes start very quickly within the first week of training. Thus, along with neural changes, various aspects of the protein metabolism in the muscle are changing in the early phases of training.

Muscle Growth Stimuli

As noted before, the number of motor units activated determines how many muscle fibers are stimulated to adapt. Thus, training will influence the stimulus for muscle growth. A well-designed resistance training program requires many important components. For example, you must consider muscle actions (isometric, concentric, and eccentric), exercise intensity, volume, and rest intervals between sets and training sessions (for a review, see Fleck and Kraemer 2014). Specific types of muscle training are discussed in greater detail in chapter 3.

Work by Dr. Gary Dudley's laboratory at the National Aeronautics and Space Administration in the early 1990s demonstrated the importance of performing both concentric and eccentric muscle actions for increasing muscle size and strength (Dudley et al. 1991; Hather et al. 1991). These studies showed that when only concentric muscle actions were used in a weight training regimen, twice the work had to be performed to get the same training effects as when eccentric actions were included. Eccentric actions clearly are an important part of a resistance training program.

Although various types of resistance training programs have been shown to elicit muscular hypertrophy, certain ranges of exercise intensity and volume appear to be optimal. Typically loads from 10 RM and lower are used for the heavier workouts in a program dedicated to increased muscle size and strength. Exercise intensity denotes the load, or weight, used during a lift, whereas exercise volume is the number of repetitions multiplied by the number of sets. Heavier intensities are needed for optimizing muscle strength and size, and the use of a periodized program that includes different intensities and volume cycles (classic or nonlinear) is very important for optimizing training effects (Peterson et al. 2004; Fleck and Kraemer 2014). This need for variation is related to the size principle. The changes in the loading of the muscle allow for some muscle to rest and recover during training. For example, if you do a light load on a given day, the motor units and associated muscle fibers are not being used directly and are recovering from the prior workout in which they were used.

The amount of rest between each exercise set also affects the muscles' responses to resistance training. Short rest periods (one to two minutes) used in accordance with moderate to high intensity and volume elicit greater acute responses of anabolic hormones compared with programs using very heavy loads and longer rest periods (three minutes; Kraemer et al. 1990, 1991). Shorter rest periods (less than one minute) are associated with greater metabolic stress (e.g., higher levels of lactic acid in the blood); metabolic stress is a stimulus for hormone release, and some of these hormones are anabolic in nature. Performing too many workouts with short rest in a given week can result in a release of predominantly catabolic hormones. Thus, variation in a workout, with longer and shorter rest periods, is important in periodization of training. The hormonal response is important because naturally occurring anabolic hormones stimulate muscle protein synthesis and contribute to signaling for other anabolic aspects of increases in muscle size. However, increases in blood concentrations of anabolic hormones are not a sole requirement for hypertrophy because heavy loading stimulates neural aspects that simply take advantage of existing anabolic hormonal environments.

Again, a concern with short-rest workouts is the need for recovery. The large increase in the catabolic hormone, cortisol, can interfere with anabolic signaling if adequate recovery is not allowed—especially day to day where resting cortisol values can increase steadily, leading to an overreaching or overtraining condition (Szivak et al. 2013). In addition, cortisol can block anabolic signaling events in the muscle and interfere with binding of testosterone on nuclear receptors (i.e., on the DNA of the muscle cell nucleus) in the myonuclei of muscle (Spiering et al. 2008a). Therefore, managing stress and allowing for recovery are key to effective and optimal training and subsequent adaptations (Spiering et al. 2008b).

Whether you have a personal trainer or you design your own resistance training program, you must keep these three issues—muscle actions, exercise intensity and volume, and length of rest periods—in mind when trying to stimulate muscle growth. Important concepts for designing resistance training programs are discussed in more detail in chapter 3.

Muscle Metabolism Supports Exercise and Tissue Growth

To understand the importance of nutrition for muscle growth, it is important to introduce the principles of muscle metabolism. Nutritional intake provides the compounds needed for energy transformation in the body. Adenosine triphosphate (ATP) is the ultimate source of energy for muscle actions. However, only a very small amount of ATP (enough to fuel approximately two seconds of intense muscle activity) can be stored within muscle. Therefore, muscle must metabolize various substrates—the carbohydrate, protein, and fat we consume—to continuously regenerate ATP.

Muscle metabolic pathways function on a continuum ranging from pathways that provide ATP very quickly (ATP-PC system) but with a small overall capacity to pathways that produce ATP relatively slowly but with a larger capacity (aerobic energy system; for a review, see Kraemer et al. 2016). At the onset of exercise, the first pathway activated is the ATP–creatine phosphate (CP) pathway (figure 2.4). As ATP is degraded, a phosphate group is removed from CP and transferred to adenosine diphosphate to regenerate ATP. Although this pathway can produce energy very quickly, its capacity is limited to producing enough ATP for approximately six seconds of exercise—for example, enough energy to sprint 40 yards (37 m).

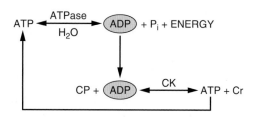

FIGURE 2.4 The cleavage of the phosphate from the ATP molecule gong to ADP allows for energy production.

Reprinted, by permission, from J. Friel, 2013, *Triathlon science* (Champaign, IL; Human Kinetics), 6.

As exercise progresses in duration to greater than six seconds, an increasing amount of energy is derived from anaerobic glycolysis (figure 2.5). *Anaerobic* means that this reaction can occur without oxygen; *glycolysis* means splitting (metabolizing) glucose. Anaerobic glycolysis produces energy quickly; however, because oxygen is not involved, lactic acid is produced at a higher rate than the muscle can metabolize it. Thus, it builds up in muscle, and the H+ ions produced must be buffered (neutralized) to limit negative effects. However, repeated exposure to higher levels of H+ than normal stresses the bicarbonate and phosphate buffering systems, leading to enhanced buffering capacities with exercise training (Kraemer et al. 2016). Workouts with short rest periods can produce high concentrations of lactic acid and H+ ions and can reduce blood pH and ATP availability. Lactic acid does not produce muscle fatigue or soreness; rather, its increased production parallels the dramatic changes in pH and H+ ion production from such workouts (Robergs et al. 2004). In fact, the lactate from lactic acid can be used as a source of energy.

Exercise of relatively low intensity and long duration relies primarily on oxidative metabolism. Oxidative metabolism (i.e., the Krebs cycle, aerobic energy system), the slowest of the three metabolic pathways, occurs in the muscle mitochondria and is capable of producing greater ATP than the anaerobic metabolic pathways (figure 2.6). One cannot gain enough energy for a 100-meter sprint using the oxidative metabolism because the energy cycle used depends on the demands of the exercise. Shorter exercise durations, such as a set of five in a resistance training workout, depend more on ATP phosphagen. As duration increases, glycolysis helps out, and as duration continues to increase, more and more oxidative metabolism contributes. For any exercise, different percentages of different energy systems are at work in each muscle as demands are placed on them. The substrates for oxidative metabolism can be glucose, fat, or protein. However, very little protein (<10 percent) is oxidized during exercise.

Metabolic pathways are active at all times on the continuum, so at any moment they are all producing ATP. However, the intensity and duration of the exercise determine which pathway will provide most of the ATP for contraction. For example, a 100-meter sprint relies primarily on ATP–CP and anaerobic glycolysis, whereas a marathon relies primarily on the Krebs cycle and aerobic energy system.

Muscles metabolize glucose, fat, and protein during exercise, and exercise causes damage to muscle structures. Therefore, it is important to ingest adequate nutrients after an exercise session in order to replenish muscle substrates and

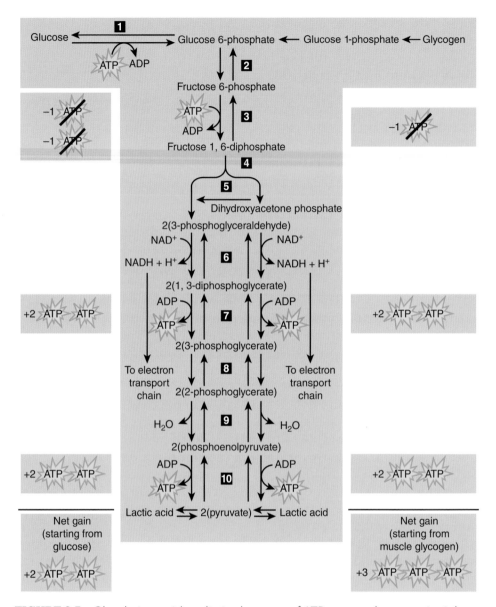

FIGURE 2.5   Glycolysis provides a limited amount of ATP energy when exercise is longer than several seconds and when exercise demands are too great for the aerobic energy cycle have time to make needed ATP to support the exercise.

Reprinted, by permission, from W.L. Kenney, J.H. Wilmore, and D.L. Costill, 2014, *Physiology of sport and exercise*, 6th ed. (Champaign, IL: Human Kinetics), 58.

promote repair. Proper hydration is also vital for optimizing recovery. Perhaps the most important fuel for continued exercise is muscle glycogen. When muscle glycogen is low, exercise intensity is dramatically reduced and, ultimately, exercise must be ceased. Fortunately, although some glycogen depletion occurs during

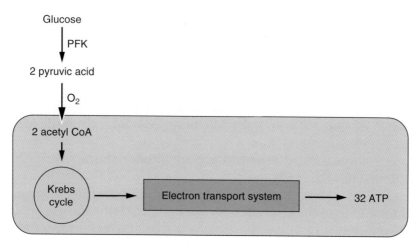

FIGURE 2.6   The Krebs Cycle also called the aerobic energy system provides a high yield of ATP energy via with the electron transport system in the mitochondria of the cell.

resistance training, it is much less than the depletion that occurs with long-duration endurance training. Additionally, after exercise, muscle must synthesize proteins to repair damage and produce new enzymes; therefore, it is important to consume adequate protein and needed carbohydrate and calories. In women, caloric intake is especially important because the losses associated with exercise demands can influence the menstrual cycle (Reed et al. 2011).

Activated Muscle Is Physiologically Supported by and Adapts to Exercise Stress

The first step necessary for increasing muscle size is to activate motor units. If a specific muscle is not stimulated to produce force, then clearly it will not respond and adapt to the stimulus. To activate a muscle fiber, an individual must apply adequate exercise intensity. This activation determines which physiological systems are brought into play and their magnitude of response. If only a small amount of tissue is stimulated, it might be supported by levels of physiological support just above resting metabolism. However, if the exercise stress is significant, various physiological systems must increase many times above resting homeostatic levels to address the exercise demands, leading to a correspondingly higher stimulus to adapt.

As discussed in chapter 1, the activation of motor units follows the size principle. You can see the size principle and its role in muscle growth by comparing endurance training, which typically uses low-intensity and high-volume exercises, with strength training, which tends to use high-intensity and low-volume exercises. Resistance training is a more prolific stimulus for muscle fiber growth than endurance training because resistance exercise provides the high-intensity stimulus necessary for recruiting Type II (fast twitch) fibers, which are more capable of increasing in size than Type I fibers. In other words, to stimulate muscles to grow, the necessary motor units have to be activated, and a relatively heavy load must be used in order to do that. Again, the high neural charges that depolarize the muscle with heavy loads stimulates the receptors and membrane dynamics to a greater extent when compared to the lower electrical neural discharge of lighter resistances. Activation of motor units and their associated muscle fibers dictates force and physiological needs for the muscle to perform and meet performance demands.

Upon activation, muscle fibers contract and produce force, which ultimately allows movement of the human body. In a curl exercise, a concentric (shortening) muscle action takes place if the muscle produces more force throughout the range of motion than the resistance provides. An isometric muscle action takes place if the resistance is greater than the force that the muscle can produce and no movement occurs. An eccentric (lengthening) muscle action takes place as the individual tries to slow the resistance as gravity takes it down in the lowering movement (Knuttgen and Kraemer 1987).

The production of muscular force sends a host of signals to all organ systems of the body, many of which support the muscles' ability to produce force and contribute to muscle recovery and growth. For example, the cardiovascular system pumps blood to the muscle to provide oxygen and nutrients and to remove waste and metabolic products, the endocrine system produces hormones that aid in force production (e.g., epinephrine, also known as *adrenaline*) and hormones that stimulate muscle growth (e.g., testosterone, growth hormone, and insulin-like growth factors), and the immune system provides signals to help coordinate the tissue repair process. In the next sections, we look more specifically at the hormonal and immune system responses to muscle activation and resistance training, and we examine how these responses activate satellite cells to effect muscle growth.

Hormonal Response to Muscle Contraction

As stated previously, the endocrine system releases hormones during and after the production of muscular force. Hormones are only signals, and their messages are realized when they bind with an appropriate receptor that mediates their signal to the target cell's nuclei. Hormones such as epinephrine help the muscles produce force. Other hormones in the body—such as testosterone, various types of growth hormone (GH), and insulin-like growth factor (IGF)—stimulate muscle protein synthesis by sending signals to produce proteins, regenerate, and grow to the muscle's genetic machinery in the myonuclei (i.e., nuclei within a muscle; for an overview, see figure 2.7). Resistance exercise naturally (i.e., without the use of drugs) increases the concentrations of anabolic (muscle building) hormones in the blood during exercise and for approximately one hour afterward. This helps signal the body to rebuild and repair body tissue, including muscle.

Testosterone, which is produced primarily in the testes in men and in the adrenal glands in women, has a dramatic effect on human physiology, including the

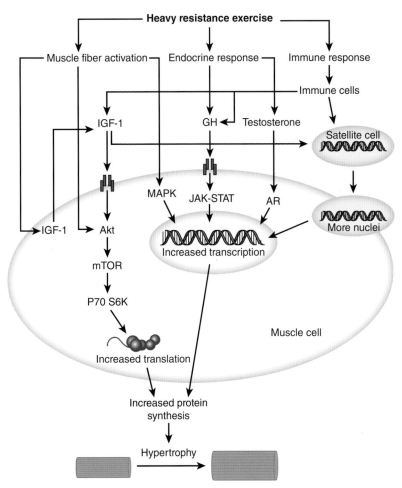

FIGURE 2.7   The muscle fiber has a host of different receptors both in the membrane and on the genetic elements in the various nuclei. A host of signals from different hormones and immune cells can influence protein synthesis and muscle fiber growth.

growth of tissue (for a review, see Vingren et al. 2010). On reaching the exercising muscle, testosterone passes through the muscle's membrane and binds to one of many testosterone-specific receptors (known as *androgen receptors*) inside the muscle cell. Once this binding occurs, testosterone sends a signal to the cell's nucleus to increase protein synthesis (i.e., make new proteins). Repeated training bouts cause the muscle fiber to increase in size or cause neural cells at the end of the motor neuron at the neuromuscular junction to increase the amount of neurotransmitter (see Kraemer et al. 2016).

Muscular force production also stimulates the release of various types of GH from the pituitary gland (a small gland in the brain). GH is the primary hormone in a superfamily of various types and forms of the primary hormone. The primary GH is a 191 amino acid hormone and in the pituitary there are shorter amino acid variants, aggregates of the GH and binding proteins all with known and unknown biological functions (for a review, see Kraemer et al. 2010). Once released from the pituitary gland, GH then binds to various receptors on the membrane of target cells in the body, stimulating the genetic machinery via intracellular signaling processes (secondary messenger molecules and pathways), which stimulate the genetic machinery in the nuclei of cells. GHs can act directly on skeletal muscle.

IGFs are another superfamily of polypeptides that has evolved as a group of hormones and binding proteins with potent anabolic functions related to growth and health (Nindl and Pierce 2010). GH also travels through the bloodstream and stimulates the production of IGF-1 (IGF-I) in the liver and muscles. IGF-I can then bind to a receptor on the outer membrane of the muscle fiber and send a signal to the muscle cell nucleus to increase the production of proteins.

A critical function of both IGF-I and testosterone is to activate a group of cells called *satellite cells*, which also contribute to muscle growth. This is discussed in detail later in this chapter.

The hormonal response to exercise is part of an integrated physiological pattern of response to an exercise stimulus created by proper program design. Over time, the hormonal response can contribute to the increase in muscle size (for a review, see Kraemer et al. 2016). Appropriately structuring a resistance training program can minimize catabolic responses and optimize anabolic hormone signaling. In general, the hormonal response to exercise is greatest when using high exercise volume (3 or 4 sets of 6-12 repetitions for each exercise), heavy loads (>80 percent of maximal strength), short rest periods (one to two minutes between sets), and exercises that target large muscle mass (squats, deadlifts, power cleans, and so forth). However, individuals must take care to not overshoot the tolerance for total work and short-rest workouts, which can promote chronic increases in cortisol. Long-term elevations in cortisol can promote a catabolic state in the body. Proper rest and periodization of the training program can minimize such negative effects. As noted previously, periodizing different volumes of work and different lengths of rest is important for optimizing recovery. (For a review of the hormonal responses and adaptations to resistance exercise, see Kraemer and Ratamess 2005; Fleck and Kraemer 2014.) The hormonal response to exercise generally is correlated with the amount of metabolic stress—that is, the higher the metabolic stress, the higher the hormonal response.

A clever experiment performed by a group of scientists in Denmark (Hansen et al. 2001) demonstrated the significance of the relationship between an increase in the anabolic hormones circulating in the bloodstream and gains in muscle strength. The scientists tested the arm strength of a group of subjects and subsequently divided the subjects into two groups. One group trained only their arms (A group), and the other group trained their arms and their legs (AL group). Both groups spent the same amount of time training their arms; however, the AL group performed additional leg exercises to increase the concentration of circulating anabolic hormones—that is, testosterone and GH. (As already mentioned, the amount of these anabolic hormones in the blood will increase more if a large amount of muscle is exercised.) At the end of the experiment, the scientists found that the A group increased their arm strength by 9 percent, whereas the AL group increased their arm strength by 37 percent! This concept was validated later in a study from a group of scientists in Norway (Rønnestad et al. 2011), who demonstrated that elevations in GH and testosterone produce superior strength training gains. These studies clearly show the importance of recruiting a large muscle mass during resistance exercise; doing so causes a large increase in anabolic hormones and a greater increase in strength and muscle size.

Disruption, Damage, and Injury Signals for Hypertrophy

During heavier concentric exercise, which also produce heavier eccentric muscle actions (maximal eccentric is about 120 percent of concentric 1RM and varies by exercise), microscopic muscle damage occurs. This muscle damage consists of a disruption of sarcomeres and cell membranes, which leads to inflammation and swelling that contribute to soreness felt after a workout (i.e., delayed-onset muscle soreness). The damage also provides an important stimulus for muscle growth and therefore is necessary for increasing muscle size.

Years ago, it was a common theory that one needed to break down muscle in order to allow the muscle to build back up and get bigger and stronger. Later it was thought that this was not true, but more recently we have come back to the original idea that disruption or some damage of the muscle is important for generating molecular signals for growth. Research of various models of delayed-onset muscle soreness has shown that damage resulting in functional impairment (e.g., difficulty moving a limb) and excessive soreness would not be optimal for positive molecular and hormonal signaling (Lewis et al. 2012; Kraemer et al. 2016). Thus, there appears to be a continuum on which an individual will see some disruption and a certain degree of damage after a resistance training workout, resulting in a positive signal for repair and growth. However, if the damage is too extreme or inappropriate for the fitness level of the individual (e.g., an untrained individual doing high-volume heavy eccentrics) and creates an injury, the repair and remodeling process will be extended into many days or even weeks. This latter end of the continuum is not typical of a properly prescribed heavy resistance training program.

Over the past decade it has also been demonstrated that tissue damage results in an immediate inflammatory response in which immune cells (e.g., neutrophils, the most common type of white blood cell) secrete both cytokines and other growth factors that stimulate growth and repair. In addition, other immune cells (e.g., phagocytes) involved with the cleanup of damaged muscle structures are stimulated and move into these areas. Reactive oxygen species that can be secreted by neutrophils can cause further muscle tissue damage if secreted in excess over time; however, reactive oxygen species secreted in just the right level can act to signal other anabolic repair mechanisms in the muscle (for a review, see Schoenfeld 2012).

The immune system is intimately involved in the muscle repair and remodeling process. The amount of inflammation experienced after exercise runs on a continuum from small to large (for a review, see Fragala et al. 2011). To help conceptualize this, go back to the 1980s when such a response was thought of as "good" or "bad" inflammation. There exists just the right amount of inflammatory response needed to stimulate and advance repair and remodeling. Although some soreness might exist the day after a workout, if too much exists, then the individual has done too much too soon and the damage and inflammatory response may be too great to quickly repair and recover from.

When muscles are damaged, an immune response follows. Immune cells (e.g., white blood cells) cause an increase in blood flow to the injured area, resulting in cell swelling. In turn, the increase in blood flow brings oxygen and nutrients to the area and helps remove the waste products. Also, similar to the hormonal response produced by resistance training, the immune response signals activation of satellite cells. This process helps muscles repair themselves and grow.

Role of Satellite Cells

The importance of satellite cells for muscle growth was first demonstrated by scientists in Sweden (Kadi and Thornell 2000). These scientists studied a group of females as they performed 10 weeks of resistance training. Before and after the training protocol, the scientists took small muscle samples from the women's trapezius (upper back) muscles. The women had a 36 percent increase in the cross-sectional area of muscle fibers at the end of 10 weeks. The hypertrophy of muscle fibers was accompanied by an approximately 70 percent increase in the number of myonuclei and a 46 percent increase in the number of satellite cells. The number of myonuclei was positively correlated with the number of satellite cells, indicating that a muscle with an increased concentration of myonuclei contains a correspondingly higher number of satellite cells. The scientists suggested that the acquisition of additional myonuclei appears to be required to support the enlargement of multinucleated muscle cells after 10 weeks of strength training. This further suggests that the number of myonuclei dictates how big a muscle fiber can become; therefore, the number is a limiting factor in muscle size development. This makes sense because nuclear domains, or the amount or area of protein that can be managed by a given myonucleus, have genetic limits and dictate the upper limits of protein accretion for that fiber.

Before getting into the specifics about how satellite cells contribute to muscle growth, let's first consider a concept called the *myonuclear domain theory*. As discussed in chapter 1, unlike most cells in the body, which have only one nucleus, muscle cells have many nuclei. The myonuclear domain theory proposes that each nucleus of a muscle cell is responsible for controlling the functioning of a finite volume of cytoplasm—the cell material outside of the nucleus. In other words, a nucleus can regulate only a certain amount of muscle fiber area. If the hormonal and immune responses stimulate a muscle to increase in size, the muscle must have a corresponding adequate number of myonuclei to regulate the increase in cytoplasm throughout the entire cell. Therefore, as the muscle fiber grows, the number of myonuclei must also increase. If growth of the cross-sectional area of the muscle fiber increases beyond an estimated 30 to 35 percent 30donated nuclei from satellite cells are needed for continual hypertrophy to occur.

How does a muscle increase its number of nuclei? That's where satellite cells come into play. As previously mentioned, one of the primary functions of the hormonal and immune responses to resistance exercise is to activate satellite cells. These cells are similar to stem cells in that they are undifferentiated, meaning that they are neither muscle cells nor any other specific type of cell, though they have the capacity to become muscle cells. They are named *satellite cells* because they are located at the periphery of muscle cells. Normally, satellite cells are quiescent (i.e., inactive). However, when muscle is damaged, the hormonal and immune responses activate the satellite cells, causing them to proliferate (i.e., to increase in number) and, finally, to differentiate (i.e., to become incorporated into the muscle fiber and actually become part of the muscle cell). Thus, after activation, satellite cells (1) produce myoblasts that can repair microtears in muscle fibers and (2) can contribute myonuclei to the muscle fiber, allowing for hypertrophy and maintenance of the size of each nuclear domain in the fiber (for a review see Bruusgaard et al. 2010). Once the satellite cells fuse to the muscle fiber, they donate their nuclei. These have been called *daughter nuclei*. This is critical because by increasing its number of myonuclei, the muscle fiber (and therefore the muscle) has an increased capacity to produce more proteins and grow (see figure 2.8). In addition, these satellite cells can regenerate in number so that they can continue to contribute to the muscle's repair the next time the muscle is injured. In fact, a single workout can activate satellite cells in the acute recovery process (Snijders et al. 2012). (For further review of muscle satellite cells, see Hawke 2005; Blaauw and Reggiani 2014.) However, as noted previously, it has been shown that hypertrophy is possible without the increase in satellite cells donating nuclei to the muscle despite their activation (Blaauw and Reggiani 2014). How and when an increased donation of myonuclei is needed from the satellite cells continues to be an important area of research.

Protein Synthesis

Upon completion of a bout of resistance exercise, the acute increase in anabolic hormones within a muscle stimulates the myonuclei to increase protein synthesis of both noncontractile and contractile proteins. More specifically, the nuclei increase production of the contractile proteins actin and myosin within the existing sarcomere. Increased quantity of contractile proteins means two things:

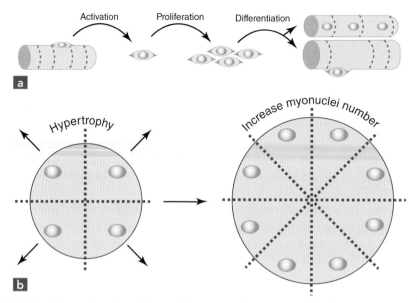

FIGURE 2.8 The role of satellite cells in muscle growth. *(a)* When a muscle fiber is damaged during resistance exercise, quiescent satellite cells are activated, causing them to proliferate and differentiate. If damage is relatively minor, as is usually the case after resistance exercise, the satellite cells will fuse to the muscle fiber to help in the repair of micro damage of the muscle fiber (bottom fiber). As noted before, if growth is increased to higher levels, then satellite cells will contribute their nuclei to allow for maintenance of the nuclear domain sizes. This process helps to repair the muscle and allows for growth. However, if muscle damage is severe, which is rare after resistance exercise, the satellite cells will fuse to one another and generate a new fiber (top fiber). *(b)* The myonuclear domain theory suggests that nuclei can "manage" only a finite amount of cytoplasm. Therefore, if a muscle is stimulated to grow, the muscle must increase its number of nuclei to manage the increase in cytoplasm. The increase in nuclei is donated by satellite cells. Note that each nucleus manages the same volume of cytoplasm before and after muscle growth.

Reprinted, by permission, from T.J. Hawke, 2005, "Muscle stem cells and exercise training," *Exercise and Sport Sciences Reviews* 66: 63-68.

1. An increase in the size of the muscle
2. An increase in the force-generating capacity of the muscle

Or, more succinctly, increased protein synthesis and protein accretion in the muscle fibers that were activated in a resistance training program means a bigger, stronger muscle.

Proteins are molecules made of amino acids. To synthesize proteins, amino acids are transported across the cell membrane and into the skeletal muscle. By increasing your amino acid intake after resistance exercise, you can increase the availability of amino acids to assist in protein synthesis; this underscores the need for an adequate diet. In total, muscle protein synthesis after resistance exercise depends highly on amino acid availability, timing of the intake of nutritional amino acid (the sooner after exercise the better), hormonal regulation (insulin, a type of GH, testosterone, and IGF-I), mechanical stress, and cellular hydration. The take-home message is this: Support protein synthesis by eating a small meal soon after exercise. This meal should contain a small amount of carbohydrate (to stimulate insulin) and protein (to increase essential amino acid availability).

In the long run, muscle hypertrophy is the result of an overall increase in muscle protein synthesis, a decrease in protein degradation (catabolism), or a combination of both. The current thought is that the summation of periods of increases in muscle protein synthesis induced by resistance exercise can chronically induce hypertrophy. It has been shown that the initial responses of muscle protein synthesis to a resistance exercise workout and to nutrition are not highly correlated with subsequent hypertrophy but rather reflect the acute metabolic demands of the exercise. It was then concluded that the early acute response of muscle protein synthesis in the hours after resistance exercise, in an untrained state, does not capture how muscle protein synthesis affects resistance-induced muscle hypertrophy (for a review, see Damas et al. 2015).

Fiber Size Increases

The coordinated responses of the endocrine system, the immune system, and the satellite cells lead to an increase in protein synthesis and, ultimately, an increase in muscle fiber size. This increase in the cross-sectional area of existing muscle fibers is attributed to an increased number of actin and myosin filaments and the addition of sarcomeres within existing muscle fibers. If enough muscle fibers are stimulated with training, an increase in the size of the whole muscle occurs.

You can observe the increase in muscle fiber size by examining a group of muscle fibers under a microscope after they have been stained. Figure 2.9 shows two pictures of a muscle sample obtained from a woman's vastus lateralis (quadriceps muscle) (a) before and (b) after an eight-week heavy resistance training program. The fibers are cut in cross-sections; the dark fibers are Type I muscle fibers, and the white fibers are Type II fibers. It is clear that this woman increased the size of all of her muscle fibers, especially the Type II (fast twitch) muscle fibers, with just eight weeks

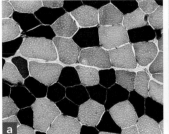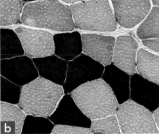

FIGURE 2.9   *(a)* A biopsy sample from the thigh muscle that was stained in the laboratory to demonstrate the changes that occur in both type and size with training. *(b)* The fibers are larger after eight weeks of heavy resistance training than they were before training. Such increases in muscle fiber hypertrophy contribute to hypertrophy of the whole muscle if enough muscle fibers are recruited through proper loading.

Courtesy of Dr. Kraemer's Laboratory.

of heavy resistance training. Logically, increases in the size of individual muscle fibers can lead to increased size of the entire muscle group. However, a significant number of fibers need to hypertrophy to see such a response for the whole muscle (figure 2.10, *a* and *b*).

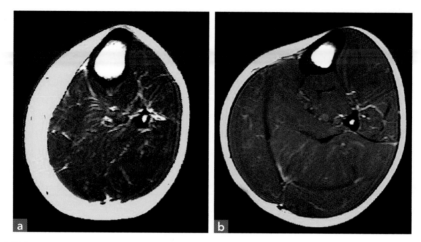

FIGURE 2.10 A magnetic resonance image of the upper arm of a woman *(a)* before and *(b)* after six months of periodized resistance training. Notice the increase in lean tissue mass of the arm and the reduction of fat around the muscle. Whole-muscle hypertrophy is a result of hypertrophy of each individual muscle fiber.

Courtesy of Dr. Kraemer's Laboratory.

Summary

As you can see, the process of muscle growth is well coordinated and is supported by several physiological systems. Now that you have an understanding of how muscle grows, you can begin to appreciate the importance of a properly designed strength training program.

3

Types of Muscle Training

William J. Kraemer, Disa L. Hatfield, and Steven J. Fleck

Strength training programs today have taken on different combinations of the acute program variables put forth more than 30 years ago in the first edition of *Designing Resistance Training Programs.* In designing a resistance training program, the needs of the individual are paramount to the program characteristics (Fleck and Kraemer 2014). Thus, optimal programs with specific goals, starting points, and progressions are designed for the individual using the basic principles overviewed in this chapter. A program for a person wishing to increase maximal strength will differ greatly from a program for a person wishing to increase local muscular endurance. In addition to outcome goals, a program design must take into account individual differences such as training experience, time allotted to train, the facilities available for training, and any special needs the person may have. The principles of any effective muscle training program are as follows:

- **Specificity of training.** Only those muscles that are trained will adapt and change in response to a resistance training program.

- **General adaptation syndrome.** Han Selye's general adaptation syndrome refers to the three stages of adaptation (Selye 1950, Selye 1976): (1) the alarm stage, caused by the onset of physiological stress (i.e., exercise training); (2) the resistance stage, in which the body begins to adapt to the demands; and (3) the exhaustion stage, which occurs with overtraining.

- **Specific adaptations to imposed demands principle.** According to the specific adaptations to imposed demands principle, the adaptation will be specific to the characteristics of the workout used.

- **Variation in training.** Programs should change the exercise stimulus over time. Periodized training is the major concept related to constructing the optimal training and recovery program.

- **Prioritization of training.** It is difficult to train for all aspects of physical development. Thus, within a periodized training program, it is optimal to focus or prioritize training goals over each training cycle, particularly for beginner athletes. In a given cycle it may be possible to focus on only one training goal. How the goals are determined and developed over time depends on the experience of the trainee and fitness level of the individual.

In this chapter, you will learn how these principles are integral to designing an effective resistance training program. In addition, this chapter outlines how to manipulate variables of a resistance training program to affect the outcomes, such as muscular hypertrophy, strength, and local muscular endurance.

Acute Program Variables

Any sound resistance training program is made up of several variables, including the exercises chosen, the order in which the exercises are performed, the intensity or load of the exercise, the number of repetitions and sets of the exercise, and how much rest you take between exercises. These are called *acute program variables* because they are variables that you can change in a single workout; they will determine the outcome of training over the long term. You can evaluate any workout by examining the choices you made for the acute program variables (Fleck and Kraemer 2014) and noting how these choices affect the training adaptations that may be associated with a resistance training program. In addition, acute program variables are what allow you to create different types of workouts.

Understanding the factors that go into creating the exercise stimulus is crucial to designing an effective training program. Figure 3.1 shows how acute program variables are one of the domains of modifiable variables that can be manipulated and help define the exercise stimuli of physiological and molecular responses and adaptations that lead to changes in muscle strength and size. Creating an effective exercise stimulus starts by deciding on the direction in which you want the training outcomes to proceed (e.g., to increase force production, power, hypertrophy, and so forth). The next step is to develop a single training session directed at these specific, trainable characteristics. The acute program variables describe the choices you can make in a single workout. The choices you make for each variable over time dictate the progression of your training program.

Choice of Exercises

The exercises you choose should reflect the areas of the body and the biomechanical characteristics of these areas that you want to target for improvement. The number of possible exercises that target specific joint angles is almost as limitless as the body's functional movements that these exercises help improve. When choosing which exercises to do, keep in mind that muscle tissue that is not activated does not benefit from resistance training (remember the size principle discussed in chapters 1 and 2). Therefore, you should first determine what you want to get out of a resistance training program and then select exercises that stress the muscles and joint angles you want to target.

Exercises can be designated as primary exercises or assistance exercises. Primary exercises train the muscles called the *prime movers* (major muscle groups

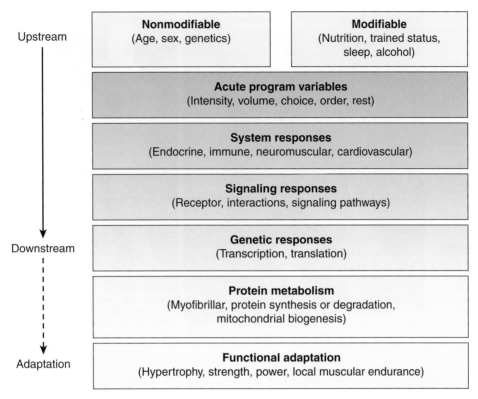

FIGURE 3.1 Upstream regulatory variables can be modifiable or nonmodifiable. The acute program variables that compose a resistance training workout are modifiable variables and affect the physiological and molecular events that mediate muscle size and functional adaptations for physical performance.

responsible for the majority of the movement made in the exercise). Examples of primary exercises include the leg press, barbell bench press, and hang power clean. Assistance exercises are those that train predominantly one muscle group that aids in the movement produced by the prime movers. The cable triceps extension and dumbbell biceps curl are two examples of assistance exercises.

Exercises can also be classified as structural (i.e., involving multiple joints) or body part specific (i.e., involving an isolated joint; see figure 3.2, *a* and *b*). Structural exercises include whole-body lifts that require the coordinated action of several muscle groups. The power clean, deadlift, and squat are good examples of structural whole-body exercises. Other structural exercises don't involve the whole body but do involve multiple joints or muscles. For example, the barbell bench press involves movement of both the elbow and shoulder joints. Some other examples of multiple-joint exercises are the lat pull-down, standing military press, and leg press. Isolation exercises are body part specific and isolate single muscle groups. The dumbbell biceps curl, leg extension, seated leg curl, and many other assistance exercises are good examples of isolation exercises.

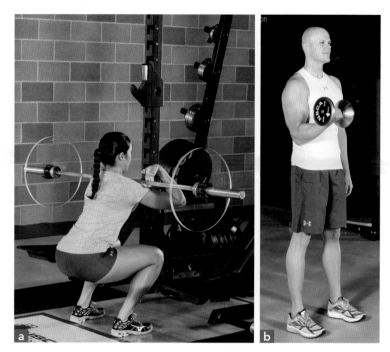

FIGURE 3.2 Some exercises, such as *(a)* the front squat, work multiple joints, whereas others, such as *(b)* the biceps curl, move just one joint.

Structural or multiple-joint exercises require neural coordination among muscles because they promote the coordinated use of movements that involve multiple joints and multiple muscle groups. It recently has been shown that multijoint exercises require a longer initial learning or neural phase compared with single-joint exercises, which likely is due to the increased neural challenge these exercises present. Many times, structural exercises involve advanced lifting techniques (e.g., power clean) that require coaching of exercise technique beyond simple movement patterns. Including structural and multiple-joint exercises in a program is especially important when whole-body strength movements are required for a particular target activity. Most sports and functional activities in everyday life (e.g., climbing stairs) depend on structural multijoint movements. Whole-body strength and power movements—in particular, running and jumping activities, making a tackle in American football, taking down an opponent in wrestling, and hitting a baseball—are the basis for success in all sports. The time saved with multiple-joint exercises is also an important consideration for an individual or team with a limited amount of time per training session. The benefits of multijoint exercises in terms of muscle tissue activated, hormonal response, and metabolic demands far outweigh those of single-joint exercises. Therefore, for best results, most workouts should revolve around multijoint exercises.

Order of Exercises

The order in which you perform your exercises affects the quality of the workout, especially if you are lifting heavy loads. (See the discussion on intensity in the next section.) Most experts believe that exercising the larger muscle groups first provides a superior training stimulus to all of the muscles involved. This is thought to be true because exercising larger muscle groups stimulates greater neural, metabolic, endocrine, and circulatory responses, which potentially augments the training of subsequent muscles later in the workout. Thus, the more complex multijoint exercises (e.g., squats) should be performed initially, followed by the less complex single-joint exercises (e.g., dumbbell biceps curls). Another rationale for sequencing multiple-joint exercises before single-joint exercises is that exercises that require the greatest amount of muscle mass and energy for optimal performance should be performed in the beginning of the workout, when the individual has the least fatigue. Thus, these sequencing strategies focus on attaining a greater training effect for the exercises involving large muscle groups. If structural exercises are performed early in the workout, you can use more resistance to do them because your muscles are not yet fatigued.

Most important, exercise order needs to correspond with specific training goals. A few general methods for sequencing exercises (for training sessions targeting either multiple or single muscle groups) include the following:

- Targeting large muscle groups before small muscle groups
- Performing multiple-joint exercises before single-joint exercises
- Alternating push and pull exercises for total-body sessions
- Alternating upper- and lower-body exercises for total-body sessions
- Performing exercises for weaker points (i.e., priorities) before exercises for stronger points
- Performing Olympic lifts before basic strength and single-joint exercises
- Performing power exercises before other types of exercise
- Performing more intense exercises before less intense exercises, particularly when performing several exercises consecutively for the same muscle group

One final consideration for exercise order is the fitness level of the person and his or her experience with resistance training. Training sessions must be designed so that they are not too stressful for the individual, especially a beginner.

Intensity or Resistance

The amount of resistance used for a specific exercise is one of the key factors in any resistance training program. It is the major stimulus related to changes in strength and local muscular endurance. Higher intensity is important for strength development in all individuals, older and younger (Peterson et al. 2004, 2005, 2010).

One of the easiest methods for determining the right resistance for an exercise is to determine your RM—the specific resistance that allows you to perform only a specific number of repetitions. Typically, to determine RM, you can choose a single training RM target (e.g., 10RM) or choose an RM target training zone (e.g., 3-5RM); you then perform each exercise at different resistances until you meet this target. As your strength level changes over time for each lift, you can adjust the resistance so that you continue to hit your specified RM target or zone. Going to failure on every repetition can be stressful on the joints, but for optimal results you should make sure that the resistance you use places you within a targeted range of reps—for example, the resistance allows you to lift the weight for only 4 or 5 repetitions compared with 14 or 15 repetitions. The training outcome for these two resistances is quite different.

Another method for determining resistance for an exercise involves using a percentage of the 1RM for a lift. For example, if your 1RM for an exercise is 100 pounds (45.4 kg), lifting 80 percent of the 1RM would mean lifting 80 pounds (36.3 kg). This method requires you to regularly evaluate your maximal strength in the various lifts so that you can adjust the resistance appropriately as you get stronger. However, if you do not test your 1RM each week, especially when beginning a program, the resistance represented by the percentage of 1RM that you use in training will decrease as your strength increases; as a result, training intensity will be reduced. From a practical perspective, using a percentage of 1RM as the resistance for many exercises may not be efficient because of the amount of testing time required. Use of an RM target or RM target zone allows you to change resistance as necessary during training in order to stay at the RM target or within the RM target zone you've chosen.

Like other acute variables, the loading intensity a person chooses depends on his or her goals and training status (i.e., whether the person is a trained athlete or a sedentary individual). The intensity of the loading as a percentage of 1RM affects the number of repetitions that a person can perform at a given load or intensity. Ultimately, the number of repetitions you can perform at a given intensity or load determines the effects of training on strength development (Hoeger et al. 1990). It is important to note that the RM at a set percentage of the 1RM can vary between free weights and machines; more repetitions can be performed when the resistance is on a set, controlled path because no balance is required (Hoeger et al. 1990; Shimano et al. 2006). If an athlete lifting a specific percentage of the 1RM can lift only a specific number of repetitions, then lifting fewer repetitions without changing the resistance would mean that the athlete is using different motor units to perform the exercise. For instance, a low-intensity (light resistance), high-repetition workout protocol would effectively activate the Type I muscle fibers (those more suited to local muscular endurance) but would not adequately activate the Type II muscle fibers (the predominant muscle fibers responsible for maximal strength and hypertrophy gains). Thus, if you want to maximize strength gains, you should lift heavier loads and therefore perform fewer repetitions. If local muscular endurance is the goal, you should use a lighter load, which in turn allows a greater number of repetitions.

Number of Sets (Volume of Exercise)

Total exercise volume (sets × repetitions × weight) is a vital concept of training progression. Using a program with a constant volume may lead you to feel stale and may cause you to discontinue your training. Varying the training volume through periodization, which enables you to use different exercise stimuli over long-term training periods, provides rest and recovery periods. We cover periodization in more detail later in this chapter.

The number of sets is a factor in the volume of exercise. Note that not all exercises in a training session need to be performed for the same number of sets. In studies examining resistance-trained individuals, multiple-set programs were found to be superior for increasing strength, power, hypertrophy, and high-intensity endurance. These findings have prompted the recommendation (Ratamess et al. 2009) to use periodized multiple-set programs when long-term progression—not maintenance—is the goal in any area (e.g., strength, endurance, hypertrophy, and so on).

No study of either trained or untrained individuals has shown single-set training to be superior to multiple-set training. It appears that both types of programs are effective for increasing strength in untrained subjects during short-term (6- to 12-week) training periods (Rhea et al. 2002; Fleck and Kraemer, 2014). However, some short-term and all long-term studies support the contention that a training volume greater than one set is needed for progressive physical development and improved performance (Peterson et al. 2005, 2010).

Still, the need for variations such as using lower volumes of training during some phases of the overall training program is also critical for continued improvement and to augment training adaptations. The key is to periodize training volume rather than just the number of sets, which represents only one factor in a volume and intensity periodization model. This model is covered in greater detail later in this chapter. Each set of an exercise presents a training stimulus to the muscle; thus, once initial fitness has been achieved, performing multiple sets (three to six) with specific rest periods between them that allow for the desired intensity is more effective than doing a single set. Some advocates of single-set programs believe that a muscle or muscle group can perform maximal exercise for only a single set; however, research has not shown this to be true (Fleck and Kraemer 2014)

The optimal number of exercises for a given resistance training goal has not been studied. Typically, the total number of sets spanning all exercises in a session is used to calculate total exercise volume. However, the type of exercises chosen (multijoint and structural exercises vs. single-joint movements) should be considered when calculating volume. Furthermore, the calculation of volume is body part specific. Thus, the appropriate volume for lower-body and upper-body exercises should be determined separately and calculated based on need.

Rest Periods Between Sets and Exercises

A major topic of study over the past 10 years has been the influence of rest periods on the stress of the workout and the corresponding amount of resistance that can be used. Rest periods between sets and exercises determine the magnitude of adenosine triphosphate–creatine phosphate energy source resynthesis and the concentrations of lactate in the blood (see chapter 2). The length of the rest period can significantly alter the metabolic, hormonal, and cardiovascular responses to an acute bout of resistance exercise as well as the performance of subsequent sets.

For advanced training that emphasizes increasing absolute strength or power, rest periods of at least three to five minutes are recommended for structural exercises (e.g., squats, power cleans, deadlifts) using maximal or near-maximal loads; less rest (one minute or less) may be needed for exercises involving smaller muscle mass or single-joint movements (Ratamess et al. 2009; Haff and Triplett 2016). Advanced lifters need so much rest because they are often lifting resistances that are closer to their genetic potential; this intensity necessitates that they maximize their recovery of energy stores for the next lift. For novice to intermediate lifters, two to three minutes of rest may suffice for structural lifts because the intensity at this level of resistance training appears to be less stressful to the neuromuscular system.

On the other hand, stressing the glycolytic and adenosine triphosphate–creatine phosphate energy systems may enhance muscle hypertrophy; thus, less rest between sets (<60-90 seconds) appears to be effective if training to increase muscle size. In addition, varying the amount of rest between sets may be effective if the goal is to optimize both strength and size, with some workouts stimulating a greater blood concentration of anabolic hormones. Research demonstrates that short-rest programs (i.e., exercises using rest periods of one minute or less) can cause greater psychological anxiety and fatigue, but these psychological mood state scale ratings are still in the normal range and are not clinically concerning or detrimental (Tharion et al. 1991). Such psychological mood state scale ratings might be related to the greater discomfort, muscle fatigue, and higher metabolic demands associated with short-rest programs with short rest when compared to longer rest workout protocols. Some of the psychological mood state elevations may be part of the arousal and preparation needed to take on a demanding workout in an effective manner and may be a positive adjustment of the psychological state before the workout.

Muscle Training Programs

You can find literally hundreds of methods of muscle strength training. However, very few of these have stood the test of time or the scrutiny of scientific research.

Of all these methods, periodization has emerged as the preferred approach to optimizing many types of training, including resistance training.

Periodization Training

Periodized resistance training has been shown to be superior to constant training methods (Fleck and Kraemer 2014). Periodization training allows for the use of many types of workouts, training programs, and modalities. In essence, it calls for varying the training stimulus (intensity or volume) over determined periods of time to allow for an optimal progression in the exercise stress and planned periods of rest.

Periodization training evolved, in part, from a principle of resistance training called *progressive resistance training* or *overload*. The principle was coined by Dr. Thomas Delorme, a U.S. Army physician working with the physical rehabilitation of soldiers in the 1940s and 1950s (Todd et al. 2012). Later, he continued his work in rehabilitation as a distinguished orthopedic surgeon at Massachusetts General Hospital in Boston. His wife came up with the term *progressive resistance training* over a dinner conversation. It was born from the specific adaptations to imposed demands principle, and it refers to the need to gradually increase the amount of physical stress placed on the body in order to continually stimulate adaptations.

Dr. Delorme's principle originally was based on a 10RM set and then percentages of that load. From there, to increase stress, he manipulated any combination of acute variables (e.g., increasing the resistance load, volume, and frequency of training and decreasing the rest time between sets) to allow adaptations to occur. Most of the approaches that Delorme tried were linear in nature and therefore hit plateaus relatively quickly. Over the decades, training methods evolved to using periodization to ensure steady improvements in performance, provide for recovery, and avoid staleness. Thus, the case for periodized training was made as athletes looked to further improve their fitness levels for competition.

Strength athletes initially relied on the classical periodization model, also called *linear periodization*. The concept of linear periodization as we know it is attributed to the work of Eastern Bloc sport programs in the early 1950s. It came about through trial and error and through mathematical modeling of how champion athletes trained as coaches tried to optimize sport performance. The coaches noticed that decreasing volume and increasing intensity (in this case, defined as a percentage of near-maximal effort) in the weeks leading up to a competition improved performance. It is important to note that the classic linear periodization programs were developed for strength and power athletes peaking for one particular contest at the end of a year, such as a world championship or the Olympics. Today, many athletes in various sports peak for multiple competitions in a single season.

These early periodization models were built around one competitive season broken into four phases: preparation, first transition (end of preseason), competition, and second transition (off-season). Today, many periodization strategies exist (for a review, see Plisk and Stone 2003). In early models, the length of each phase depended on the length of the competition season, the mode of training, and individual differences of the athletes. The preparation phase involved increasing strength and muscle mass; in this phase, exercise volume was high and intensity was low. In the first transition phase, volume decreased as intensity increased, and the goals were to optimize muscular power and increase skill proficiency. The competition phase was also referred to as *peaking*. The characteristics of the competition phase differed depending on the sport; however, training during this time was always sport specific, or designed based on the demands of competition. The off-season was spent performing activities that would aid in recovery and rehabilitation but not lead to complete detraining.

Periodization has its own terminology. The longest cycle is the multiyear plan, which can range from two years to a four-year period leading up to an Olympic Games. In this plan is a macrocycle of several months to a year. The macrocycle is then divided into smaller cycles, called *mesocycles*, which range from two to six weeks for a year. Finally, the smallest cycle, called a *microcycle*, ranges from several days to two weeks.

Linear Periodization

The phases of linear periodization often use progressive overload, which calls for gradual and linear increases in intensity and a reduction in volume as the cycle progresses. For example, in a mesocycle of six weeks, two-week microcycles will start light and become progressively heavy by the third microcycle. The volume will continue to decrease as the intensity of the resistance increases. Then, after the six-week mesocycle, an active rest cycle of varying length may occur depending on the athlete's background and training level. Then, the program may repeat for another mesocycle.

In linear periodization, a typical goal over the macrocycle is to increase the body's muscle hypertrophy and strength toward the theoretical genetic maximum. Thus, the basis of a linear method of periodization consists of developing muscle hypertrophy followed by improved nerve function and strength. If this is repeated again and again with each microcycle and in each phase, loading would progressively increase from workout to workout. You can see in table 3.1 that some variation exists in each cycle because of the range of repetitions for each cycle. Still, the general trend for the 16-week program is a steady linear increase in intensity.

Volume also varies in a linear periodization program. The program starts with a higher volume, which gradually decreases as the intensity of the program increases. As athletes become stronger, they can tolerate higher volumes of exercise during the heavy and very heavy microcycles. Linear periodization can help beginners get used to the training stress because it starts off with relatively light weights and higher volume. The linear periodization program may also be designed based on RM target training zones (see table 3.2).

TABLE 3.1 Typical Periodization Format for a Training Program

Goal	Preparation phase (4 wk)	First transition (4 wk)	Competition phase (4 wk)	Second transition (off-season)
	Muscle growth (hypertrophy)	Maximal strength and power	Peak	Recovery (light physical activity)
Reps	8-10	4-6	1-3	12-15
Sets	4-5	3-4	3-5	3-5
Intensity	Low	Moderate	Very high	Low
Volume	High to moderate	Moderate	Low	Low

TABLE 3.2 Linear Periodized Program Using Repetition Training Zones*

Mesocycle	Repetition training zone
1	3-5 sets of 10-12RM
2	4-5 sets of 8-10RM
3	3-4 sets of 4-6RM
4	3-5 sets of 1-3RM

*Each cycle is 4 wk long.

You must be very careful not to progress too quickly to high volumes of heavy weights. Pushing too hard can lead to injury, overuse strain, and overtraining syndrome, all of which can compromise progress for months. Although it takes a great deal of excessive work to produce such an overtraining effect, young and highly motivated trainees easily can make this mistake out of sheer desire to make gains and see progress in their training. To avoid progressing too quickly, you can first do 6 to 12 weeks of a general preparation phase to get ready for a more formalized periodized program. This phase would involve using light weights, learning the exercises, and progressing to the starting RM percentage range that will be used in a program.

In any periodized training program, the purpose of the high volume of exercise in the early microcycles (often called the *off-season training* for a given sport) is to promote the muscle hypertrophy needed to eventually enhance strength in the later phases of training (toward peaking). Thus, the late cycles of training are linked to the early cycles, and these cycles enhance each other because strength gains are related to changes in muscle size. Programs designed for gaining strength without the needed muscle tissue have limited potential.

The increases in the intensity of the periodized program then start to focus on developing the needed nervous system adaptations for enhanced motor unit recruitment. Heavier weights demand that high-threshold motor units become involved in the force production process. Force production of the motor units is further enhanced with the associated increase in muscle protein from the earlier cycles of training. You can see in table 3.2 how different parts of the 16-week program build on one another.

Nonlinear Periodization

Periodization has evolved beyond the linear method, and more modern forms can be manipulated to meet the special needs of particular athletes. In the past decade, *nonlinear periodization* (sometimes referred to as *undulating periodization*) has replaced the classical, linear approach for many athletes dealing with an academic schedule or individuals interested in basic strength fitness (Rhea et al. 2003a and b; Kraemer and Fleck 2007; Miranda et al. 2011). Rather than sequentially increasing or decreasing the volume and intensity, nonlinear periodization calls for more frequent (i.e., weekly and sometimes daily) changes to maintain variation in the training stimulus. Recent research comparing it with linear periodization has shown that making more frequent variations to a program elicits greater gains in as little as 15 weeks. Nonlinear periodization is thought to be effective because the constant variation of the acute variables demands that physiological adaptations take place constantly (as opposed to a gradual increase in intensity or volume that causes plateaus in gains to occur). The newer concept of flexible nonlinear periodization asks the question "Is the athlete or individual ready to train with this training session today?" for each predesigned workout in a planned mesocycle (Kraemer and Fleck 2007).

Another important aspect of nonlinear periodization is the volume and intensity of the assistance exercises. The primary exercises typically are periodized, but with the nonlinear approach you can also use a two-cycle program to vary the exercises involving small muscle groups. For example, in the cable triceps extension, you could rotate between moderate (8-10RM) and heavy (4-6RM) cycle intensities. This would provide the hypertrophy needed for isolated muscles of a joint but also provide the strength needed to support heavier workouts of the large muscle groups.

Individual differences in schedule or competitive demands are also of great consideration when designing this type of program. In the nonlinear approach, athletes can train both for increases in muscle size (hypertrophy) and for making gains in neural aspects of strength in the same 7- to 14-day period of the longer mesocycle. This may be more convenient for many individuals' schedules, especially when competition, travel, or other schedule conflicts make the traditional linear method difficult to adhere to.

In this approach, workouts rotate among very heavy, heavy, moderate, and light training sessions. If you were to miss a workout, you simply would perform that workout on the next day and continue with the rotation. Rather than letting a certain number of weeks dictate the length of a mesocycle, a mesocycle is completed when a certain number of workouts are completed.

Table 3.3 provides an example of a nonlinear periodized training program over 5 weeks from a 16-week macrocycle for the lower-body muscles. You will notice that the variation within each week of training is much greater than in a linear program and ranges from 1RM sets to 12RM sets. You can also add a power training day in which loads may range from 30 to 45 percent of 1RM and release of the mass being lifted is allowed if no deceleration occurs with the movement of the joints (e.g., as in bench press throws). Variations such as this may also be considered a "down" day in which the physiological stress of the workout is not high because of the lack of the eccentric portion of the lift, thus allowing the athlete more recovery time.

Table 3.4 shows a nonlinear program using an RM target training zone for each of the different workouts. In this program, the variation in training is much greater within the week and ranges from 1RM to 15RM. To add variation to the program and allow some recovery from higher-intensity exercise, medicine ball plyometrics and other lower-body plyometrics are also performed. An active rest break occurs after 12 weeks of training, which would correspond to the second transition phase in the classical periodization model. Interestingly, one complete day of rest per week may eliminate an overreaching syndrome.

Whether you use a linear or a nonlinear periodization program, the overall effects appear to be the same: training for both hypertrophy and neural gains. Periodized programs are effective and used in different sports and within different training cycles. For example, when a sport has a long season, nonlinear

TABLE 3.3 Example of a Nonlinear or Undulating Form of Progression in Resistance Training*

	Wk 1	Wk 2	Wk 3	Wk 4	Wk 5
Day 1	82% × 3 × 3	87% × 2 × 3	75% × 6 × 3	85% × 3 × 3	90% × 1 × 3
Day 2	60% × 8 × 3	50% × 3 × 9	53% × 12 × 3	62% × 8 × 2	55% × 5 × 5
Day 3	Optional day: active rest and recover or very light assistance work				

*Intensity (as a percentage of 1RM) × repetitions × number of sets.

TABLE 3.4 Nonlinear Periodized Program Using the RM Training Zone Approach

Day	RM training zone
Monday	4 sets of 12-15RM
Wednesday	4 sets of 8-10RM
Friday	3-4 sets of 4-6RM
Monday	4-5 sets of 1-3RM
Wednesday	Power day
Friday	2 sets of 12-15RM

periodization is superior in season. Use of the appropriate program is dependent on the situation. However, any periodized program is superior to a constant training program.

Other Strength Training Protocols

Although periodization training has become the predominant method of training in both the athletic and fitness worlds, many other forms of training can be useful in attaining goals and adding variation to the normal routine. Many of these programs are simple to follow, and beginners tend to find some of them (e.g., circuit training) less intimidating. Furthermore, most of these programs have been shown to elicit gains in short-term training (up to eight weeks), after which periodized training is superior.

Circuit Training

Circuit training gained popularity as strength training machines (e.g., Universal, Nautilus, Marcy, and Pyramid) became more commonplace in the 1970s. In circuit training the athlete choses 8 to 12 exercise stations, performs the exercises in a circuit (one after the other), and then repeats the circuit one to three times.

Circuit training primarily aims to address cardiovascular endurance as well as local muscular endurance. It also promotes some moderate gains in strength. Chapter 7 covers circuit training in more detail.

This type of program can be time and space efficient when large numbers of people are training because each piece of equipment is in virtually constant use. It is also very effective for an individual with a limited amount of training time because most circuit protocols use light weights and short rest for about 8 to 10 exercises (Fleck and Kraemer 2014).

One-Set Program

Like circuit training, most one-set programs evolved from the commercial advertising for weight machines of the 1970s and were popularized because of the ease of use and inflated claims of efficacy. One-set programs are often done in a circuit fashion in which one set of 8 to 12 repetitions of each exercise is performed to failure.

These programs, also sometimes erroneously referred to as high-intensity training, have not been proven to be as effective as periodized programs or even progressive overload programs that use multiple sets (Tan 1999; Peterson et al. 2004, 2005). Nevertheless, they can provide a fast change-up routine in even a nonlinear workout and might be categorized as a one-set circuit workout.

Multiple-Set System

The multiple-set system originally consisted of two or three warm-up sets of increasing resistance followed by several work sets at the same resistance. This training system became popular in the 1940s and was the forerunner of the multiple-set and repetition systems of today. Considerable research has been done to determine the optimal resistance and number of repetitions for developing strength using a multiple-set system. For some multijoint exercises, a 5RM or 6RM performed for a minimum of three sets (with a range of three to six sets) appears to be optimal for increasing strength in beginner to advanced trainees.

You can perform a multiple-set system at any desired resistance and for any number of repetitions and sets to meet the desired goals of a training program. However, performing a multiple-set system for a long period of time without changing other training variables normally results in plateaus in strength and power gains. The majority of resistance training systems use some variation of a multiple-set system. If gaining strength and power is the objective of training, you can optimize the multiple-set system by periodizing training.

Super Slow System

The super slow system involves performing very slow repetitions that range from 20 to 60 seconds per repetition. Proponents say that strength development is enhanced by the increased amount of time the muscle is under tension. To date, little data are available to support this theory. The amount of force that a muscle can produce dramatically decreases with time; to move a weight slowly, you have to significantly reduce the resistance you use, which in turn recruits more endurance muscle fibers (Hatfield et al. 2006). Individuals in the Hatfield et al. (2006) study performed fewer repetitions of super slow movements, although the time under tension during a repetition was longer. The results of that study indicated that a very slow velocity (10-second eccentric and 10-second concentric actions) may not elicit appropriate levels of force, power, or volume to optimize strength and athletic performance. Super slow sets appear to have some potential efficacy in developing slow-velocity muscular endurance.

This system of resistance training typically is used for isolated-joint exercises or machine exercises in which the movement can be controlled throughout the range of motion. Usually, super slow sets are performed for only one or two sets in an entire workout. The resistance varies depending on a person's muscular endurance fitness level; therefore, it is not related to the resistance used for a repetition at normal speed. As the time to complete the repetition increases, the amount of resistance that can be lifted decreases. Thus, each point in the range of motion receives a strength stimulus that is less than optimal.

Pyramid or Triangle Routine

Popularized by powerlifters, the pyramid method of resistance training uses a gradual increase in resistance—and thus a decrease in repetitions—with each set of a single exercise. Once you perform a very low number of repetitions (one to five), you decrease the resistance and increase the number of repetitions in increments until you reach your starting point. An example of this would be performing a 10RM, 8RM, 6RM, 4RM, 2RM, 4RM, 6RM, 8RM, and 10RM with the resistance set to allow only the listed number of repetitions. This method often is performed as a half pyramid (e.g., going up to only a specific resistance, such as the peak 2RM set in the previous example). The heavier the resistance, the longer the rest you need. Therefore, this type of program is very time intensive, and it typically is used for only two or three exercises in a workout. Pyramid routines are discussed in more detail in chapter 7.

Super Setting

Super setting is a term used to describe alternating between two exercises for two different target muscle groups. These muscle groups can be opposing groups (e.g., biceps and triceps) or groups at different joints (e.g., quadriceps and deltoids). Bodybuilders commonly use super setting to stimulate definition and burn fat. Scant data exist on the efficacy of using super sets, yet many programs use various types of super sets to maximize the metabolic intensity (i.e., to improve the hormonal profile for specific gains such as hypertrophy) of a body part being trained (e.g., biceps and triceps). Proponents hypothesize that super setting ensures that all the muscles of a particular joint are exercised, thus allowing symmetry of size to be maintained among the muscles around a joint. Super setting may be created in a number of ways. Here are two examples:

1. Biceps curl 10RM, triceps push-down 10RM. Repeat three times with no rest between exercises.
2. Lat pull-down 10RM, seated cable row 10RM, bent-over row 10RM. Repeat three times with one minute of rest between each exercise.

The first example focuses on two opposing muscle groups and uses the push–pull approach. The second example concentrates on one particular body part or joint (in this case, the back muscles). Super sets often are placed within a workout or at the end of a workout when local muscular endurance and definition are the primary goals of the program. This type of workout protocol can be very demanding given the short rest periods. Super sets are discussed in more detail in chapter 7.

Negative Resistance Training

For most resistance exercises, the lowering of the weight during the repetition is called the *negative* or *eccentric* portion. During this phase, the muscles involved are actively lengthening so you can lower the resistance in a controlled manner. Conversely, the lifting of the resistance during the repetition of an exercise is called the *positive* or *concentric* portion.

A person normally is able to handle more weight in the lowering phase of a repetition than in the lifting or positive portion of the repetition. Negative resistance training involves lowering more weight than you can lift in the concentric phase of the repetition. You can perform this type of training by having spotters help you raise the weight and then lowering it on your own. You also can perform negative resistance training on some resistance training machines by lifting the weight with both arms or legs and then lowering the resistance with only one arm or leg. On some machines, it is possible to lift the weight with both the arms and the legs and then lower the weight using just the arms or just the legs. Be sure to use proper exercise and safety spotting techniques when performing heavy negative resistance training.

Advocates of negative training believe that using more resistance during the negative portion of the exercise results in greater increases in strength. However, studies show that using 120 percent of the concentric (positive) 1RM for negative training does not result in greater gains in strength compared with normal training with concentric repetitions. Optimal eccentric resistances for particular muscle groups and for populations using different equipment are quite variable (Fleck and Kraemer 2014). Ranges of 105 to 140 percent of the concentric 1RM have been proposed, but such resistances may depend on whether a machine or free weights are being used. Machines reduce the amount of balance required and the involvement of assistance muscles; thus, heavier eccentric (negative) resistances may be possible. It has been shown that a repetition that uses a heavier eccentric resistance (105 percent of the concentric 1RM) immediately before the concentric phase of the repetition results in achieving a heavier concentric 1RM. Therefore, eccentric training may enhance the neural facilitation of the concentric movement. Further study is needed to determine whether such training affects gains in strength. For free weights, 105 to 110 percent of the concentric 1RM probably represents the upper limit of effective eccentric resistances for most exercise movements.

Split Routine System

Many bodybuilders use a split routine system. Bodybuilders perform many exercises for the same body part in the same exercise session to encourage hypertrophy. Because this is a time-consuming process, not all parts of the body can be exercised in a single training session. Solving this predicament has led to training various body parts on alternate days, or a split routine. A typical split routine system entails training the arms, legs, and abdomen on Monday, Wednesday, and Friday and training the chest, shoulders, and back on Tuesday, Thursday, and Saturday. This system helps minimize the time spent per session, but it means training six days per week.

You can develop variations of a split routine system so that training sessions take place four or five days per week. Even though training sessions are still quite frequent, this allows sufficient recovery of muscle groups between training sessions because body parts are not trained on successive days. The split routine system allows you to maintain a higher intensity of training for a particular body part or group of exercises; these higher intensities would not be possible if the four to six training sessions were combined into two or three longer sessions. Maintaining a higher intensity (i.e., heavier resistances) should result in greater gains in strength. Split routines allow you to pay more attention to the assistance exercises needed to enhance strength development.

Forced Repetition System

Forced repetitions are an extension of the exhaustion set system and the cheat system used by some powerlifters and other trained individuals (Ahtiainen et al. 2004). After you have performed a set to exhaustion, your training partners assist you by lifting the resistance just enough to allow you to lift three or four additional repetitions. You can use this system with many exercises after you have performed a set to exhaustion. This system forces the muscle, which is partially fatigued, to continue to produce force. This may benefit those attempting to increase local muscular endurance. In experienced strength athletes, the forced-repetition protocol for leg extensors was found to enhance the acute neural and hormonal responses to a greater extent than a traditional set protocol. Thus, it might be a viable change-up workout to use in a training program. The efficacy of forced repetitions for increasing strength remains unclear, but such protocols may well be of some value in more advanced strength-trained individuals as a variation in the workout protocol (Ahtiainen et al. 2004).

Take care when using this system because it can cause increased muscular soreness. Because the forced repetitions are performed under conditions of fatigue, the lifter must concentrate on lift technique and never give up during a movement. The spotters need to be extremely attentive and capable of lifting the weight if the lifter loses exercise technique.

Functional Isometrics

The functional isometrics system attempts to take advantage of the joint angle specificity of strength gains from isometric training. Training usually is performed in a power cage, and the pins often are placed at the sticking point of the exercise being performed. However, functional isometrics also can be performed by a partner holding a weight at a certain angle or by two individuals pushing against one another. Functional isometrics entail performing a dynamic contraction for four to six inches (10.2-15.2 cm) of a movement; at that point, the resistance hits the pins in a power rack. The lifter then continues to attempt to lift the resistance with maximal effort for five to seven seconds.

The objective of this system is to use joint angle specificity to produce increases in strength at the weakest point in the range of motion. The maximal resistance for any exercise is determined by the amount of resistance that can be moved through the sticking point or weakest point in that movement. The use of functional isometrics in conjunction with normal resistance training (i.e., dynamic and constant) has been shown to cause significantly greater increases in 1RM for the bench press compared with normal resistance training alone.

Many powerlifters use this system without a power rack during the last repetition in a heavy set (e.g., 1-6RM). They attempt to perform as much of a repetition as possible, and when they cannot move the weight, they continue to produce force isometrically for five to seven seconds at the exact angle where the sticking point occurs. This type of training requires very attentive spotters. To optimize this training, you must know where the sticking point is in the range of motion. These sticking points can change with training. This system is appropriate when the major goal of the program is to increase 1RM capabilities for a particular exercise.

Rest-Pause System

The rest-pause system involves using near maximal resistances (1RM) for multiple repetitions. This is made possible by taking a 10- to 15-second rest between repetitions. For example, you may perform one repetition of an exercise with 250 pounds (113.4 kg), which is near the 1RM for the exercise. You put the weight down and rest for 10 to 15 seconds and then perform another repetition with 250 pounds. You repeat this four or five times. If you cannot perform a complete repetition, spotters lend just enough assistance to allow you to complete the four or five repetitions. You perform only one set of an exercise, but you may perform two or three exercises per muscle group in the same training session. The goal of this system is to use the maximal resistance possible; proponents of the system believe that this allows for the greatest possible gains in strength (Fleck and Kraemer 2014).

Priority System

The priority system can be applied to virtually all types of resistance training programs. This system involves using an exercise order in which exercises that apply to the major goals of the training program are performed first; this way, you can perform these exercises with maximal resistances or intensity. If you perform the high-priority exercises late in the training session, fatigue may prevent you from using maximal resistances or intensity, which may limit your adaptation to the training.

For example, a bodybuilder's weakest muscle group in terms of definition and hypertrophy may be the quadriceps group. Using the priority concept, this bodybuilder would perform exercises for the quadriceps group at the beginning of a training session. A basketball coach may decide that a power forward's biggest weakness is lack of upper-body strength, which results in being pushed around under the boards. Therefore, this player would perform major upper-body exercises at the beginning of the training session. A football player may want to develop strength and power in the thighs, hips, and lower back; therefore, this player would perform heavy hang cleans and squats in the beginning of the workout.

Complex, Concurrent, Contrast, and Cross-Training

Complex, concurrent, contrast, and cross-training all have been used to train all three energetic pathways concurrently. This is necessary for sports that rely on different metabolic pathways, such as speed strength, muscular endurance, or power. Depending on the requirements of the individual training, concurrent training goals may or may not conflict with each other. For instance, it has been shown that aerobic training can affect maximal strength gains. Aerobic training up to a specific threshold (around 75 percent of maximum heart rate for 20-30 minutes two or three times per week) appears to have no effect on strength gains, but anything more than that can negatively affect strength gains. Although heavy resistance training, such as what a strength athlete or bodybuilder performs, may lead to muscular adaptations that normally would be disadvantageous to an aerobic athlete, studies have shown that strength training does not impair maximal oxygen consumption.

Concurrent training may be mutually beneficial to different goals. For instance, it has been shown that concurrent strength and power training increases measures of power, such as throwing velocity and vertical jump height. Often, these two variables are trained together in one workout (sometimes called the *contrast method*). By alternating heavy loads with lighter loads performed at maximal speed, you can develop both maximal strength and power.

This type of training fits very well into a periodized scheme of training. Once you have established your goals, you can develop the meso- and microcycles for obtaining the primary objectives. Secondary objectives can then be added to the existing program to make a complete, well-rounded training program. For instance, speed and power may be the primary goals of a football running back, but maximal strength may be a secondary objective. Thus, the contrast method would work well for this athlete.

Training Modalities

It is clear from the many methods of training that many different training tools (e.g., free weights, machines, medicine balls, and so on) are available. All of these tools fit into a specific modality of training, and all have inherent strengths and weaknesses. For instance, many power athletes use both free weights and medicine balls or plyometric training. In addition, even powerlifters use some machine training to supplement their free-weight training.

Constant-Resistance Devices

With constant-resistance devices, the absolute load does not change during the course of the exercise. These devices include barbells, dumbbells, medicine balls, and other freestanding objects that do not require a pulley or lever to move.

The primary drawback of these devices is that they do not correct for the increase in musculoskeletal leverage during a movement. Thus, the top end or lock-out of a movement may be easier than the initial portion of the concentric motion. However, these devices do require other muscles to act as stabilizers, thus increasing the total amount of physiological work the body must perform during the exercise. Secondary benefits of using such devices are that the range of motion is not limited and that any exercise can be adapted to account for individual differences, such as a person's size or physical capabilities. Furthermore, these devices can easily be adapted to fit into the scope of an individual's functional movements (i.e., mimicking an individual's sport-specific or everyday movements) and allow for progression in weight, range of motion, and modality as skill capabilities improve.

Variable-Resistance Devices

Variable-resistance devices include most resistance exercise machines, cable systems, and rubber tubing. These devices are characterized by a change in load somewhere in the range of motion. For instance, machine levers increase the absolute load at the point in the range of motion where the musculoskeletal system is at a mechanical advantage. Rubber devices such as bands and surgical tubing have become popular because they offer more resistance at the top end of a movement as the band or tubing comes under greater stretch. Although it may be advantageous to overload the musculoskeletal system throughout the whole range of motion (e.g., to increase lock-out strength in the bench press exercise), using machines to strength train presents some notable disadvantages:

1. Machines are not always designed to fit the proportions of all individuals. People who are taller or shorter than the norm, those with special physical considerations, and people who are obese often cannot use machines with ease.
2. Machines use a fixed range of motion; thus, the individual must conform to the movement limitations of the machine. Often, these movements do not mimic functional or athletic movements.
3. Most machines isolate a muscle or muscle group, thus negating the need for other muscles to act as assistant movers and stabilizers; this subsequently decreases the total amount of physiological work.
4. The misconception that machines provide extra safety may lead an individual to not pay attention to the exercise. It is still possible to become injured when using machines.

Despite these drawbacks, variable-resistance devices are still a good tool for training. They do isolate particular muscle groups, which may be necessary in the case of an injury or a special physical need (e.g., vertigo problems). These devices are also useful for beginners because they are perceived to be less intimidating. However, for midlevel and advanced lifters and athletes, machines and other variable-resistance devices should be used only to supplement training. The benefits of constant-resistance devices (i.e., free weights) far outweigh the benefits of variable-resistance devices.

Static-Resistance Devices

Static-resistance devices are rarely used. These are devices in which a person pulls or pushes against an immovable apparatus for isometric exercises. Isometric contraction is not practical for most sports or for everyday functioning. However, as discussed earlier in this chapter, pushing a barbell against the safety racks, or using a wall or partner for an isometric contraction, occasionally is used to overcome a sticking point in a range of motion.

Plyometric Training

Plyometric training is a popular form of training for speed, power, and starting strength. The term *stretch–shortening cycle exercises* is starting to replace the term *plyometrics,* and it describes this type of resistance exercise more accurately (Knuttgen and Kraemer 1987).

The stretch–shortening cycle (SSC) refers to a natural part of most movements; the cycle is a sequence of eccentric, isometric, and concentric actions. It is characterized by an eccentric motion leading into a ballistic concentric motion. For example, in the bench press exercise, if you were to start the lift from your chest, you would use an isometric and then a concentric action only. However, if you were to start the lift with the bar at arm's length, you would use an eccentric, then isometric, then concentric action. Depending on the length of the isometric action, the concentric portion of the lift can be much easier because of the SSC. That is, the longer you isometrically hold the weight before the concentric action, the larger the decrement in the SSC and therefore the more difficult the concentric portion of the lift will be.

Bounding, leaping, and medicine ball throws are common plyometric or SSC exercises (figure 3.3). The key to plyometric training is using the SSC to allow

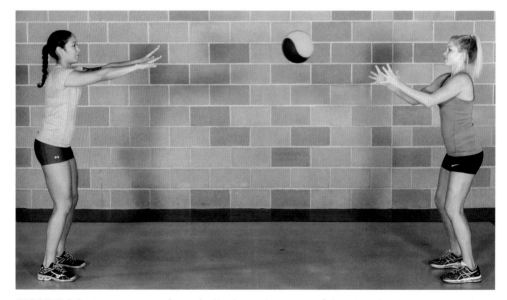

FIGURE 3.3 Passing a medicine ball takes advantage of the stretch–shortening cycle to help increase your power output.

for an enhanced concentric contraction mediated by the preactivation during the eccentric action. Thus, the speed of the eccentric muscle action is vital to the concentric repetition. The ability of the SSC to increase power output depends on load, time, and the ability of the muscle to induce a force-enhancing prestretch of the muscle.

When the sequence of eccentric to concentric actions is performed quickly, the muscle is stretched slightly before the concentric action. The slight stretching stores elastic energy. This elastic energy is added to the force of a normal concentric action, which is one of the common explanations given for why more forcible concentric action results after an SSC. The other common explanation is that a reflex results in quicker recruitment of muscle fibers or recruitment of more muscle fibers involved in the movement.

It is easy to demonstrate how an SSC results in a more powerful concentric action. Perform a normal vertical jump (i.e., a countermovement jump). During this type of jump, you bend at the knees and hips (eccentric action), then quickly reverse direction and jump (isometric followed by concentric action). A countermovement jump involves an SSC. Now perform a jump by bending at the knees and hips, stopping for three to five seconds in that position, and then jumping. This is called a *noncountermovement jump*; it does not involve an SSC and results in a jump that is not as high as a countermovement jump (i.e., a jump involving an SSC). You can also demonstrate the effect of an SSC by throwing a ball for distance with a normal overhand throwing motion. Then throw a ball for distance starting from the end of the wind-up position (no SSC). The normal throwing motion will produce a throw of greater distance.

Training Recommendations

These recommendations are general and are within the scope of what the scientific research stipulates as being general domains to work within. Other recommendations also only set general guidelines for the domains of the acute program variables, but ultimately each program must be designed to meet the goals of the individual. Additionally, each type of workout is used within a periodized training program.

To design an effective training program, you must perform a needs analysis. Such an analysis can help you determine what type of training modality is best for you (e.g., free weights vs. machines vs. plyometrics), what exercises to select, what energy pathways to use in your training, how to manipulate the acute variables of training, and how to work around existing injuries and prevent future ones.

Chapter 7 provides more guidelines for determining your workout goals and building your program from those goals. Briefly, the following are some general recommendations for achieving specific goals with resistance training during a peaking portion of a macrocycle.

- **Maximal strength.** In general, to best achieve maximal strength heavy loads (>85 percent of 1RM) should be performed with few repetitions (2-6).

A moderate to high number of sets with two to five minutes of rest between sets is recommended for maximal strength gains. For advanced lifters, a split routine (i.e., workouts spread over four to six days per week) is best for achieving these goals. Elite Olympic weightlifters are known to perform three to six workouts per day, thus increasing the frequency and overall volume of training. You should train for each muscle group two or three days per week, organized in a periodized manner. Multiple-joint exercises with free weights should make up the primary exercises, and machines and single-joint movements should be used as complements.

- **Muscular hypertrophy.** Understanding that heavier loads are needed to activate all motor units and, therefore, muscle fibers, one needs to use muscular hypertrophy workouts within a periodized training program which includes each of the different loading schemes. For muscular hypertrophy workouts, exercises that use both concentric and eccentric muscle actions are best. Use moderate to heavy loading (70-85 percent of 1RM) for 6 to 10 repetitions per set, with 3 to 6 sets per exercise. Advanced lifters, such as bodybuilders, may increase the load and the number of sets and may decrease the rest time (one to two minutes between sets in some workouts). It is important to carefully reduce rest so as not to overshoot the individual's toleration of the workout as noted by symptoms of dizziness and nausea. Both single- and multiple-joint exercises should be included. Keep frequency similar to when training for maximal strength: Work each major muscle group one to three days per week, depending on training status.

- **Muscular power.** When training for muscular power, velocity of the movement is very important. Power is developed across the entire force velocity curve. Thus, loading can be used across the entire range of intensities. There is a power output associated with every resistance when movement occurs. The number of repetitions should range from 3 to 6, and repetitions should not be performed to failure. It appears that sets of 3 repetitions for more sets (e.g., 3-6) is better as fatigue sets in with large-repetition sets. Rest of three to five minutes between sets is also needed in order to provide recovery for optimal performance in the power output of each repetition. Frequency and rest time between sets are similar to that when training for strength. Note that you can enhance power development through concurrent training for maximal strength. You should plan power training in a periodized fashion, paying attention to developing maximal strength along with power. When training for maximal power, you can use a variety of training modalities, such as plyometric exercises (e.g., depth jumps and bounding), medicine ball throws, resistive running devices (e.g., parachutes), and free weights (e.g., hang pulls, hang snatch lifts, power cleans, and snatch lifts).

- **Local muscular endurance.** Local muscular endurance is best trained using lighter loads using one or two sets for higher repetitions (15-25). Keep rest time between sets short—one to two minutes for sets with higher repetitions and less than one minute for sets with moderate repetitions. Frequency and exercise selection are similar to that when training for muscular hypertrophy and strength.

Summary

You can use many different methods to train and enhance muscle, and the program you design should be specific to your needs, training goals, and the event for which you are training. The possibilities for creating a new resistance training program are almost infinite.

It is easy to design many distinctly different programs by manipulating acute program variables. Popular or "fad" training systems should be evaluated in terms of their acute program variables and their ability to address the needs of an individual or sport. The choice of which training system or systems to use depends on the goals of the program, time constraints, and how the goals of the resistance training program relate to the goals of the entire fitness program. A major goal of any program is to bring about physiological adaptations while providing the rest and recovery needed to prevent nonfunctional overreaching or, at worst, an overtraining syndrome.

4

Nutrition for Muscle Growth

William J. Kraemer, Maren S. Fragala, and Jeff S. Volek

A balanced and sufficient diet is essential in order for intense resistance training to produce gains in muscle strength and size. It is estimated that 2,300 to 3,500 calories are required to build one pound (0.45 kg) of muscle. Dietary approaches can vary, but it is vital for the individual to take in adequate calories and the necessary nutrients to support the repair and remodeling of the body after a workout. Additionally, proper hydration is mandatory for every bodily function, including optimal metabolism.

The ultimate goals of optimal nutritional intake during resistance training are to maximize protein synthesis, minimize protein degradation, restore muscle fuel stores, and maintain euhydration (Volek et al. 1997). This is achieved by creating an environment in the body that promotes the development of tissues, including muscle and bone. Creating this environment involves ensuring the availability of enzymes (which are catalysts for biochemical reactions) and amino acids (which are the building components of muscle). As you learned in chapter 2, it also requires hormonal actions that signal and facilitate the building of muscle, as well as sufficient exercise intensity to stimulate the growth and development of protein. Adenosine triphosphate (ATP), the body's energy source, is needed for many functions. It is needed for the muscle contraction process mediating the interactions of actin and myosin to produce force well as for many chemical reactions that occur in the body, including protein synthesis. ATP is available in limited supplies in the body's stores, and you need to replenish these supplies from the foods you eat.

Nutrition can influence both the workout intensity and the recovery process between weight training sessions, which in turn affects the intensity of the following exercise session. Consuming the proper proportion of nutrients at critical times around any single resistance training session optimizes the postworkout recovery process in the muscle—and therefore maximizes muscle strength gains.

Without adequate energy stores in the muscle, the muscle may not be able to generate adequate force during a muscular contraction when called on to do so. Furthermore, without adequate availability of amino acids, protein synthesis and recovery after training may be compromised.

In this chapter, we review some of the basics of muscle metabolism as they relate to nutritional intake as well as the role of hormones in that metabolism. We discuss macronutrients, micronutrients, and supplements and how these and the timing of their intake affect the gains brought on by resistance training.

Muscle Metabolism

Muscle proteins are constantly undergoing remodeling through physical and chemical processes. This is referred to as *muscle metabolism*, which encompasses the building or synthesis (anabolism), maintenance, and breakdown (catabolism) or degradation of protein, some of which is used for energy.

Net protein synthesis (i.e., when the amount of protein synthesis exceeds breakdown) occurs when energy demands are adequate to support the stimulus created for muscle growth. When energy requirements are not adequate, protein degradation can occur to produce energy. However, the contribution of protein to energy requirements to meet exercise demands typically is less than 10 percent. Because protein plays important roles in the body, it generally is spared as a source of energy production, and the body relies primarily on carbohydrate or fat to produce energy for exercise, depending on the intensity, duration, and type of training. Carbohydrate is stored in the muscle and liver in the form of glycogen. (Interestingly, during resistance exercise women use less glycogen and more fat than do men; Volek et al. 2006). This glycogen is broken down into glucose molecules and is then metabolized to produce ATP. During longer-duration or lower-intensity training, the body can metabolize fat through a process called *lipolysis* to generate energy. Evidence is growing that individuals who are adapted to a ketogenic (low carb) diet can utilize fat for longer periods of time to meet exercise demands (Noakes et al. 2014).

Protein synthesis needs to be understood in terms of acute versus chronic responses. Acute responses, such as changes in protein balance or glycogen degradation and synthesis, occur in the short time after a single training session. Chronic responses are long-term effects seen from long-term training, such as increases in muscle strength and size. Numerous studies have examined the immediate environmental effects of nutrition and training on the muscle after an acute bout of exercise. However, few have examined the long-term effects on muscle size increases and strength. Thus, the acute effects of nutritional practices in strength training, such as glycogen repletion and protein synthesis, are assumed to result in long-term gains in muscle strength and size. Acute and chronic muscle protein synthesis responses vary in response to resistance exercise and training (Damas et al. 2015). Although acute increases in protein synthesis take place, protein synthesis alone is not indicative of the amount of muscle hypertrophy that will occur. Recently, it has been proposed that protein requirements are decreased as the muscle meets its genetic limits for size. When the size of the fiber reaches its genetic limit for further production of protein, it would be wasteful because it could not be incorporated into the muscle. Thus, the amount of protein synthesis is reduced in order to not waste the energy required for synthesis. This might be consistent with the reduction in muscle protein synthesis and protein intake requirements that come when an individual is fully trained. The time frame in which this occurs appears to be related to the gain potential for muscle size, which subsequently may be related to the number of muscle fibers activated with training as well as the type of muscle fiber that makes up the motor units (see chapter 2).

During fasting or in the absence of nutritional intake after training, the muscle is in a state of negative protein balance, indicating that protein degradation exceeds protein synthesis and that little glycogen repletion is occurring. Even without training, consuming a meal results in a positive energy balance and increases in both lean body mass and fat mass. The goal for strength athletes is to maintain a net positive protein balance, meaning that protein synthesis exceeds protein breakdown and the muscle is in an anabolic or muscle-building state. Accordingly, strength athletes want to avoid a net negative protein balance, where muscle protein breakdown exceeds synthesis and the muscle is in a catabolic or muscle-breakdown state. To do this requires appropriate dietary intakes of the macronutrients: carbohydrate, protein, and fat.

Role of Hormones

Nearly every physiological function in the body is regulated by hormones—chemical messengers that travel via the bloodstream to target tissues in the body (e.g., muscle). Figure 4.1 provides an overview of the roles that hormones play. Because resistance exercise dramatically affects hormonal responses in the body and in part stimulates the development of tissues (including muscle and bone), you need to understand how the food you eat affects these hormones. Hormones play a significant role in metabolic balance. They largely are responsible for the fuel selection, partitioning of nutrients, and gene regulation that ultimately affect body composition and muscle mass.

As you learned in chapter 2, an acute bout of resistance exercise (considering the load, number of sets, number of repetitions, and number and length of rest intervals) creates a stimulus that generates a hormonal response. Muscle actions trigger a series of mechanical and chemical events in the muscle that signal hormones to regulate enzymes, which in turn regulate the genetic formation of proteins. For anabolic actions, just the muscle fibers that are activated as part of the motor unit used to perform the exercise will be affected. Conversely, catabolic factors (e.g., reactive oxygen species, cortisol, and so on) can target all muscle fibers. Some nutrients, such as the branched-chain amino acid leucine, can stimulate protein synthesis directly in muscle. Exercise increases blood flow and thus increases the delivery of hormones and nutrients to the target receptors

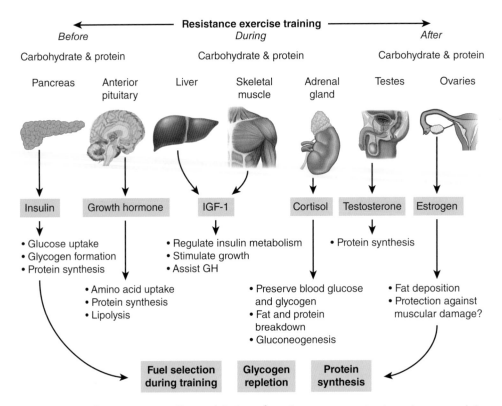

FIGURE 4.1 The quantity, quality, and timing of nutrient consumption in resistance training may have a large influence on the hormones that regulate fuel selection during training, glycogen repletion, and protein synthesis. Proper consumption of nutrients can result in optimal gains in muscle strength and power.

on and in the muscle cells. The anabolic environment is enhanced by the exercise stimuli along with the availability of nutrients and hormones. Consumption of carbohydrate and protein appears to affect the responses of hormones involved in muscle metabolism—including insulin, testosterone, growth hormone, cortisol, estrogen, and insulin-like growth factor-1—thus affecting muscle protein and glycogen balance. Although the role of insulin in response to exercise and diet is understood, the influence of the other hormones listed remains unclear. Metabolic context is the important factor related to the role of certain hormones and their effects.

• **Insulin** is released from the pancreas in response to high concentrations of circulating blood glucose. This hormone promotes glucose and amino acid uptake by the tissues, glycogen formation, and protein synthesis in the presence of sufficient amino acids. Its importance as a trigger for protein synthesis remains under study and most likely is related to overall dietary practices (e.g., high- or low-carbohydrate diets).

- **Growth hormone** (GH) is group of polypeptide hormones made up of the primary monomer (191 amino acids) and aggregates of it. GHs of different sizes are secreted from the anterior pituitary gland (located at the base of the brain) in response to exercise, sleep, stress, and low plasma glucose. Different isoforms function metabolically to cause the muscle cells to take up amino acids, leading to an increase in protein synthesis, lipolysis (fat metabolism), and glucose conservation. This ultimately contributes to anabolic processing in the body, although connective tissue may be targeted more than muscle. The larger aggregates of GH, called the *bioactive forms,* make up the greatest amount of GH in the blood (Nindl et al. 2003; Kraemer et al. 2010; see figure 4.2). Thus, one must view GH as a much more complex superfamily that includes binding proteins to which the GH forms attach. An increased amount of GH is released in response to exercise, likely contributing to metabolic fuel adaptations during exercise and tissue repair after exercise. However, GH concentrations decrease

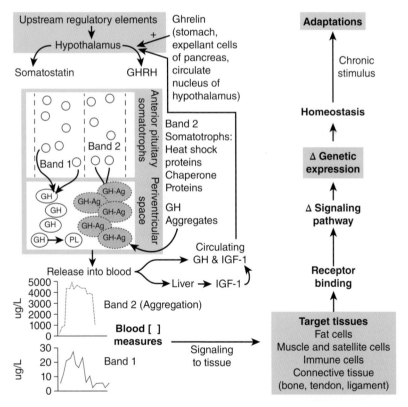

FIGURE 4.2   Resistance exercise stimulates the anterior pituitary gland to secrete GH in its various forms arising from two types of somatotrophs called band 1 and band 2 granules. Band 1 cells secrete the familiar 191-amino acid form of GH and smaller molecular weight peptides, and band 2 cells secrete larger bioactive aggregate forms of GH. The larger bioactive aggregates make up more than 20 to 40 times the amount of GH in the blood and most likely are responsible for many of the functions of GH, thus a super family of biologically active peptides; (PL = prolactin).

in response to increased blood glucose from carbohydrate consumption. Conversely, GH concentrations increase in response to the hypoglycemia (low blood glucose levels) created after the body cells take up glucose from the blood in the hours after carbohydrate ingestion. Furthermore, circulating fatty acids inhibit GH secretion. An increased amount of GH is released in response to greater activation of anaerobic glycolysis and lactate formation. In both men and women, GH concentrations are elevated in the 30 minutes after resistance training.

- **Insulin-like growth factor (IGF)** is an anabolic hormone and a group of binding proteins produced in the liver and skeletal muscle that mediate different anabolic functions and metabolic reactions. GH can stimulate the production of IGFs in the liver (Matheny et al. 2010; Nindl and Pierce 2010). IGFs stimulate the growth of most body tissues, including skeletal muscle, and concentrations are substantially increased in response to progressive overload resistance exercise. IGF-1 (IGF-I) does not appear to be immediately affected by metabolic stressors of glucose and insulin (i.e., exercise and feeding), but it does appear to regulate glucose during the fasted state.

- **Testosterone** is an anabolic (tissue building) and androgenic (responsible for masculine characteristics) hormone produced primarily in the male testes but also in the adrenal glands in both men and women. It is the most anabolic stimuli in men and is present in much larger quantities in men than in women. Decreases in testosterone with feeding or after initial increases with resistance exercise represent an increased uptake of testosterone by the androgen receptors. With increased androgen binding, anabolic signaling occurs. These androgen receptors are located on the DNA in the nuclei of the muscle and other cells (e.g., neurons) that mediate the anabolic signals of testosterone (Vingren et al. 2010). When testosterone binding is inhibited, the development of muscle size and strength is compromised even though other anabolic signaling mechanisms are operational (Kvorning et al. 2006a and b, 2007).

- **Estrogen** is a sex hormone produced primarily in the ovaries in females (males produce small amounts of estrogen in the testes) and is responsible for fat deposition and female sex characteristics. Although estrogen rarely is considered an important hormone for muscular development and strength, understanding the role estrogen plays in energy metabolism and protein synthesis is critical to the female athlete. Many researchers avoid studying female athletes because controlling or accounting for these athletes' monthly fluctuations in hormone is difficult, and animal models are used in many studies of female hormones and muscle metabolism. Nevertheless, researchers recently have recognized that estrogen has a potential protective effect against skeletal muscle damage, which may have important consequences for female muscular responses to resistance training. Females have been shown to have lower blood concentrations of creatine kinase (a marker of muscle damage) compared with males, suggesting that female muscle may sustain less damage from resistance exercise. The mechanisms for this protective effect are not completely understood, but estrogen may play an antioxidant role or a role in the inflammatory response. Some evidence in vitro and in rats indicates that ovarian hormones inhibit muscle protein synthesis. How these findings apply to humans and how they affect nutritional considerations for the female strength athlete are unclear.

- **Cortisol** is a steroid hormone (i.e., it can pass through a cell membrane without a receptor to reach the nucleus) produced in the adrenal glands above the kidneys in response to exercise, injury, or stress. Cortisol preserves blood glucose and glycogen concentrations by increasing fat and protein breakdown in the liver, which fuels the production of new glucose (gluconeogenesis). Cortisol also breaks down proteins (by inhibiting protein synthesis) to form amino acids that can be taken up by the liver, stimulating the mobilization of free fatty acids from adipose (fat) tissue. This then stimulates the liver enzymes for glucose synthesis and blocks the entry of glucose into tissues, encouraging those tissues to use fatty acids as fuel. Because cortisol is related to an increased rate of protein catabolism, it has an inhibiting effect on skeletal muscle hypertrophy. Cortisol concentrations fluctuate regularly throughout the day and are significantly increased during an acute bout of resistance exercise in both men and women. Protein appears to have the greatest stimulatory effect on cortisol levels. Cortisol causes immune cells to be nonfunctional due to their use of glucose as a primary energy source (Fragala et al. 2011) and blocks molecular signaling systems in muscle (Spiering et al. 2008a). High concentrations of resting cortisol are associated with sequences of training and lack of recovery. Cortisol plays a catabolic role due to its effects on protein metabolism and competitive binding on parts of the upstream regulatory receptor for testosterone on the DNA in the nuclei of cells. With acute resistance exercise, cortisol receptors in the activated skeletal muscles with resistance exercise do not change within men (Vingren et al. 2009).

Macronutrients

All three of the major energy-yielding macronutrients (i.e., dietary nutrients) required by the body in large quantities—carbohydrate, fat, and protein—are essential to muscular development. Protein provides amino acids, which are the chief structural material of protein that in turn helps protein synthesis. Carbohydrate is the primary energy source that fuels training, and the presence of carbohydrate in the body stimulates muscle growth. Fat is essential for maintaining an adequate hormonal environment for muscle development. The quantity and quality of these macronutrients and when you consume them affect how the nutrients are used by muscle tissue. When muscle tissue takes up these macronutrients, hormones are released in response. These hormones interact with receptors on target tissues, resulting in gene transcription and translation for protein, fat, and carbohydrate metabolism. The muscle protein metabolism response occurs in the 24 to 48 hours after resistance exercise. Thus, any meals consumed during this time will affect muscle hypertrophy (i.e., increase muscle size).

Protein

Muscle comprises primarily protein (about 22 percent) and water (about 70 percent). The remainder of muscle comprises glycogen, fat, vitamins, and minerals. Similar to fat and carbohydrate, protein is made up of carbon, hydrogen, and oxygen. However, unlike fat and carbohydrate, protein contains nitrogen. This molecular difference gives an indication of the metabolic state of muscle tissue. Nitrogen balance is the difference between the amount of nitrogen taken in and the amount excreted or lost. When nitrogen supplies do not meet nitrogen demands, protein tissue is broken down due to catabolism and nitrogen is lost in the urine (i.e., negative nitrogen balance). If more nitrogen is consumed than excreted, you will be in an anabolic or muscle-building state (i.e., positive nitrogen balance).

Amino acids, which are the building blocks of protein, contain carbon, hydrogen, oxygen, nitrogen, and in certain cases sulfur. Every alpha amino acid has a carbon atom called an alpha carbon, C , bonded to a carboxylic acid, –COOH, group; an amino, $-NH_2$, group; a hydrogen atom; and an R group that is unique for every amino acid. Adequate quantities of amino acids must be available for protein synthesis to occur. At least 20 different amino acids are used to synthesize proteins, each differing in molecular structure, shape, and properties (see table 4.1). Typically, nine amino acids are considered essential for adults, meaning that they must be consumed in the diet because they cannot be synthesized in the body from other precursors. In contrast, nonessential amino acids can be synthesized in the body from the essential amino acids. Essential amino acids are vital for muscle building and metabolism (for a review see Kraemer et al. 2016). Additionally, some amino acids, such as histidine and arginine, are considered semiessential because the ability to produce them is reduced in infants and children. Furthermore, some amino acids, such as arginine and glutamine, are considered conditionally essential because their requirements are increased during times of catabolic stress.

Proteins are rated by their biological value as complete (high biological value) or incomplete (low biological value) depending on whether they contain all of the essential amino acids. Typically, proteins from animal sources (i.e., eggs, meat, fish) contain all of the essential amino acids and are thus considered complete. Most proteins in grain and vegetable products do not contain all of the amino acids and are considered incomplete. These plant-based incomplete sources of protein can be combined to provide all of the amino acids.

Although protein contains about four calories per gram of energy, typically it is not considered a primary energy source like carbohydrate and fat. The amino acids—especially the essential amino acids supplied by dietary protein—allow the body to synthesize the protein it needs for tissues, hormones, and enzymes. In addition, protein is inefficient at providing energy. Protein has a high thermic effect, meaning that for the amount of calories provided per gram of protein (compared with fat or carbohydrate), much of the energy is used for metabolic processes, resulting in a lower energy density.

TABLE 4.1 Nonessential and Essential Amino Acids

Nonessential	Essential
Alanine	Isoleucine
Asparagine	Leucine
Aspartic acid	Lysine
Carnitine	Methionine
Citrulline	Phenylalanine
Cysteine	Threonine
Cystine	Tryptophan
Gamma-aminobutyric acid	Valine
Glutamic acid	
Glutamine	
Glutathione	
Glycine	
Hydroxyproline	
Ornithine	
Proline	
Serine	
Taurine	
Tyrosine	

How Muscles Use Protein

Intense training increases the rate of both muscle protein synthesis and degradation. The rate of muscle protein synthesis exceeds the rate of protein degradation, resulting in net protein accretion, or growth. Research has shown that in the 4 hours after training, muscle protein synthesis activity is 50 percent greater than before training. In the 24 hours after training, muscle protein synthesis activity is 109 percent greater than before training. Muscle protein synthesis varies with resistance training, and acute protein synthesis is not indicative of the amount of muscle hypertrophy taking place (Damas et al. 2015). Also, as muscle reaches its maximal genetic size dimensions, muscle protein synthesis might slow down; however, this may vary among muscles and individuals. How muscle fibers grow may also vary by fiber type. Type I and Type II muscle fibers vary in their emphasis on protein synthesis and reduction in degradation. Increases in synthesis and less reliance on reducing degradation are typical of Type II fibers, whereas lower increases in protein synthesis and greater reductions in degradation are typical of Type I fibers.

Ingesting amino acids through food or supplements before and after exercise stimulates the transportation of amino acids into skeletal muscle and therefore stimulates protein synthesis. Similar results have been observed when individuals consume amino acids either one or three hours postexercise. Furthermore, some evidence suggests that consuming amino acids immediately before resistance exercise increases protein synthesis even more than does consuming them after training. This possibly is attributable to the increased blood flow to muscle that occurs during training, which then results in increased delivery of amino acid to the muscles. Muscle anabolism occurs whether amino acids or carbohydrate alone are consumed at one and two hours after exercise. However, evidence shows an additive effect, to some extent, if amino acids and protein are combined.

High-volume resistance training or overreaching heavy training (i.e., when training volumes are higher than normal but not quite to the point of over-training) followed by inadequate recovery initially reduces muscle strength and power. These reductions are moderated with amino acid supplementation. Additionally, during periods of energy deficit, such as in a fasted state or after a workout, a high-protein diet has been shown to be effective in increasing lean body mass and strength.

How muscles use protein is also related to why some athletes turn to using steroids even though they are dangerous and banned from most competitive sports. The use of steroids appears to reduce the protein requirements necessary for nitrogen balance and anabolism; this results from an increased ability to recycle the amino acids from broken-down proteins in order to synthesize new muscle protein.

Daily Protein Requirements

Typically, the amount of protein needed to promote a positive nitrogen balance (an indicator of whole-body protein use) and to grow and develop skeletal muscle is between 1.2 and 2.2 grams per kilogram of body weight per day. However, this amount depends on the amount of muscle mass stimulated with the workout. For muscle to grow, even in older adults, more than the typical recommended dietary allowance of 0.8 gram per kilogram of body weight per day is required. As muscle increases in size, the amount of protein needed regresses to a lower level—that is, use of amino acids may be more efficient in strength athletes. Generally, a diet comprising 25 to 30 percent protein—which typically is greater than 0.8 gram per kilogram per day—is recommended for strength athletes. If the individual follows a typical diet, this proportion should allow for the consumption of adequate amino acids as well as sufficient quantities of carbohydrate and fat. Again, the type of training and the amount of muscle fibers stimulated during training may influence protein requirements; higher amounts of protein are required when training stimulates a larger amount of muscle fibers.

It is important to remember that essential amino acids are more critical than nonessential amino acids. Essential amino acids have been shown to be primary regulators of muscle protein synthesis, whereas nonessential amino acids show little contribution. In particular, branched-chain amino acids (e.g., leucine) appear to be the most important stimulators of muscle protein synthesis.

Carbohydrate

Similar to protein and fat, carbohydrate molecules contain carbon, hydrogen, and oxygen. Like protein, carbohydrate provides four calories of energy per gram, but carbohydrate does this much more efficiently than protein. Many foods contain carbohydrate in combination with other macronutrients. Some foods containing primarily carbohydrate are bread, rice, pasta, potatoes, cereals, and crackers.

The carbohydrate an individual consumes ultimately is converted to glucose, a simple sugar that is transported to all body tissues for energy. When this energy isn't used immediately, it is stored in the form of glycogen, a more complex sugar. When a person consumes a typical diet, glycogen is the major energy source during resistance exercise of moderate repetitions (8-12). Glycogen is stored primarily in the muscle and the liver, and some amounts are found circulating in the bloodstream.

How Muscles Use Glycogen

The muscles use glycogen by first breaking it down into glucose, which is then broken down to produce ATP through a process known as *glycolysis*. About 82 percent of the ATP used during a set of biceps curls taken to the point of failure is derived from glycolysis. Because of its proximity and availability to the mitochondria (the site of aerobic ATP production in the muscle cell), glycogen is readily and quickly available to fuel the muscle during resistance training. Thus, if the athlete is on a typical diet and glycogen stores are low, exercise performance can be impaired.

Glycogen stores are depleted to varying extents after exercise. Muscle glycogen is depleted by about 30 to 40 percent after resistance exercise, particularly in Type II (fast-twitch anaerobic) muscle fibers. Furthermore, muscle damage resulting from the eccentric, muscle-lengthening phase of isotonic exercises, such as lowering the weight in a biceps curl, reduces the ability of the muscle to store glycogen. This reduced storage capacity is caused by a decreased rate of entry into the muscle cell which is mediated by the hormone by insulin interactions with its cellular receptors. Thus, the daily dietary carbohydrate requirement for strength athletes to promote optimal muscle glycogen resynthesis is increased when muscle is damaged. Strength athletes should replenish those glycogen stores as soon as possible. Interestingly, depletion of glycogen with resistance training does not inhibit the anabolic signaling for muscle growth (Camera et al. 2012).

Because insulin release is triggered by circulating blood glucose, ingesting carbohydrate leads to elevated insulin levels. Glycogen repletion is faster when carbohydrate is consumed after exercise. Glycogen repletion is similar whether carbohydrate is consumed alone or in combination with protein or amino acids. Some evidence suggests that certain amino acids (e.g., leucine) can increase insulin secretion, leading to attempts to enhance postexercise glycogen resynthesis and protein anabolism by combining carbohydrate with amino acids. This postexercise consumption of combined carbohydrate and amino acids has been shown to increase glycogen resynthesis after submaximal cycling exercise, likely because of increased insulin secretion. However, its effects after resistance training are unknown.

Consuming a carbohydrate and protein supplement before and during resistance exercise is recommended because it maximizes the effect of insulin and enables a person to benefit from increased blood flow for amino acid delivery. Carbohydrate appears to be most effective in leading to muscle glycogen repletion when consumed immediately after training (compared with two hours after training) at a rate of 1.2 grams per kilogram per hour at 30-minute intervals for four hours. Furthermore, consuming carbohydrate before and during exercise has been shown to attenuate the decrease in muscle glycogen during training and improve the volume and intensity of a second training session within the same day. Some studies have also shown that supplementation of protein and carbohydrate before, immediately after, or two hours after resistance training enhances the acute GH response and the GH response during late recovery compared with a placebo.

Although feeding does not appear to affect total levels of insulin-like protein-I binding protein (IGFBP-I), another protein that travels in the blood and is bound to IGF-I, IGFBP-I appears to contribute to glucose regulation by countering the glucose uptake of free IGF-I. IGFBP-I concentrations gradually decrease after feeding and increase in the three to four hours after feeding. IGFBP-I concentrations are reduced in response to carbohydrate feeding (compared with no supplementation) during and after endurance exercise; however, these reductions were not correlated with blood glucose concentrations during feeding, suggesting that factors other than blood glucose and insulin regulate IGFBP-I. These other factors may include liver glycogen depletion because a high correlation between liver glycogen and IGFBP-I responses to exercise has been observed.

Compared with fasting, consuming nutrients before and after resistance training results in a prolonged decrease in blood testosterone levels. This is related to the production, secretion, or metabolic clearance of testosterone. In men, total testosterone concentrations acutely increase in response to resistance training; in women, some research shows an elevation but other research shows no change. Supplementation of carbohydrate and protein appears to attenuate the testosterone response to exercise. Postexercise feeding leads to increased muscle-specific protein synthesis during recovery that is testosterone dependent. Therefore, these observed decrements in circulating testosterone likely are attributable to the increased uptake in skeletal muscle that results in protein synthesis. Furthermore, testosterone concentrations are significantly decreased in response to a glucose tolerance test, where blood is sampled and evaluated at periods after the consumption of a given amount of glucose.

Consuming a carbohydrate solution during exercise has been shown to decrease the acute cortisol response and to increase muscle hypertrophy over 12 weeks of training. Carbohydrate supplementation during exercise may reduce the need for gluconeogenesis during exercise, thus potentially reducing the need for cortisol. Again, all of the information put forth in this section is based on the use of a typical high-carbohydrate diet (55-60 percent of total calories) and not a low-carbohydrate, high-fat (i.e., ketogenic) diet (15-20 percent of total calories; Volek et al. 2015). Sensitivity to carbohydrate as it relates to negative clinical responses varies among individuals (Volk et al. 2014).

Daily Carbohydrate Requirements

Carbohydrate with a high glycemic index is more effective at increasing the rate of glycogen repletion. *Glycemic index*, which refers to how quickly carbohydrate is metabolized, is a numerical rating of how much of an increase in circulating blood sugar is triggered by the consumption of a food. Carbohydrate sources with a high glycemic index, such as fruits and processed sugar, are metabolized quickly. Carbohydrate sources with a low glycemic index, such as starches and cellulose, are metabolized more slowly. *Glycemic load* is another term used when referring to the increase in blood sugar that a specific food causes. Unlike glycemic index, glycemic load takes into consideration the amount of the food that is consumed. (See table 4.2 for some typical glycemic index values.) Despite the ability to increase glycogen resynthesis, carbohydrate with a high glycemic index is more detrimental for fat loss because the insulin response inhibits fat-breakdown enzymes and promotes fat deposition and maintenance. Recently, this has led to questions on the overuse of high-carbohydrate diets and drinks to promote athletic performance (Paoli et al. 2013; Noakes et al. 2014).

TABLE 4.2 Glycemic Index of Select Foods

High (GI > 69)	Medium (56 < GI < 69)	Low (GI < 56)
White bread	Wheat bread	Rye bread
Corn Flakes cereal	Life cereal	All-Bran cereal
Rice cakes	Ice cream	Peanuts
Jelly beans	PowerBar protein bars	Apples
Popcorn	Sweet corn	Milk
Pretzels	Baked potatoes	Baked beans
Gatorade	Raisin Bran cereal	Yams

Glycemic index (GI) is a rating of the time and amount in which a given food causes an increase in blood sugar in relation to pure glucose, which has a glycemic index of 100.

Fat

Like carbohydrate, fat comprises carbon, hydrogen, and oxygen. However, fat is the most energy-dense macronutrient, providing about 9 calories per gram. One pound (0.45 kg) of body fat contains 3,500 calories of energy. Thus, fats increased utilization during exercise can limit the rate of glycogen use. Recent studies have demonstrated that when individuals start a dietary program, fat and protein better align together and protein and carbohydrate better align together, and issues appear to occur when fat and carbohydrate are used together. A low-carbohydrate diet consists of normal protein intake and restricted carbohydrate intake, and a high-carbohydrate diet consists of normal protein intake and restricted fat intake. Most of the diet literature is based on findings in which subjects consumed high-carbohydrate diets, but such findings are now being re-examined, and more data are coming out regularly (Noakes et al. 2014, Volek et al. 2015).

Based on a high-carbohydrate diet, dietary fat is often classified as good or bad depending on its effects on blood cholesterol. Saturated fat, derived mainly from animal products (e.g., butter, cheese, ice cream, red meat), and trans fat, found most often in commercially packaged snack foods, are usually considered to be bad fats because they elevate blood cholesterol levels. Unsaturated fat, derived from plant sources (e.g., vegetable oils, nuts, and seeds), is considered to be good fat because it improves blood lipid profiles. Unsaturated fats include polyunsaturated fat (e.g., sunflower, corn, and soybean oils) and monounsaturated fat (e.g., canola, peanut, and olive oils).

Although dietary fat is required in order to maintain concentrations of circulating testosterone in the body, a high-fat diet appears to impair the ability to perform exercise at a high intensity compared with a high-carbohydrate diet. Research shows that eating a diet very low in fat (<10-15 percent of total calories) reduces testosterone concentrations in healthy men. In a high-carbohydrate diet, a moderate level of fat (15-20 percent of daily energy consumption) and some saturated fat (<10 percent) is often recommended for the strength athlete.

Low-Carbohydrate Diets

The preferential use of ketones as an energy source consequent to adaptation to a properly formulated low-carbohydrate diet has now been shown to have many positive benefits for health and performance in diets for athletes (Volek et al. 2015, 2016). Keto-adaptation is a dietary approach that can enhance the athlete's ability to cope with stress and can reduce recovery time between high-stress sport events and workouts. Once the body is in ketosis, a stable and sustainable source of fuel for the brain rather than glucose is provided. The major circulating ketone body, beta-hydroxybutyrate, recently has been shown to act as a signaling molecule that is capable of altering gene expression, thus eliciting complementary effects of keto-adaptation that could extend human physical and mental performance. Thus, beyond weight loss, this dietary method is a major advancement in dietary approaches for individuals with various morbidities (e.g., diabetes, metabolic syndrome, epilepsy) as well as athletes who want to enhance their performance.

Water

The human body comprises about 40 to 75 percent water, depending on body composition and age. Water is essential to muscular strength because it composes about 70 percent of muscle. Fat is only 20 to 25 percent water, making it a lighter form of energy storage than muscle. The water molecule is an essential link between glucose molecules in glycogen as well as between amino acids in protein. For every gram of carbohydrate stored in the body, 2.7 grams of water is stored. Therefore, for every pound (.45 kg) of carbohydrate, 3.7 pounds (1.7 kg) of water is stored. Dehydration of as little as 1.5 percent of body weight has been reported to decrease muscular endurance and performance on the 1RM bench press.

Without exercise and under normal environmental conditions, a typical adult loses about 2.5 liters of water per day, mostly from urine. However, high temperature and exercise can increase a person's water loss to as much as 7 liters per day. Generally, you should replace water at a rate of 1 to 1.5 milliliters per calorie of energy expended. However, because this is difficult to track, approximately 8 to 16 ounces (237-473 ml) of water should be consumed per hour before, during, and after training to avoid dehydration.

Micronutrients

Vitamins and minerals are called *micronutrients* because they are required by the body in small amounts and are essential for facilitating various body functions and biochemical reactions, including muscular contraction. Vitamins are organic substances, meaning they contain carbon, yet they do not contain calories (energy). They trigger reactions in the body. Vitamins are classified into two types: water soluble and fat soluble. Water-soluble vitamins are not stored in the body; these include the B vitamins and vitamin C. Fat-soluble vitamins are stored in the adipose (fat) tissue in the body; these include vitamins A, D, E, and K. Vitamins are required only in small amounts by the body's tissues; however, they are metabolized, so they must be replaced by what is consumed. Vitamins play critical roles in energy metabolism and tissue formation. See table 4.3 for a complete list of vitamins and minerals and their dietary sources and functions.

Minerals are inorganic substances found in water and soil, and they enter our bodies from the foods we eat—that is, from the plants that take up the minerals and from the animals that eat the plants. Minerals are all the chemical elements in the body besides carbon, hydrogen, oxygen, and nitrogen. Twenty-two minerals compose 4 percent of our total body weight. Minerals are classified as macrominerals and microminerals. Macrominerals (major minerals) include calcium, phosphorus, magnesium, sulfur, sodium, potassium, and chloride; these minerals exist in the body in quantities of about 35 to 1,050 grams, depending on mineral and body size. Trace minerals include iron, iodine, fluoride, zinc, selenium, copper, cobalt, chromium, manganese, molybdenum, arsenic, nickel, and vanadium; these exist in the body in quantities of less than a few grams. Both macro- and microminerals are critical to metabolic processes and the synthesis of glycogen, protein, and fat. Although few studies show beneficial effects of vitamin or mineral supplementation above recommended levels, vitamin or mineral deficiencies may impair strength and training. Thus, a multivitamin often is recommended for athletes to ensure they are consuming adequate amounts and have no deficiencies.

Supplements

Several nutritional supplements are marketed with claims of increasing muscular strength and size, but many of these claims lack scientific support. Investing in these ineffective supplements may be a waste of money for the strength athlete.

TABLE 4.3 Vitamins and Minerals

Vitamin or mineral	Major dietary source	Major function
Fat-soluble vitamins		
Vitamin A	Dairy products Liver Carrots Sweet potatoes Green leafy vegetables	Antioxidant (protects cells from oxidation) Gene expression
Vitamin D	Dairy products Egg yolks Fish oil Sunlight exposure	Promotes absorption and use of calcium and phosphorus
Vitamin E	Vegetable oils Nuts Seeds	Antioxidant (protects cells from oxidation)
Vitamin K	Spinach Eggs Cauliflower Liver	Assists in protein formation (particularly essential to blood clotting)
Water-soluble vitamins		
Vitamin B_1 (thiamin)	Pork Peanuts Legumes Whole grains	Coenzyme (assists enzymes) in energy metabolism
Vitamin B_2 (riboflavin)	Dairy products Meats Enriched grains Beans Green leafy vegetables	Coenzyme in energy metabolism
Niacin	Nuts Meats Beans	Coenzyme in energy metabolism
Vitamin B_6	Meats Fish Poultry Legumes	Coenzyme in amino acid metabolism
Folic acid	Green vegetables Legumes Nuts Grains	Coenzyme in DNA and RNA metabolism
Vitamin B_{12}	Animal products	Coenzyme in DNA and RNA metabolism
Pantothenic acid	Animal products Whole grains	Coenzyme in energy metabolism

Vitamin or mineral	Major dietary source	Major function
Biotin	Meats Whole grains Vegetables	Coenzyme in energy metabolism
Vitamin C (ascorbic acid)	Citrus fruits Broccoli Strawberries Cantaloupe	Antioxidant Improves iron absorption
Macrominerals		
Calcium	Milk Dark green vegetables Legumes	Muscle contraction Nerve transmission Bone formation
Phosphorus	Milk Meats Poultry Whole grains	Bone formation Acid–base balance Component of coenzymes
Magnesium	Whole grains Green leafy vegetables	Protein synthesis Coenzyme Glucose metabolism
Sulfur	Protein	Component of protein
Sodium	Salt Soy sauce	Regulates body water Nerve function
Potassium	Meats Milk Fruits Vegetables	Regulates body water Nerve function
Chloride	Salt Soy sauce	Acid–base balance Gastric secretion formation
Trace minerals		
Iron	Meats Eggs Whole grains Green leafy vegetables	Hemoglobin formation Coenzyme component Myoglobin formation
Iodine	Fish Dairy Iodized salt	Thyroid hormone formation
Fluoride	Drinking water Tea Seafood	Tooth and bone structure
Zinc	Meats Seafood Whole grains Vegetables	Component of enzymes involved in protein synthesis and energy metabolism

> continued

TABLE 4.3   > *continued*

Trace minerals		
Vitamin or mineral	**Major dietary source**	**Major function**
Selenium	Meats Nuts Seafood Whole grains	Component of enzymes Antioxidant enzyme
Copper	Organ meats Seafood Nuts Legumes	Component of enzymes Assists in use of iron and hemoglobin in the body
Chromium	Seafood Meats Whole grains Asparagus	Involved in glucose and energy metabolism Enhances insulin function
Manganese	Vegetables Fruits Nuts Whole grains	Component of enzymes
Molybdenum	Legumes Cereal Vegetables	Component of enzymes

Vitamins and minerals are essential to the diet of strength athletes because they have critical functions in the biochemical processes responsible for energy metabolism and protein synthesis. DNA = deoxyribonucleic acid; RNA = ribonucleic acid.

However, evidence supports the use of some supplements, such as creatine, branched-chain amino acids, and L-carnitine; these supplements may be beneficial to the strength athlete when used correctly. In a survey of Division I athletes, 89 percent had used or currently were using nutritional supplements, including sport drinks and bars. Additionally, about 47 percent consumed a multivitamin, and 37 percent used a creatine supplement.

Creatine

Creatine is an amino acid derivative (from arginine, glycine, and methionine) that is available in meats and fish and is synthesized in the liver, pancreas, and kidneys. Because creatine plays a critical role in ATP metabolism, creatine supplementation theoretically increases the bioavailability of phosphocreatine (PCr) in skeletal muscle cells, enhancing muscle performance. Having more available PCr facilitates the resynthesis of ATP to provide energy for brief, high-intensity exercise (e.g., resistance training). This results in a better match between ATP supply and demand. PCr may also increase the force of muscular contraction and delay fatigue during anaerobic exercise by buffering the intracellular hydrogen ions formed with lactate production.

The amount of creatine in human skeletal muscle normally ranges between 90 and 160 mmoles per kilogram of muscle in dry muscle. The effectiveness of creatine supplementation appears to vary with these baseline levels; the greatest advantage is observed in those with the lowest baseline levels. Although anecdotal evidence suggests that increased muscle cramping occurs with creatine supplementation, no serious side effects have been scientifically verified.

More than two dozen studies have reported that creatine supplementation enhances the development of lean body mass and muscle strength in response to resistance training. This increased muscle strength and mass could be attributable to several mechanisms, including an effect on protein metabolism, synthesis, and transcriptional expression at the genetic level. Research supports this theory: Five-day oral dosages of 20 grams per day have been shown to increase muscle creatine availability by 20 percent and significantly accelerate PCr regeneration after intense muscle contraction. Significant enhancement of performance—both brief, high-intensity work and total time to exhaustion—has been observed in male athletes using creatine supplementation of 20 to 30 grams per day.

Long-term creatine supplementation has been shown to enhance the progress of muscle strength during resistance training in sedentary males and females. Twelve weeks of creatine supplementation enhances fat-free mass, physical performance, and muscle morphology in healthy men in response to heavy resistance training. This likely is attributable to higher-quality training sessions. Short-term creatine loading results in enhancement of both maximal strength and weightlifting performance. Therefore, part of the ergogenic (performance enhancing) effect of creatine shown in studies is likely attributable to this acute effect and part likely is attributable to the ability to train with higher workloads (although the relative contributions of these mechanisms remain unclear).

Branched-Chain Amino Acids

Branched-chain amino acids include three essential amino acids (leucine, isoleucine, and valine) that are needed to maintain muscle and preserve glycogen. Branched-chain amino acids are found naturally in foods such as dairy products, meat, whey, and eggs. Because of their role in muscle metabolism, branched-chain amino acids sometimes are isolated and consumed as a dietary supplement. In a study of branched-chain amino acid supplementation during four weeks of resistance training overreaching (defined earlier), initial reductions in strength and power were attenuated.

L-Carnitine

Carnitine is synthesized in the human liver and kidneys and is found in meats and dairy products. L-carnitine (the supplement form of carnitine) is thought to benefit exercise performance because it spares muscle glycogen by increasing free fatty acid transport across mitochondrial membranes, thus increasing fatty acid oxidation and use for energy. L-carnitine also appears to delay fatigue by reducing muscle lactate accumulation associated with exercise.

Some studies have shown a decreased respiratory exchange ratio—the ratio of carbon dioxide expired to oxygen consumed at the level of the lungs—with L-carnitine supplementation (2-6 grams per day) during exercise, suggesting that fatty acids rather than carbohydrate were used for energy. However, another study measuring muscle glycogen and lactate concentrations directly through biopsy and serum analysis failed to demonstrate any glycogen-sparing effect or reductions in lactate concentrations while supplementing with 6 grams per day of L-carnitine. Supplementation of L-carnitine L-tartrate (a source of L-carnitine when split into L-carnitine and L-tartaric acid in the body) in healthy men for three weeks has been shown to reduce the amount of exercise-induced muscle tissue damage, leave a greater number of receptors intact for hormonal interactions, reduce the level of muscle soreness, and result in less of an increase in markers of muscle damage and free radicals (atoms or compounds with unpaired electrons, which are thought to cause cellular damage).

Summary

To maximize the acute anabolic response to nutrition, strength athletes must consider the stimulus of resistance training combined with the availability of amino acids, the timing of supplement or macronutrient ingestion immediately before and after training, and the presence of insulin. To create a hormonal environment that enhances recovery from training, an athlete should ingest both protein and carbohydrate immediately before and after training.

Although more research is needed on the chronic adaptations to resistance training and nutrition, existing evidence suggests that protein and carbohydrate supplementation enhances the development of lean body mass in response to training. Several supplements are marketed with claims of increasing muscular strength and size; however, the only supplement with convincing scientific evidence to support its benefits to the strength athlete is creatine, which has been shown to improve the quality of the workout stimulus.

PART II

Resistance Training Guidelines

In this part of the book you will discover the proper methods for strength training and how to develop a program that will result in the greatest gains. You'll learn how to follow appropriate testing procedures to assess your strength; from there you will discover how to make the correct choice of training method to maximize output while minimizing risks.

Chapter 5, "Strength Assessment," lays the foundation for strength and power testing to help you define your strength training goals. These test results are interpreted so you can understand your strengths and weaknesses and then use this information to determine what areas to spend the most time on to improve your strength performance.

Chapter 6, "Types of Strength and Power Training," delineates the ways you can train in and out of the gym. There are a myriad of choices in the real world for training muscle, and this chapter helps you choose the one that suits your needs and time limitations.

Chapter 7, "Workout Schedule and Rest," organizes your workout into specific sections and details the purpose of each. Your workout should be a function of your goals and provide steps to accomplishing everything you want for strength and power. This chapter will allow you to adjust your variables in such a way to achieve maximum results.

Finally, chapter 8, "Safety, Soreness, and Injury," provides information on strength training in a manner that allows you to realize your goals without incurring injury. It also discusses muscle soreness, which is inevitable in some forms of resistance training, but you can minimize and control it by following proper guidelines. Finally, you can easily identify any injuries before they become serious, and proper form and methods of training can eliminate them altogether.

5

Strength Assessment

Kylie K. Harmon, Dustin D. Dunnick, and Lee E. Brown

Before beginning any exercise program, you must have a proper understanding of your current level of fitness. Your level of fitness has many aspects, including strength, power, and muscular endurance. In turn, these aspects are affected by a multitude of factors, including age, body mass index, and prior training experience (i.e., training age).

This chapter discusses how to assess certain aspects of your fitness level—in particular, muscular strength and power. Proper assessment is a critical step in developing an effective resistance training program because it allows you to see your areas of strength and weakness. You can then use this information, coupled with your personal goals, to develop an appropriate program. Furthermore, repeated assessments allow you to track your progress and determine which aspects of your training program are effective and which can be improved. Regardless of your current level of fitness, resistance training can be a fun and effective way to improve your overall health and well-being.

Strength and power can be measured using valid, accurate, and reliable assessment tests and an individual self-assessment. In this chapter, we detail how to perform the most commonly used assessment tests to help you measure your individual strength and power.

Setting Goals

When a person begins any exercise program, he or she usually has a set of goals to achieve. These can include losing weight, improving overall fitness, increasing muscle strength, or gaining an edge in a particular sport. Collecting some baseline data on where you are can help determine the types of exercises that will assist you the most in achieving your goals. This is especially true for strength and power training. Given the wide variety of resistance training methods available, it is important to decide which training methods to focus on and which are best suited for you.

The authors acknowledge the significant contributions of Daniel P. Murray, Sagir G. Bera, and Brian W. Findley to this chapter.

Your resistance training goals should be specific to what you want to accomplish through training. Before setting your goals, ask yourself, "Why am I doing this?" If you want to improve general strength, then you should focus on increasing the amount of weight you can lift. If, on the other hand, you want to achieve something more specific, such as being a better basketball player, you should focus on improving your performance in the components of that specific game.

Goals should also be realistic and attainable. This is not meant to discourage you from having lofty goals. On the contrary—setting the bar high for yourself can help keep you focused and motivated. Remember, though, that the loftier the goal, the longer and harder you will likely have to work to achieve it. In other words, it is not realistic to want to be able to bench press 200 pounds (90.7 kg) after six weeks of training if your current maximum is 100 pounds (45.4 kg). The goal will be difficult to achieve but not impossible. The short time frame, however, makes such a goal unrealistic.

Avoid setting unrealistic goals because they can lead to frustration and discouragement. Appropriate and realistic goals, on the other hand, can create satisfaction and a feeling of achievement. Once these initial goals are accomplished, you can change them to reflect the progress that you've made. Creating a sense of accomplishment through goal setting is vital because it gives you positive reinforcement for resistance training and can help you stick with the activity for the long haul.

Assessing Strength

The choice of strength assessments may be determined by your goals. If your goal is to improve overall physical fitness, then a self-assessment may be the best choice. However, if your goal is to improve a specific aspect of your performance, then more sophisticated tests such as the 1RM or computer-based assessments may be more beneficial. In addition, anthropometric measurements, such as height and weight, can be utilized by all individuals. Overall, the more assessments you make of your strength and conditioning level, the more you will understand your baseline fitness. However, completing more tests will require more time.

Note that some of the assessments in this chapter require more experience on the part of both the exerciser and the tester. For example, for 1RM tests, the exerciser must have a moderate level of strength and experience lifting in the gym, and spotters must be experienced to provide a safe testing environment. Computer-based tests may require expensive equipment and well-trained testers, whereas anthropometry and self-assessments may be done with minimal expense and experience.

Self-Assessment

Perhaps the easiest and most convenient way to evaluate your strength is to do a simple self-assessment. Even though many test protocols assess strength and power, a simple self-assessment remains one of the most effective ways to understand your personal strength capabilities. This is because only you can feel your muscles at work. Thus, a quick measurement of your overall strength and power may be very valuable to eventually achieving your exercise goals.

The beauty of doing a self-assessment is that there is no single right way to complete one. Basically, all you have to do is compare your current level of strength with the level you had before; this enables you to assess whether you need to make changes to your strength training program. Or, if you are beginning an exercise program, you simply determine whether you are at an appropriate strength and power level for achieving the types of gains you wish to make.

The first step is to determine why you need or want to increase strength or power. Some questions you might ask yourself include "Am I consistently having trouble doing everyday tasks?" and "Do I find it increasingly difficult to pick up items that previously were easy to lift?" Perhaps you feel that you are not getting as much as you would like out of your body during physical activity, or maybe you want to be able to run faster and jump higher when competing in sport. For any of these situations, you want to determine how much strength you feel you are lacking or would like to gain; deficiencies can be designated simply as "a lot," "a little," or "an average amount." A simple, subjective self-evaluation can be a useful supplement to a comprehensive strength and power testing protocol. If after performing your self-assessment you still have questions regarding your strength level, consult a certified strength and conditioning specialist for further evaluation.

1RM Protocol

One of the most universally accepted and used methods for testing strength is the 1RM protocol. Essentially, a person's 1RM for a specific exercise is the maximum amount of weight they can lift for no more than one complete repetition while maintaining correct form.

The 1RM test is an important tool because it allows you to establish a baseline that can be used to determine subsequent exercise intensities and loads for your workouts. In fact, the majority of the time, when people talk about doing a strength and power assessment, they are referring to doing a 1RM test. Usually, only the major muscle groups of the body are tested. Maximal upper-body strength is measured using a bench press, whereas lower-body strength is measured using the back squat. Maximum muscular power can be measured using a power clean.

Determining a 1RM for any exercise is a comprehensive process. Many sets of the exercise are performed, ultimately leading to the actual 1RM determination. (This process is detailed in the following procedures.) Performing the 1RM test properly means taking appropriate safety precautions. Before performing any of these procedures, you must have an understanding of the proper form and technique for safely completing the exercise you choose to use (refer to part III for detailed exercise instructions). Sturdy equipment must be used to ensure

1RM Test—Barbell Bench Press

Refer to chapter 9 for detailed instructions for the barbell bench press.

1. Begin with a warm-up set in which the resistance is low enough to allow you to complete 5 to 10 repetitions easily. Rest for one minute. Perform another warm-up set with a resistance that allows you to complete 3 to 5 repetitions. This usually means increasing the weight about 10 to 20 pounds (4.5-9.1 kg) or 5 to 10 percent of the previous set. Rest for two minutes.

2. Perform another warm-up set with a resistance that allows you to complete 2 to 3 repetitions.

3. Rest for two to four minutes.

4. Estimate another load increase of 10 to 20 pounds (5-10 percent) that allows you to perform only 1 repetition of the exercise with correct form. If you were able to complete the rep, go to the next step; if you were not able to lift the weight, go to step 6.

5. Rest for two to four minutes and then estimate another moderate increase in weight (10-20 pounds or 5-10 percent). Repeat the trial.

6. If you are unable to lift the weight, rest for two to four minutes, decrease the weight by 5 to 10 pounds (2.3-4.5 kg), and repeat. Continue increasing or decreasing the weight as needed until you determine your actual 1RM. Try to complete the process within 5 sets after completing the warm-up sets.

Procedures for the 1RM back squat and 1RM power clean are very similar to those for the 1RM bench press. The same procedures are followed for the number of warm-up sets and repetitions. The difference is that you should increase the weight in 30- to 40-pound (13.6-18.1 kg; 10-20 percent) increments instead of 10- to 20-pound (5-10 percent) increments. During the actual 1RM determination, the same increases in weight and rest periods apply. However, for a failed back squat or power clean 1RM attempt, the weight is decreased in increments of 15 to 20 pounds (6.8-9.1 kg; 5-10 percent).

that the participant and the weights are properly secured and supported. Use benches or squat racks with safety bars, and enlist the help of a spotter to ensure proper form and technique, as well as safety, during testing. Finally, be sure to use adequate rest periods to allow for recovery and to promote proper form.

As you can see from the instructions for the barbell bench press 1RM test, completing 1RM testing protocols takes a lot of time and effort. This is one of the drawbacks of the test. Fortunately, the results of the 1RM test are well worth obtaining. Competitive sport teams often use these tests to measure an athlete's strength and power. If only one test could be performed to determine strength or power, the 1RM would be the test to use.

Still, some people find the 1RM test to be more intense than their bodies are able to handle. As an alternative to a 1RM test, you can perform a multiple RM test and then convert the results into an estimated 1RM value using any of a variety of prediction equations. Table 5.1 lists some predicted 1RM values based on the weight used and repetitions completed. To use the table to estimate your 1RM, use the top row to find the number of repetitions you completed. Follow down the column until you find the load you lifted for the number of repetitions you indicated at top. Following the row to the far left, your predicted 1RM value is indicated in the first column. For example, if you were able to perform 5 repetitions

TABLE 5.1 Estimating 1RM Training Loads

Maximum repetitions	1	2	3	4	5	6	7	8	9	10	12	15
% RM	100	95	93	90	87	85	83	80	77	75	67	65
Load (lb or kg) 10	10	9	9	9	9	8	8	8	8	7	7
20	19	19	18	17	17	17	16	15	15	13	13
30	29	28	27	26	26	25	24	23	23	20	20
40	38	37	36	35	34	33	32	31	30	27	26
50	48	47	45	44	43	42	40	39	38	34	33
60	57	56	54	52	51	50	48	46	45	40	39
70	67	65	63	61	60	58	56	54	53	47	46
80	76	74	72	70	68	66	64	62	60	54	52
90	86	84	81	78	77	75	72	69	68	60	59
100	95	93	90	87	85	83	80	77	75	67	65
110	105	102	99	96	94	91	88	85	83	74	72
120	114	112	108	104	102	100	96	92	90	80	78
130	124	121	117	113	111	108	104	100	98	87	85
140	133	139	126	122	119	116	112	108	105	94	91
150	143	140	135	131	128	125	120	116	113	101	98
160	152	149	144	139	136	133	128	123	120	107	104
170	162	158	153	148	145	141	136	131	128	114	111
180	171	167	162	157	153	149	144	139	135	121	117
190	181	177	171	165	162	158	152	146	143	127	124
200	190	196	180	174	170	166	160	154	150	134	130
210	200	195	189	183	179	174	168	162	158	141	137
220	209	205	198	191	187	183	176	169	165	147	143
230	219	214	207	200	196	191	184	177	173	154	150
240	228	223	216	209	204	199	192	185	180	161	156
250	238	233	225	218	213	208	200	193	188	168	163
260	247	242	234	226	221	206	208	200	195	174	169

> continued

Reprinted, by permission, from National Strength and Conditioning Association, 2015, Program design for resistance training. In *Essentials of strength training and conditioning*, 4th ed., edited by G.G. Haff and N.T. Triplett (Champaign, IL: Human Kinetics), 455-456.

TABLE 5.1 > *continued*

Maximum repetitions	1	2	3	4	5	6	7	8	9	10	12	15
% RM	100	95	93	90	87	85	83	80	77	75	67	65
Load (lb or kg)	270	257	251	243	235	239	224	216	208	203	181	176
	280	266	260	252	244	238	232	224	216	210	188	182
	290	276	270	261	252	247	241	232	223	218	194	189
	300	285	279	270	261	255	249	240	231	225	201	195
	310	295	288	279	270	264	257	248	239	233	208	202
	320	304	298	288	278	272	266	256	246	240	214	208
	330	314	307	297	287	281	274	264	254	248	221	215
	340	323	316	306	296	289	282	272	262	255	228	221
	350	333	326	315	305	298	291	280	270	263	235	228
	360	342	335	324	313	306	299	288	277	270	241	234
	370	352	344	333	322	315	307	296	285	278	248	241
	380	361	353	342	331	323	315	304	293	285	255	247
	390	371	363	351	339	332	324	312	300	293	261	254
	400	380	372	360	348	340	332	320	308	300	268	260
	410	390	381	369	357	349	340	328	316	308	274	267
	420	399	391	378	365	357	349	336	323	315	281	273
	430	409	400	387	374	366	357	344	331	323	288	280
	440	418	409	396	383	374	365	352	339	330	295	286
	450	428	429	405	392	383	374	360	347	338	302	293
	460	437	428	414	400	391	382	368	354	345	308	299
	470	447	437	423	409	400	390	376	362	353	315	306
	480	456	446	432	418	408	398	384	370	360	322	312
	490	466	456	441	426	417	407	392	377	368	328	319
	500	475	465	450	435	425	415	400	385	375	335	325
	510	485	474	459	444	435	423	408	393	383	342	332
	520	494	484	468	452	442	432	416	400	390	348	338
	530	504	493	477	461	451	440	424	408	398	355	345
	540	513	502	486	470	459	448	432	416	405	362	351
	550	523	512	495	479	468	457	440	424	413	369	358
	560	532	521	504	487	476	465	448	431	420	375	364
	570	542	530	513	496	485	473	456	439	428	382	371
	580	551	539	522	505	493	481	464	447	435	389	377
	590	561	549	531	513	502	490	472	454	443	395	384
	600	570	558	540	522	510	498	480	462	450	402	390

with 104 lbs, your estimated 1RM would be 120 lbs. Although prediction equations are not as accurate as an actual 1RM measurement, a prediction value may be adequate for the average individual. And, as discussed throughout this chapter, a variety of other tests can also be used, individually or collectively, to properly determine strength and power.

Anthropometric Measurements

Anthropometric measurement is another simple way to measure strength, albeit indirectly. *Anthropometry* can be defined as the scientific measurement of the body. The only instrument you need to make these measurements is a simple, flexible tape measure, not unlike the one that a tailor would use.

Every few weeks, use the tape measure to measure the circumference of a variety of big muscle groups, such as those of the thighs, upper arms, chest, and calves (figure 5.1). By taking the measurements every few weeks, you can chart the progress of gain or loss in muscle size. Note that an increase in muscle size often comes with slight increases in fat mass because concerted effort to increase muscle hypertrophy requires excess caloric consumption. This potentially can confound muscle mass assessments. However, generally speaking, the larger the circumference of the muscle, the stronger it is.

Although anthropometric measurements may seem primitive, they can be a great way to identify changes in strength. However, we recommend that anthropometric measurements be used only as a supplement to other strength and power assessment tools.

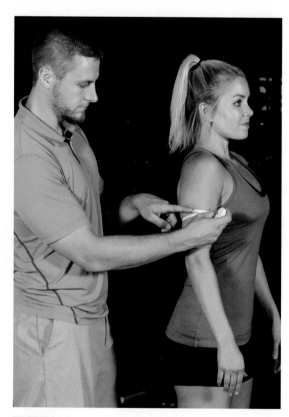

FIGURE 5.1 Increases in a muscle's circumference tend to indicate an increase in that muscle's strength.

Computerized Measurements

On one end of the strength assessment spectrum is the simple, low-tech self-assessment. On the other end of the spectrum are a variety of available computerized measurement tools. Computers have the ability to quantify a person's actual strength and power, which can't be done with a normal self-assessment. With computers, you have the option of performing a large number of tests and getting very accurate results. In addition, computers can precisely measure muscle strength and power in all sorts of positions and movements. The most frequently used tools are electromyography equipment, isokinetic dynamometers, and force plates.

Electromyography (EMG) measures electrical signals in the muscle to determine general levels of strength. As you learned in chapter 1, each muscle in your body is innervated or connected by a set of nerves, or motor neurons. These motor neurons ultimately are controlled by your central nervous system, including your brain. Muscular strength is partially determined by the neuromuscular control that you have over those muscles. In fact, the initial adaptations to resistance training exercise are mostly neuromuscular adaptations (refer to chapter 2). (That's one reason why you do not see huge gains in muscle mass until after the first few weeks of regular training.) Strength training forces your nerves to learn how to best and most efficiently send a signal to the muscles, causing them to contract. As a person's muscles get stronger, the electrical activity of the muscles increases. EMG pads placed on various locations on the surface of the muscle, or fine wires inserted directly into the muscle, are connected to an EMG machine or computer, and the electrical activity of that muscle can be measured as it contracts. When this process is repeated after a few weeks of resistance training, it can be used to determine increases in neuromuscular activity and thus gains in muscle strength.

An isokinetic dynamometer is another piece of equipment that can be used to measure strength and power (see figure 5.2). Dynamometers look like large exercise machines that are connected to a computer. They measure the torque (force or strength) that is produced

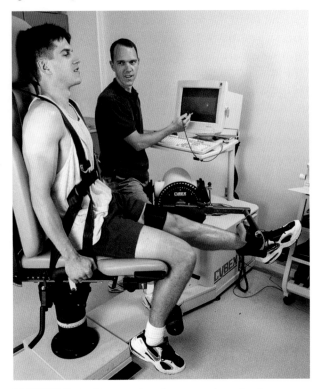

FIGURE 5.2 By exerting force against the lever arm of the isokinetic dynomometer, the strength of the participant's left leg is measured.

© Human Kinetics

when someone pushes or pulls on the dynamometer lever arm; a computer program then analyzes the data and provides a measure of the torque and power that was produced. The collected information gives you some of the most precise, accurate, and quantifiable assessment data available on strength and power.

With a few adjustments to the dynamometer, almost every major muscle in the body can be tested. These machines can measure muscle strength through the muscle's entire range of motion, otherwise known as the *dynamic strength* of the muscle. Isokinetic training is discussed in more detail in chapter 6.

Isokinetic dynamometers can also measure isometric or static strength at specific angles of a joint. This can be especially useful as a clinical tool in identifying areas of strength deficiency or imbalance. For instance, an athlete recovering from knee surgery can be tested to determine whether the quadriceps of the leg that was operated on is as strong as the quadriceps on the opposing side. The results of the test can be used to help determine whether this athlete is ready to return to the field of play or needs more time to rehabilitate.

Another kind of dynamometer is the hand-grip dynamometer (see figure 5.3). The hand-grip dynamometer is used to measure grip strength. Hand-grip dynamometers are compact, relatively inexpensive, and simple to use. First, the dynamometer is adjusted to fit the participant's hand-grip size. The participant then stands with arms at the sides and holds the dynamometer with a neutral grip. Without excess body movement, the participant squeezes the dynamometer as hard as possible for several seconds. The dynamometer then gives a reading of the force produced.

Another computerized method of strength assessment, the force plate, allows an individual to measure various force outputs, such as peak force, as well as how quickly force is produced. Essentially a giant bathroom scale, a force plate detects body weight as well as any changes in force output due to movement. Like the dynamometer, a force place commonly is used to measure isometric strength. A typical example of this type of assessment is the isometric midthigh pull. To perform this assessment, a power rack is positioned over the plate and a barbell is fixed in the rack at midthigh level. The participant stands on the plate and grasps the bar with both hands, keeping the thighs close to the bar and the knees slightly bent. When instructed to do so, the participant pulls forcefully on the bar, pushing through the heels. A computer connected to the force plate collects the force that the participant exerts into the ground.

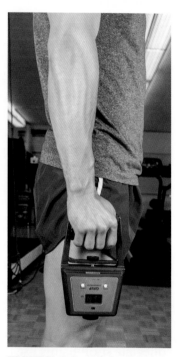

FIGURE 5.3 While standing in a neutral position, the participant squeezes the dynomometer with maximal force.

For a precise measurement of strength and power, isokinetic dynamometers, EMG, and force plates are the way to go. Unfortunately, that accuracy comes at a price—literally. Many of these machines are very expensive and usually are found only in clinical or laboratory settings. Prior background knowledge is required to operate such machines. Also, a medical referral may be required. Much of the time, the strength and power measurements from isokinetic dynamometers or EMG are more elaborate than what is needed by an individual. Thus, for most people, we recommend simpler and more routine assessment tests.

Assessing Power

As with strength assessments, the test you choose to assess your power will depend on your specific goals. The 1RM, vertical jump, and 40-yard dash protocols described in this section require relatively simple equipment. Be aware that measures of strength relate to the maximum weight you can lift, whereas measures of power relate to your explosiveness (see chapter 12).

1RM Protocol

The 1RM protocols for strength assessments can also be applied to power assessments. The techniques and procedures for performing the tests are essentially the same; the only difference is the way the exercise is performed. The repetitions performed during strength assessments are done more slowly, and the weight is controlled throughout the entire range of motion of the exercise. In contrast, power exercises are performed ballistically, and the individual attempts to move the weight as fast as possible. Typical power exercises that are performed during 15RM protocols are weightlifting movements or Olympic lifts (discussed in chapter 12).

Vertical Jump Test

You probably have heard sportscasters talk about a basketball player with a "48-inch vertical" or a football player with a "36-inch vertical." They are referring to these players' vertical jump test scores. The vertical jump test is routinely used to measure lower-body power. A vertical jump test does not determine exact power measurements for individual muscles. Instead, the test is used to compare an athlete's power (or vertical jump height) with that of others taking the same test or to measure an athlete's improvements over time. Many professional and collegiate sport teams use the vertical jump test to determine the power level of their athletes and to determine whether an athlete needs to improve lower-body power for his or her specific sport.

Like many power assessment tests, the vertical jump is a simple test that almost anyone can perform. The vertical jump height of an athlete can be measured in two ways. The first way is to use a commercially available vertical jump test device, such as the Vertec (figure 5.4a). Alternatively, the test can be performed using a wall and some chalk to put on the jumper's fingertips (figure 5.4*b*). A commercial device usually will give more accurate results because testing conditions remain uniform for each trial. Nonetheless, a wall and some chalk are fairly precise, simple, and inexpensive.

Essentially, the vertical jump test consists of an athlete jumping as high as they possibly can. The test begins with the athlete standing directly underneath the device or six inches (15.2 cm) to the side of a wall. An initial measurement is taken with the athlete reaching as high as possible with their feet flat on the ground. If using a wall, a mark is made at this point with the chalk. If using a commercial device, the device is adjusted so that the athlete can just reach

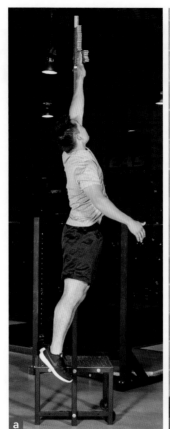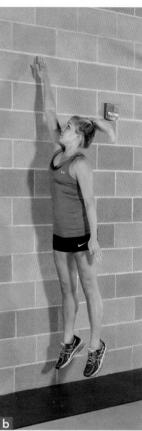

FIGURE 5.4 *(a)* The athlete taps the vanes of the jump device at the highest point of his vertical jump. *(b)* The athlete taps the wall with her fingertips at the highest point of her vertical jump. The chalk on her fingertips marks the wall, indicating her jump height.

the lowest vane. For either test setting, the athlete bends down, swings both arms down and back, quickly swings both arms forward and up, and jumps as high as possible. At the highest point in the jump, the athlete leaves a chalk mark on the wall or taps a vane on the vertical jump device. Vertical jump height is defined as the distance between the initial standing mark and mark left at the top of the jump. Athletes should perform three trials, recording the highest jump. A brief recovery period is allowed between each trial.

An athlete can determine his or her level of lower-body power by comparing the vertical jump test score with descriptive data for the test (see table 5.2). Maximum vertical jump height is an important variable that applies directly to performance in many sports, including basketball and volleyball. Unfortunately, vertical jump height cannot readily be compared with quantitative power measurements from tests such as the 1RM power clean. Thus, vertical jump tests should primarily be used to measure and compare vertical jump height. As with many strength

TABLE 5.2 Vertical Jump, Static Jump, and Broad Jump Descriptive Data*
for Various Groups

Group, sport, or position	Number of athletes	Vertical jump		Static jump		Broad jump	
		in.	cm	in.	cm	in.	cm
College soccer (women) (118)	51	16.1 ± 2.2	40.9 ± 5.5				
High school soccer (women) (118)	83	15.6 ± 1.9	39.6 ± 4.7				
College lacrosse (women) (118)	79	15.8 ± 2.2	40.1 ± 5.6				
Under 18 Gaelic football (men) (22)	265	17.0 ± 2.0	43.3 ± 5.1			78.0 ± 8.1	198.2 ± 20.7
National soccer (women) (17)	21	12.4 ± 1.6	31.6 ± 4.0	11.9 ± 1.5	30.1 ± 3.7		
Under 19 soccer (women) (17)	20	13.5 ± 1.5	34.3 ± 3.9	12.9 ± 1.1	32.8 ± 2.9		
Under 17 soccer (women) (17)	21	11.4 ± 0.8	29.0 ± 2.1	11.1 ± 1.0	28.2 ± 2.5		
Under 21 soccer (men) (17)	18	15.9 ± 1.7	40.3 ± 4.3	14.6 ± 1.5	37.0 ± 3.9		
Under 20 soccer (men) (17)	17	15.8 ± 1.9	40.2 ± 4.7	15.0 ± 1.9	38.0 ± 4.9		
Under 17 soccer (men) (17)	21	16.1 ± 2.0	40.9 ± 5.1	14.7 ± 1.9	37.3 ± 4.7		
Division I Spain soccer (women) (99)	100	10.3 ± 1.9	26.1 ± 4.8				
National ice hockey (women) (89)	23	19.8 ± 2.2	50.3 ± 5.7#			84.6 ± 4.3	214.8 ± 10.9
National soccer (women) (42)	85	12.1 ± 1.6	30.7 ± 4.1				
Division I Norway soccer (women) (42)	47	11.1 ± 1.6	28.1 ± 4.1				
Ice hockey National Hockey League draftees (men) (15)	853	24.4 ± 3.0	62.0 ± 7.6#			100.0 ± 7.0	254.0 ± 17.8
College wrestling (men) (109)	20	220.5 ± 3.13	52.0 ± 8.0#				
National weightlifting (men) (32)	6	23.9 ± 1.5	60.8 ± 3.9				
National soccer (men) (123)	17	22.2 ± 1.6	56.4 ± 4.0				

Group, sport, or position	Number of athletes	Vertical jump		Static jump		Broad jump	
		in.	cm	in.	cm	in.	cm
National soccer (men) (124)	14	22.3 ± 2.6	56.7 ± 6.6				
National soccer (men) (124)	15	20.9 ± 1.6	53.1 ± 4.0				
National soccer (men) (106)	270	17.8 ± 0.7	45.1 ± 1.7	17.4 ± 0.5	44.1 ± 1.3		
National handball (women) (40)	16	15.1 ± 1.7	38.4 ± 4.4				
National handball (men) (39)	15	19.0 ± 2.8	48.2 ± 7.2				
Under 16 rugby league (men) (114)	67	18.0 ± 2.0	45.7 ± 5.2				
Under 17 rugby league (men) (114)	50	19.3 ± 2.3	49.1 ± 5.8				
Under 18 rugby league (men) (114)	56	19.9 ± 2.2	50.6 ± 5.7				
Under 19 rugby league (men) (114)	45	20.7 ± 2.2	52.5 ± 5.5				
Under 20 rugby league (men) (114)	25	20.8 ± 2.1	52.8 ± 5.4				
High school volleyball (women) (98)	27	18.5 ± 3.3	47.1 ± 8.5#				
NCAA Division I volleyball (women) (98)	26	20.8 ± 2.5	52.8 ± 6.3#				
National rugby league forwards (men) (20)	12	14.7 ± 1.7	37.3 ± 4.4				
National rugby league backs (men) (20)	6	15.9 ± 2.5	40.3 ± 6.4				
National rugby league (men) (35)	26	20.0 ± 2.9	20.0 ± 2.9				
National rugby league (men) (34)	58	24.7 ± 2.2	62.8 ± 5.7#				
National rugby union (men) (21)	30					101.6 ± 7.9	258.0 ± 20.0

> continued

TABLE 5.2 > *continued*

Group, sport, or position	Number of athletes	Vertical jump		Static jump		Broad jump	
		in.	cm	in.	cm	in.	cm
National rugby union (women) (10)	15	15.0 ± 1.6	38.0 ± 4.0	13.8 ± 1.2	35.0 ± 3.0		
High school track and field (women) (75)	8					83.4 ± 6.3	212.0 ± 16.0
NCAA Division I soccer (women) (67)	15	12.2 ± 2.0	31.0 ± 5.0			57.9 ± 4.3	147.0 ± 11.0
High school rugby league (men) (112)	302	16.3 ± 2.1	41.3 ± 5.3				
Junior national volleyball (men) (33)	14	21.5 ± 0.9	54.6 ± 2.2#				
Junior national volleyball (women) (33)	15	18.0 ± 0.6	45.7 ± 1.6#				
Under 18 Australian rules football (men) (127)	177	23.9 ± 2.2	60.6 ± 5.5#				
NCAA Division I lacrosse (women) (117)	84	15.8 ± 2.2	40.2 ± 5.6				
NCAA Division I soccer (men) (102)	27	24.3 ± 2.8	61.6 ± 7.1#				
National soccer (women) (1)	17	12.0 ± 0.5	30.5 ± 1.2				
National soccer (women) (76)	17	12.8 ± 1.5	32.6 ± 3.7				
National soccer (men) (76)	17	17.2 ± 0.9	43.7 ± 2.2				
National junior soccer (women) (76)	17	11.2 ± 0.8	28.4 ± 2.0				
National junior soccer (men) (76)	17	17.3 ± 1.9	43.9 ± 4.8				
National soccer (men) (2)	214	15.4 ± 2.0	39.2 ± 5.0	14.8 ± 1.9	37.6 ± 4.8		

*The values listed are means ± standard deviation. The data should be regarded as only descriptive, not normative.

#Jumps performed with arm swing.

Reprinted, by permission, from National Strength and Conditioning Association, 2016, Adaptations to anaerobic training programs, D. French. In *Essentials of strength training and conditioning*, 4th ed., edited by G.G. Haff and N.T. Triplett (Champaign, IL: Human Kinetics) 300-301.

and power measurements, vertical jump tests should make up just one portion of an overall testing protocol.

To calculate peak power in watts from vertical jump height, use the following equation (Harman et al. 1991):

[(61.9 × jump height in centimeters) + (36.0 × body mass in kilograms)] + 1822

To calculate average power, use the following equation (Johnson and Bahamonde 1996):

[(21.2 × jump height in centimeters) + (23.0 × body mass in kilograms)] − 1393

To calculate relative power, simply divide the resulting peak power and average power values by body mass in kilograms.

Margaria-Kalamen Stair Climb Test

A Margaria-Kalamen may sound like a fancy cocktail, but it is actually a useful test for calculating an individual's lower-body power (Margaria et al. 1966; Kalamen 1968). The test is easy to administer and requires very little equipment—just steps and a timer.

You can perform a Margaria-Kalamen test on any staircase that has at least nine steps and at least 20 feet (6 m) of flat area leading up to the staircase (figure 5.5). Each step should be about 7 inches (17.8 cm) tall. Perform the test using the following instructions:

1. An electronic start timer is placed on the third step, and a stop timer is placed on the ninth step. (A simple timer will suffice if no electronic timer is available, though the results may not be as accurate. In such a case, it is better to have a second person also timing and then average the results of each trial to get the time measurement.)

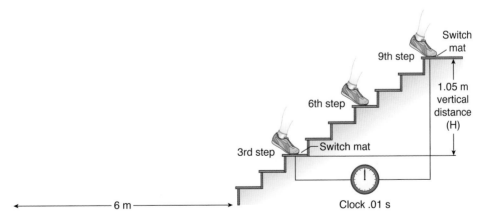

FIGURE 5.5   The Margaria-Kalamen stair sprint test is a simple method for assessing your level of power relative to others in your age group.

Adapted from M. Foss and S.J. Keteyian, 1997, *Fox's physiological basis for exercise and sport*, 6th ed. (New York: McGraw-Hill Companies). By permission of S.J. Keteyian.

2. The participant takes three warm-up runs up the stairs.

3. The participant then stands, facing the staircase, exactly 20 feet (6 m) from the base of the staircase. He or she begins to sprint from a standstill.

4. On reaching the staircase, the participant steps on the third, sixth, and ninth steps only. Timing begins immediately after stepping on the third step and ends after reaching the ninth step.

5. The time is recorded to the nearest hundredth of a second.

6. The following formula is then used to calculate power in watts:

$$power = [(M \times D) \times 9.8]/t$$

where M is body mass in kilograms, D is vertical height in meters between the first and last steps, and t is time from the third step to the ninth step.

7. The calculated power for the participant can be compared with the information in table 5.3, a standardized chart used to determine the level of power.

For people who do not have the facilities or resources to do other power assessment tests, the Margaria-Kalamen stair sprint test offers a simple but universally accepted power testing protocol. Because little equipment is required to perform this test and to make the power calculations, most people can perform this test correctly without prior training. Although the Margaria-Kalamen test

TABLE 5.3   Margaria-Kalamen Stair Sprint Test Guidelines

Classification	Age group (yr)				
	15-20	21-30	31-40	41-50	Over 50
Men					
Poor	<113	<106	<85	<65	<50
Fair	113-149	106-139	85-111	65-84	50-65
Average	150-187	140-175	112-140	85-105	66-82
Good	188-224	176-210	141-168	106-125	83-98
Excellent	>224	>210	>168	>125	>98
Women					
Poor	<92	<85	<65	<50	<38
Fair	92-120	85-111	65-84	50-65	38-48
Average	121-151	112-140	85-105	66-82	49-61
Good	152-182	141-168	106-125	83-98	62-75
Excellent	>182	>168	>125	>98	>75

Units are kilogram-meters per second. To calculate watts (newton-meters per second—a more standard unit of power), multiply the values by 9.807.

Adapted from M. Foss and S.J. Keteyian, 1997, *Fox's physiological basis for exercise and sport*, 6th ed. (New York: McGraw-Hill Companies). By permission of S.J. Keteyian.

can be used to estimate power, it is best suited for classifying the level of power into categories, including *poor, average,* and *excellent.* If you simply are looking to compare your level of power with that of others in your age group rather than to determine an exact numerical power measurement, the Margaria-Kalamen stair sprint test may be good for you.

40-Yard Dash

The 40-yard dash, which measures lower-body power, is simple and easy to administer. To perform this test, clearly mark 40 yards (36.5 m) on a flat grass or turf surface, setting a cone several yards beyond the finish line. The participant gets several practice runs and should run the distance with increasing intensity. Once fully prepared, the subject begins with their foot just behind the starting line. On the signal, the subject runs with full speed through the cone at the finish line. (Running through the cone ensures that the participant does not begin to decelerate prematurely.) Although timing gates should be used for optimal accuracy, handheld timing devices such as a stopwatch can work well. If using a handheld device, the tester should stand at the end of the 40 yards to ensure that timing stops at the moment the participant crosses the 40-yard line.

Once the sprint time is recorded, lower-body power can be calculated using the following:

1. Convert distance to meters by multiplying by 1.09.
2. Calculate velocity by dividing meters by time.
3. Multiply body mass in kilograms by 9.8 to obtain newtons.
4. Multiply newtons by velocity to get power in watts.
5. Divide watts by body mass to obtain relative lower-body power.

Wingate Anaerobic Power Test

The Wingate anaerobic cycle test uses a cycle ergometer to measure lower-body power. Due to the strenuous nature of this test, it should be used primarily with individuals who are accustomed to intense exercise. Before testing the participant is fitted to the cycle, and the seat is adjusted to produce 5 degrees to 10 degrees of knee flexion at the bottom of the range of motion. After a two- to three-minute warm-up at a self-selected pace interspersed by several short sprints, the participant quickly ramps up to top speed. Once top speed is reached, a preselected weight of 7.5 percent of body weight is physically dropped. The weight is instantly added to the flywheel resistance. The participant pedals against this resistance. The participant must give maximum effort for the entirety of the test. The connected computer software then analyzes the test and provides peak power, average power, and percentage fatigue (Brown and Weir 2001). The results of this test are most valid for cyclists, who are used to this specific mode of exercise.

Interpreting the Results

Regardless of which specific assessments you choose to perform, the reason for completing them is the same. Primarily, these tests give you a personal baseline from which to start building a program. Although it is important to measure self-improvement, you may also wish to compare your performance against established norms. Charts and books containing normative data (e.g., Hoffman 2006) will allow you to compare your strength and power levels against established norms and give you the means to create goals to work toward. Your goals will keep you focused on your reason for resistance training and help you construct an appropriate program.

The answers you get from your assessments, coupled with your goals, tell you which types of exercises to include in your program. For instance, a high school football player who scores well on a 1RM bench press test but achieves a mediocre score on a vertical jump test would want to tailor his program more toward improving his lower-body power, even if the rest of his team is working more on upper-body strength. A middle-aged woman who is just starting resistance training might score poorly on a 1RM barbell bench press test but do well on a similar squat test. If her goal is to develop more overall strength, these results may lead her to include more upper-body training than lower-body training in her program.

Summary

This chapter describes a broad selection of strength and power assessment protocols. Some tests are relatively simple, such as the self-evaluation, vertical jump test, and 40-yard dash, whereas other tests are more complicated, such as the 1RM and computer-controlled tests. There is no wrong or right test. Rather, test selection should be based on the needs of the participant and the availability of equipment. For example, if you want to compare your level of power with that of others, you may choose the Margaria-Kalamen stair sprint test. If you are looking for accuracy, an isokinetic dynamometer test may be appropriate. Vertical jump, 1RM, and power tests are staples of the competitive sport industry. No matter which test you choose, you must always look out for your health and safety by using proper form and following the procedures precisely. The results from your assessment should help you determine which resistance training exercises will aid you in ultimately reaching your goals.

Types of Strength and Power Training

Dustin D. Dunnick, Kylie K. Harmon, and Lee E. Brown

Almost everyone has had the experience of walking into a gym or fitness center for the first time and seeing hundreds of different pieces of equipment. You hear fellow exercisers talking about working out on the fitness machines or with free weights, or using medicine balls or exercise rubber bands. The gym can be an intimidating place for a person who does not know what types of exercises to perform and what equipment to use.

This chapter helps explain some of the different types of training often used for strength or power, including isotonic, isometric, and isokinetic training; plyometric and medicine ball training; resistance bands and cords; and kettle-bell and suspension training. As you recall, strength is the maximum force that your muscles can generate at a particular speed, whereas power is the force that is produced over a range of velocities. Thus, you would expect to have quick, explosive movements incorporated into power exercises (e.g., the power clean) as opposed to the steady movements performed in strength exercises (e.g., the leg extension or Romanian deadlift). We discuss some of the advantages and disadvantages of each of the main categories of training. In addition, we make recommendations on how to incorporate these into an overall training program. You may find it helpful to refer to chapter 5 to properly assess your level of strength as you choose the types of training that are right for you.

Isometric Training

Exercises intended to improve muscle strength and power come in many forms. In the past, isometric exercise was the most common form used to improve strength. However, people trying to increase their strength have gradually

The authors acknowledge the significant contributions of Sagir G. Bera, Daniel P. Murray, and Brian W. Findley to this chapter.

shifted their focus to other types of exercise that are more functional in nature. Nonetheless, isometric exercise is still an effective training method for gaining strength.

Isometric exercises are those in which the exercising muscle or limb does not move. In other words, contraction of the involved muscle occurs with no apparent movement of the joint. The force of the muscle contraction causes tension in the muscle without a noticeable change in its length. Isometric exercises usually are performed by mimicking a pushing or pulling action in the various joint positions. An example of an isometric exercise is pushing a fixed object, such as a wall or a bar or weight machine attached to the floor (figure 6.1a). Another example of an isometric exercise is holding a weighted object in a stationary position with muscles contracted, such as holding a dumbbell in place with your arm slightly bent (figure 6.1b). Linemen in American football must be proficient in holding a two-, three-, or four-point stance for a few seconds before exploding off the line; thus, they can benefit from isometric training followed by an explosive movement. An example would be holding a medicine ball at chest level in a half squat for five seconds and then exploding forward and throwing the ball against a wall.

Research has shown that isometric exercise can significantly increase the tension of the muscle. Thus, in contrast to regular isotonic weight training (discussed in the next section), a person can achieve maximum muscular contractions by

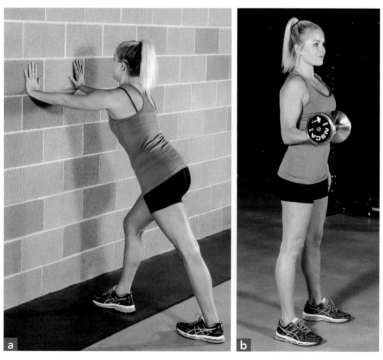

FIGURE 6.1 An isometric exercise can be done by (a) pushing against an immovable object or (b) holding a weight in a stationary position with the muscles contracted.

performing isometric exercises. In addition to gains in muscle strength, isometric exercise can lead to an increase in muscle mass and improvements in bone strength. It also provides all the benefits associated with muscle strength, including elevated muscle metabolism (energy use by the body), which is important when trying to increase caloric expenditure and burn fat.

You don't need to have free weights or a weight machine to do isometric exercises; therefore, it is an easy and convenient form of strength training that you can perform anywhere, such as a hotel room or bedroom. All you need is a fixed or stationary object that you can push or pull against. Typically, you perform this type of exercise by holding a muscle or joint in a set position for six to eight seconds. However, to produce noticeable improvements in strength, each exercise needs to be repeated between 5 and 10 times per session over a period of four to eight weeks.

Although isometric exercise can be a very effective strength training method, it has numerous drawbacks, many of which are associated with the nonfunctional adaptations to this mode of training. For example, because isometric exercises are performed in a position in which the limbs are set, the involved or contracting muscle will achieve gains in strength primarily at that position. This type of gain in muscle strength is a good example of exercise specificity, wherein you improve mainly within the movement patterns and range of motion that you are training. If you wanted to become better at cycling, you would not spend the majority of your time running; rather, you would spend most of your time cycling because that is the specific activity that you are training for. With isometric exercise, you are strengthening your muscles in a static position, so you would expect improvements in strength in that particular position only. As a result, you would have to perform isometric exercises through the whole range of motion of the limb to get equal improvements in muscle strength across this range. Furthermore, given that isometric exercises are performed in a static position, a person may experience a reduction in dynamic speed and athletic performance. This can be contrasted with the dynamic movements performed in isotonic training.

Another drawback of isometric exercise is that it can dramatically increase blood pressure due to the large increase in muscle tension and an increase in intra-abdominal pressure that may be achieved with isometric exercise. Unfortunately, the increase in blood pressure can be dangerous and lead to damaged or ruptured blood vessels in addition to an irregular heartbeat. Thus, it is recommended that individuals with high blood pressure and heart problems refrain from performing isometric exercise. Additionally, muscular endurance can decrease because blood is not constantly pumped through the muscle (as it is in isotonic exercise).

This decrease in athletic performance and muscle endurance makes isometric training a less appealing form of strength training exercise compared with some other forms. Isometric contractions are used primarily in a rehabilitative or physical therapy setting. Because of their shortcomings, isometric exercises should be treated as only one part of a larger overall program rather than the sole workout type in a strength training program.

Isotonic Training

Usually, when you hear people talking about strength and power exercises, they are referring to isotonic training, or simply resistance training, with free weights or machines. Unlike isometric training, isotonic training involves an exercise movement using a constant load—that is, the weight being lifted remains the same regardless of the movement performed or the speed used during the exercise. This is in contrast to what you typically see with other types of resistance training. Like every form of resistance training, isotonic training has many physical and physiological benefits as well as some disadvantages.

Compared with other resistance training methods, isotonic training may be the most beneficial to overall health. Routine resistance training can lead to the development of muscle strength, power, and muscular endurance, but these are not the only benefits of isotonic training. Routine isotonic exercise also has been shown to improve tendon and ligament strength. A person can improve joint stability and posture by combining stronger tendons and ligaments with overall muscle strength. This important quality can help reduce the risk of injury during normal physical activity and decrease the chances of experiencing the effects of common problems such as arthritis and lower back pain.

Some additional benefits of isotonic training include improvements in bone strength, energy, and fat loss. Continuously loading the body or placing a force on the body is necessary for building bone density (see figure 6.2). Lifting a weight forces the bones in the body to support a load that they are not used to supporting, causing more minerals to be deposited in the bones, thereby increasing their strength. Increased muscle mass from isotonic weight training has

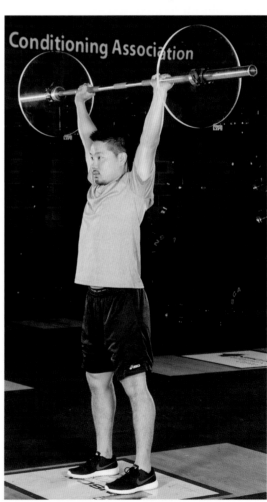

FIGURE 6.2 Isotonic exercises such as this barbell overhead press can condition the body to more easily perform everyday activities.

also been shown to improve fat loss. Some believe that the added muscle mass improves metabolism, although this topic is still highly contested. In addition, a person may feel that increased muscle mass gives them more energy to carry out normal acts of daily living. These health benefits are supplementary to the primary purpose of resistance training, which is to improve the characteristics of the muscles.

Muscles grow in response to stresses being placed on them. Progressive resistance training overloads the muscles, or forces them to work at a higher intensity. The overload principle is the basis of all types of training. Overload from resistance training can cause microscopic tears in the muscles; these tears are part of the normal muscle-building process. As these tears occur, the natural muscle-rebuilding process is stimulated. Protein molecules are laid down to generate more muscle filaments. Accordingly, the size and makeup of muscles will adapt to the exercise and grow. (See chapter 1 for a discussion of the types of muscle fibers.) Essentially, working at a level to which it is not accustomed forces the body to adapt to the extra stresses, resulting in an improvement in that specific activity (as is expected with exercise specificity). In the case of resistance training, the specific adaptation to an overload is for the muscles to increase in size, strength, muscular endurance, and power.

Adjusting the Load to the Goal

Whether you are a seasoned athlete, someone recovering from a recent injury, or a chronic couch potato, we recommend that you partake in some form of resistance training. Isotonic exercises are perfect for almost any population because they can be personalized to fit specific needs. Altering intensity, number of sets, and repetitions of an exercise is enough to influence how the muscles will adapt and grow in response to that exercise. However, with any exercise, it's also important to become familiar with what to do, how to do it, why you are doing it, and when you should do it. This will ensure that you know the risks and benefits of what you are doing and can correctly plan how to achieve your exercise goals. (Chapter 5 discusses exercise goals and how to determine them.)

Although you may see improvements in muscular strength, power, hypertrophy, and muscular endurance for any given exercise, it is best to focus specifically on improving one at a time.

You can accomplish this by adjusting the level of intensity or the number of sets and repetitions performed for each exercise, also known as the *training program*, to suit the desired area of improvement. The intensity of isotonic training commonly is defined as a percentage of an individual's 1RM weight lifted for a particular exercise. Note that a person's 1RM can vary dramatically depending on the exercise, muscles used, and exercise mode (e.g., free weights vs. machine).

As discussed in chapter 3, to improve muscle strength, you should attempt to perform between 2 and 5 sets of approximately 2 to 6 repetitions at an intensity of at least 85 percent of your 1RM for that specific exercise. For individuals trying

TABLE 6.1   Adjusting Training Load to Training Goals

	Frequency (times/wk)	Intensity (% RM)	Volume	Rest
Power	1-2	30-60	3-6 reps 3-6 sets	2-5 min
Strength	3-5	>85	2-6 reps 2-5 sets	2-3 min
Hypertrophy	4-6	67-85	6-12 reps 3-6 sets	30-90 s
Endurance	5-7	<65	15-25 reps 2-3 sets	<30 s

to improve muscle power, the ideal is to perform 3 to 6 sets of 3 to 6 repetitions at 30 to 60 percent of 1RM. A lighter percentage (30-45 percent of 1RM) should be used with power exercises that allow for the release of the mass being lifted (e.g., bench press throws). The proper rest period between each set for both strength and power exercises is between two and five minutes.

Improving muscular endurance requires approximately 2 or 3 sets of 15 to 25 repetitions. Muscular endurance exercises are performed at intensity levels below 65 percent of 1RM, with short rest periods of one to two minutes for sets with higher repetitions and less than one minute for sets with moderate repetitions. Finally, those looking to improve muscle mass (hypertrophy) should do 3 to 6 sets of 6 to 12 repetitions at 67 to 85 percent of 1RM, with rest periods of between 30 and 90 seconds. Table 6.1 provides a summary of these numbers.

Choosing Equipment

Training load is only one of the many variables in isotonic training. Another variable is the type of exercise equipment used during training. Generally, the two types most readily available in public gyms are free weights and machines. In addition, a variety of inexpensive exercise equipment (e.g., resistance bands, kettlebells, and suspension training systems) can be found at many retail stores.

Although both free weights and machines can be used effectively to improve muscle attributes, each has certain advantages over the other. Resistance training machines are much more expensive than free weights. Moreover, because of the fixed nature of their movement, several machines are necessary in order to target every major muscle group in the body. Conversely, free weights (e.g., dumbbells, barbells, and weight benches) are relatively inexpensive, and these weights and associated benches usually are interchangeable and stackable so that a variety of muscles can be worked in many different positions. If you do not have access to a gym or if you are looking for a convenient isotonic workout at home, a free weight or suspension training system is the way to go.

Free weights and machines also physically work the muscles in slightly different ways, making each ideal for different groups of people. For example, because the way machines can move is fixed, they are highly recommended for people who are new to resistance training, recovering from an injury, or lacking in adequate muscle strength. Machines encourage proper form by limiting the range of motion that is needed for the exercise (see figure 6.3). The risk of injury is further reduced by built-in safety mechanisms. Machines can be used to work almost every major muscle group via exercises such as dumbbell biceps curls, abdominal crunches, shoulder presses, leg curls, and leg presses. Additionally, machines can be used to train isolated muscles.

Conversely, free weight systems, as the name implies, involve freestanding exercises in which the lifter can move the weights in any plane of movement. For that reason, free weights are better suited for people with adequate strength and proper training experience. The added benefit of lifting with a free-moving system is that it not only forces the primary muscles to work but also recruits the adjoining muscles that aid in supporting the movement (figure 6.4). For instance, the bench press is used primarily to strengthen the chest, but it can also strengthen the triceps because they aid in the movement of the exercise. This can vastly improve overall strength and joint stability, but the benefits can come at a price: If you use incorrect form and mechanics during a free weight exercise, you may put yourself at increased risk of injury. As you'll see in part III, a wide array of muscles can be trained using free weight exercises.

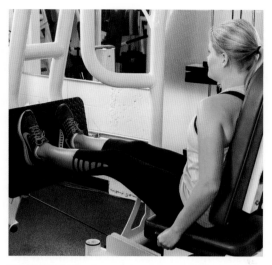

FIGURE 6.3 Exercising on a weight training machine helps ensure safety for the beginning lifter. In this exercise, the risk of injury is reduced because the machine keeps the back stationary.

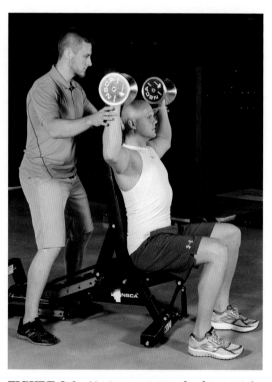

FIGURE 6.4 Having a spotter for free weight exercises helps ensure safety and proper form.

One of the advantages of using a suspension training system is the high variability in work intensity that can be achieved simply from changing foot placement to change the angle of the exercise. This can allow novice lifters to work on strength movements without the use of free weights but with some stability work that machines cannot provide.

When training for muscle strength, hypertrophy, or endurance, free weights, machines, or suspension training can be used effectively. However, training for muscle power should be performed almost exclusively with free weight systems. Power exercises such as squats, hang cleans, and snatches are difficult to perform and should be done only with proper training and supervision. These movements often require large loads and strenuous body movements. Power training is primarily used in competitive athletic environments in order to improve physical performance, although it can be utilized as a total-body workout for those with limited time and excellent technique.

Isotonic training is important if you are trying to improve the strength, power, endurance, and size of your muscles as well as your overall health. In general, isotonic exercises are the type of resistance exercise best suited for most people. After age 25, muscle mass gradually starts to shrink (atrophy) as levels of inactivity increase. Thus, people should participate in isotonic and resistance training not only to maintain muscle strength but also to maintain the strength needed for everyday functional ability and complete independence. Nevertheless, whether you are training for hypertrophy, strength, or other reasons, you must set goals for your training and then choose the types of exercises necessary to reach those goals. The majority of any strength and power training program should consist of isotonic exercises, with other types of training integrated to work on specific deficiencies. You will start noticing and feeling the benefits of isotonic training within weeks of regular training.

Isokinetic Training

The third main category of strength training is isokinetic exercise. This is the type of strength training least known to the general public, and it is rarely seen in a community fitness setting. In isokinetic training, the speed of movement is held constant throughout the entire exercise (as opposed to the constant length and constant load experienced with isometric and isotonic exercise, respectively).

Specialized machines known as isokinetic dynamometers (see chapter 5) are required to perform these types of movements. Dynamometers are bulky, expensive pieces of equipment, and unique training and knowledge are required in order to operate them. As a result, isokinetic dynamometers typically are found only in health care or rehabilitation settings. However, if you are fortunate enough to work out on an isokinetic dynamometer, you can take advantage of quite a few strength training benefits not offered by isotonic or isometric training alone.

Isokinetic training combines some of the best features of the other types of strength training: The high-tension contractions of isometrics are combined with the range of motion of isotonics. To accomplish this, the dynamometer electronically controls the speed at which it moves regardless of how much or how little someone pushes. This is known as *accommodating resistance,* and the muscle experiences overload as a result. Using the computer or control panel of the machine, you set the desired exercise speed, which typically ranges from 30 to 500 degrees per second. The slower speeds are more intense than the faster speeds. Range of motion can also be limited to a preset range, which can be useful in limiting the movement of a person who is injured. Also, dynamometers come with interchangeable attachments so they can be used to isolate and exercise almost every muscle group in the body. Isokinetic dynamometers are able to provide maximum resistance throughout the entire range of motion of a limb and the speeds at which the muscle contracts.

Strength training on an isokinetic machine is perhaps the most efficient method of exercise for gaining strength. You can gain maximum strength throughout the entire movement range along with some of the added benefits of isotonic and isometric exercise. In addition, a lot of research has been done on how isokinetic training can improve the speed with which a person can move a limb through a range of motion, which has applications for improving running or throwing speed. Also, isokinetic dynamometers are very safe because they have built-in safety features such as safety stops. The ability of isokinetic dynamometers to completely control the various parameters, such as range of motion and speed, makes this form of exercise desirable in a physical therapy and rehabilitation setting.

Unfortunately, isokinetic exercise has various disadvantages as well. First, because isokinetic dynamometers are so expensive, they rarely are found in a public fitness facility. Additionally, most isokinetic machines isolate movements during exercise, thereby eliminating most of the supplementary strength gains found with free weights. Moreover, a good deal of background knowledge is required to properly use the complex computer program and the various attachments of the dynamometer.

Isokinetic exercise can be a good way to gain strength, but its many limitations may make it less desirable to the average person than some other methods. Isometric and isotonic exercises are much more convenient to perform. People can achieve maximal strength gains using isokinetic machines, but doing so requires a lot of time, money, and effort. Unless you have an isokinetic machine readily available, we recommend that you stick with forms of strength training that are more convenient and cost effective.

Plyometric Training

Have you ever wanted to dunk like LeBron James? Or throw a punch like Mike Tyson? Or even run as fast as Usain Bolt? If you answered yes to any of these questions, then you'll want to make plyometric exercise an important component of your overall training and conditioning program. Most elite athletes use some form of plyometric exercise to improve the agility, speed, and power necessary for explosive movements.

Plyometrics is a training protocol used to get your muscles to create the greatest amount of force in as little time as possible. Plyometric exercise is based on the stretch–shortening cycle of the muscles (also discussed in chapter 3). You can generate more force by prestretching a muscle immediately before a concentric muscle contraction than you can when performing a concentric muscle contraction alone. To better understand the physiology of the stretch–shortening cycle, think of your muscle as a rubber band. When you stretch a rubber band, you create an elastic force in the band. Because of the rubber band's elasticity, the strain created by the stretch causes the rubber band to return to its original shape. Similarly, your muscles have an elastic component and will attempt to return to their original state in response to any sort of stretch (see figure 6.5). This is how the stretch–shortening cycle works in the body.

Plyometrics combines the physiological characteristics of the stretch–shortening cycle in the muscles with strength and power to create a truly explosive movement. To better describe how plyometric activity works, consider the example of a two-leg standing long jump, focusing primarily on the quadriceps muscle group on the top of the thighs. (Other muscles are used in this movement, but for the purpose of simplification we do not discuss them.) Before the initial takeoff, the long jumper dips down a bit, forcing the quadriceps to eccentrically contract and stretch. Soon after, the quadriceps concentrically contract, causing the leg to straighten out and spring off the ground. (See chapter 1 for a review of eccentric and concentric contractions.) Plyometrics focus on training the period of time between the eccentric and concentric phases.

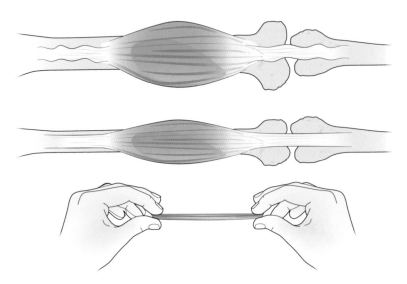

FIGURE 6.5 Similar to a stretched rubber band, a muscle stretched quickly will attempt to return to its natural state. This phenomenon, known as the stretch–shortening cycle, provides the basis for plyometric training.

The transition period between the eccentric and concentric phases is known as the *amortization phase.* Quickly transitioning through the amortization phase enables the body to generate a powerful concentric contraction using the stretch–shortening cycle. However, the body can produce this additional power only when the amortization period is short—typically in the hundredths of a second. This short time frame allows the elastic component and the stretch reflex to add power to the strength of the muscle. By minimizing the amortization phase and improving the stretch–shortening cycle, you can learn to run faster, jump higher, and perform better than you have before.

Plyometrics usually are performed in an athletic strength and conditioning setting but are more frequently being used in a public fitness setting. Fortunately, a variety of plyometric exercises can be performed with various pieces of equipment that are easy to find, such as sturdy wooden boxes or crates and weighted balls. One of the most popular plyometric exercises is the depth jump. For this exercise, you begin by standing on a small box. You then step off the box, and upon landing on the ground you push up and jump as high as you can with both feet (figure 6.6, *a* through *c*). Depth jumps frequently are used to train basketball or volleyball players to jump higher.

A variety of plyometric exercises can also be performed with the upper body. These commonly involve medicine balls. (We discuss medicine balls in the next

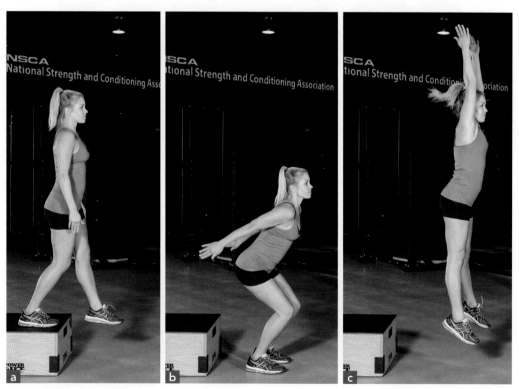

FIGURE 6.6   The depth jump is an ideal plyometric exercise for athletes who wish to improve their vertical jumping power.

section.) The chest pass is one example of a medicine ball plyometric exercise; it can be performed either with two people passing the ball back and forth (figure 6.7, *a* and *b*) or with one person throwing the ball against a wall. To perform the exercise, you use a chest pass to throw the ball to another person or the wall, and when the ball is returned to you, you immediately throw another chest pass back. This plyometric drill focuses on training the upper body to produce powerful throwing or pushing movements, such as those used when passing a basketball or when blocking in football.

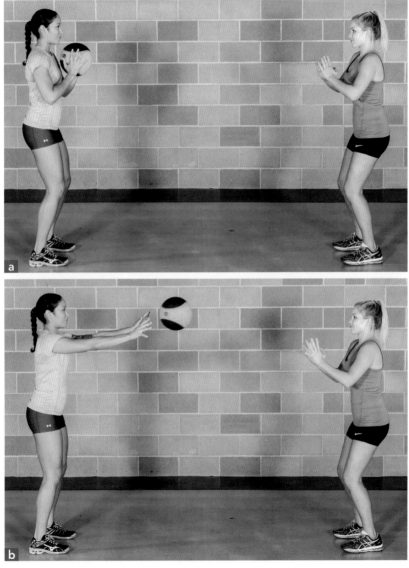

FIGURE 6.7 A properly performed chest pass requires that the athlete pass the medicine ball back to her partner immediately upon catching it.

Like any other type of resistance training, plyometric training has many benefits, including increases in muscle and bone strength. Additionally, because the movements performed during plyometric drills mimic those used during athletic activities, such drills produce improvements in power and performance that transfer to those activities (i.e., functional power). This is one of the main reasons why plyometrics are done primarily in athletic strength and conditioning settings. With proper plyometric training, athletes can learn to use the maximum power their body generates on the court, track, or playing field.

Plyometrics have drawbacks and limitations. First, public fitness settings may not have the appropriate space and equipment for plyometric training (although, as previously mentioned, you can create your own equipment from items such as sturdy wooden boxes). Also, because of the highly intensive nature of plyometrics, they should not be performed without a proper foundation of strength. Build up a routine training program and develop a minimum base of strength before adding plyometrics. Then, learn the proper techniques for performing these exercises from a trained professional. In addition, these activities should be performed no more than two or three times per week so that your muscles have time to rest and recover from the activity.

As you can see, plyometrics can be very beneficial to people trying to maximize the power their muscles can generate. These exercises can help you improve your athletic performance while giving you an active, high-intensity workout. Realistically, plyometrics need to be performed only if you are taking part in competitive sport and you want to exploit every last bit of power your muscles can generate.

Medicine Ball Training

Medicine balls are not spherical containers of prescription drugs, as the name may imply. Rather, they are weighted balls that typically come in a variety of weights, ranging from .5 to 30 pounds (.2-13.6 kg); colors; and sizes, ranging in diameter from 3.5 to 10.6 inches (8.9-26.9 cm). Although medicine balls come in many forms (figure 6.8a), the two most distinct forms resemble a dodgeball from your childhood years and an extremely old leather basketball. Most public fitness gyms carry medicine balls and make them readily available to members.

Medicine balls can be used in a variety of ways for strength and power training. Because medicine balls are available in specified weights, they can be used in ordinary isotonic or isometric training, similar to the way dumbbells, barbells, or weight plates are used. In fact, some medicine balls come with handles that allow you to easily mimic many of the exercises you could perform with dumbbells (figure 6.8b). Although medicine balls can be useful as a tool for gaining strength, they are most often used to train for power.

The texture and composition of most medicine balls allow them to be easily handled and used for a variety of exercises. For example, they can be thrown up in the air or against the wall and caught with relative ease, as shown in the chest pass example. Many basketball players and boxers use this type of exercise

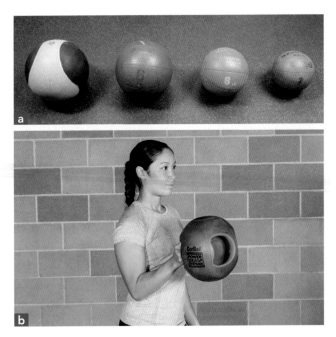

FIGURE 6.8 *(a)* Medicine balls vary in style, weight, and size. *(b)* Some medicine balls have handles that allow them to be used as dumbbells.

to develop the ability to quickly pass the ball or throw a punch. Additionally, medicine balls can be used to build core strength and stability. The core muscles (abs, lower back, and muscles of the trunk) are often neglected, but they play an essential role in any power training program. Although strengthening the muscles surrounding the abs will not directly lead to gains in power, core training with a medicine ball will help you better transfer the power of the movement from your body to whatever action you are performing. For example, stronger abs can help a baseball pitcher transfer power from the legs to the abs and, ultimately, to the arms to throw the ball. This kind of strength allows pitchers such as Aroldis Chapman to throw a baseball at 100 miles per hour.

Be aware that using medicine balls in your training program has some disadvantages. First, many gyms do not have enough space to allow people to safely throw medicine balls against the wall or in the air, which limits the number and type of exercises that can be performed. This is one reason why power training with medicine balls is seen more often in collegiate or professional athletic settings and rarely seen in public settings.

Second, medicine balls raise safety concerns similar to those of isotonics or isometrics, although the material medicine balls are made of decreases the amount of damage that people or surroundings may suffer if the ball is accidentally mishandled. To minimize the risk of injury, people using medicine balls to train for power must ensure that they have adequate strength to be taking part in power exercises and that they use correct form and technique when performing the exercises.

Training with medicine balls can greatly improve and diversify any strength and power training program. Medicine balls are relatively inexpensive and can be a convenient type of training to perform at home. Medicine balls should always be used in conjunction with other types of exercise to achieve your ultimate training goals. Again, safety must always be your primary concern when performing this type of exercise. If you have appropriate facilities in which to use medicine balls in your workout, this type of training can add variety and enjoyment to your normal exercise regimen.

Kettlebell Training

The use of kettlebells as a training implement has grown in popularity over the years, although kettlebells have been around since the 1700s. Although they were first used as a measurement device for grains, farmers started to use kettlebells as a way to show off their strength. Most modern kettlebells simply look like cannon-

balls with handles and range from 5 to 200 pounds (2.3-90.7 kg). Kettlebell training has advantages when it comes to swinging movements and stability work because the weight is below the handle instead of on the outside, like on a dumbbell.

Due to the recent popularity of the kettlebell, the variety and availability is quite large. They can be as simple as a solid piece of iron or steel that is rubberized so they can be dropped without much worry about damaging floors. Kettlebells have become very popular with home gyms and smaller gyms and athletic facilities because they are portable and because relatively little space is required for storage.

Kettlebells can be used for various training goals but often are used to accomplish multiple goals simultaneously. However, research on kettlebell training is relatively new, and data on strength (Manocchia et al. 2013), power (Lake and Lauder 2012), and endurance (Thomas et al. 2014) are limited.

One of most popular uses is the kettlebell swing. The kettlebell's lower center of mass increases the distance of the weight from

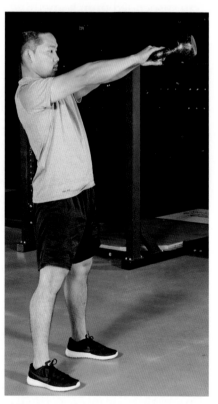

FIGURE 6.9 The kettlebell swing takes full advantage of the kettlebell shape, increasing posterior chain activation.

the body, thus increasing the work done by the posterior chain more than if the work was performed with a dumbbell (see figure 6.9). Use of kettlebells is also popular in core and stability work. Holding a kettlebell in one arm while performing a lunge forces the lifter to keep their core tighter in order to keep the spine vertical. In addition, holding the kettlebell above the head can make the movement more difficult while adding stabilizing demands on the shoulder joint. The use of proper technique is critical when working with kettlebells to help develop stabilization, and novice lifters should use lighter weights. The beauty of using a kettlebell overhead is the ability to hold the weight with the bell up or down. Keeping the weight vertical increases the stabilizing requirement and demands more grip strength.

Suspension Training

Suspension training systems (STSs) have gained a lot of popularity in recent years due to their versatility, simplicity, and ease of use. Although multiple types and brands are available on the market, STSs simply require some sort of rope or strap suspended from something solid enough to hold a person's body weight. In addition, the mobility and easy setup of these systems have made them a popular personal training tool.

The bread and butter of the STS is its ability to use a person's body weight in multiple angles and positions to make an exercise either easier or more difficult. An example is using an STS for push-ups. If a person were to stand fairly vertical, there would be very little resistance; however, if a person were to move their feet farther back and lower the angle of their body, the intensity of the movement would increase (see figure 6.10a). This makes STSs a great tool for training people who may not possess the strength to do a regular push-up. Additionally, increasing the intensity also requires a higher demand from the shoulders for stabilization compared with doing push-ups on the floor. Further challenge can be adding by placing the feet instead of the hands in the handles (see figure 6.10b).

The added stabilizing requirement of the STS makes it well suited for abdominal exercises. Increasing or decreasing the body angle can change the intensity of the abdominal exercise. Furthermore, whereas a traditional plank is performed with both the feet and the arms on the ground, with an STS you can suspend either the upper body (essentially a push-up position) or the lower body (see figure 6.11). Research has shown that activation of the rectus abdominis is greater when performing a plank with an STS compared with performing a traditional plank (Atkins et al. 2015).

Although STSs are great for novice lifters or those without access to free weights, their ability to stimulate strength gains may be limited. If someone uses only an STS and can already do more than 30 bodyweight pushups, the lack of ability to add resistance beyond body weight will cause strength gains to stagnate. However, an intermediate to advanced lifter who uses only free weights

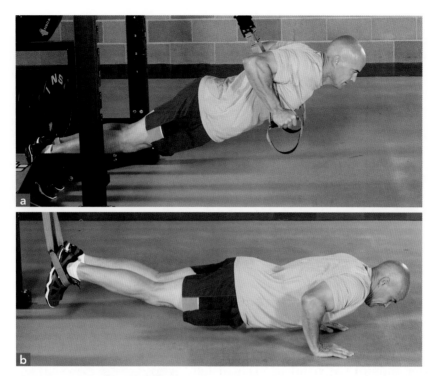

FIGURE 6.10 *(a)* Placing the hands in the STS gives the user the freedom to make the push-up more or less difficult by moving their feet forward or backward. *(b)* Placing the feet in the STS increases the stabilization requirement from both the shoulders and the abdominals.

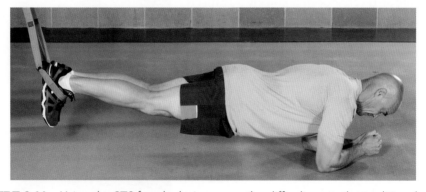

FIGURE 6.11 Using the STS for planks increases the difficulty over the traditional plank.

and machines may benefit from the stabilizing requirements of an STS or the simple variety it can add to a workout.

As with most workout equipment, safety and proper technique are very import-ant to consider when using any STS. Because an STS suspends a person's body weight, whether fully or partially, the placement and anchoring of the device are important. Make sure it is suspended from a sturdy surface that is strong enough to support more than the lifter's weight and is secured in a spot that provides little to no room for the STS to slide. If using a freestanding structure, such as a squat rack, make sure it does not tip over. Avoid securing the STS to structures that are top heavy.

Resistance Band Training

The use of resistance bands and cords as a form of exercise is becoming increasingly popular. These are not regular rubber bands from your local office supply store. Rather, exercise bands and cords come in a variety of bright colors and in either flat sheets (resistance bands) that are approximately four inches (10.2 cm) wide by 6 feet (1.8 m) long or longer cables (resistance cords). Each color corresponds to a particular degree of tension. As with normal rubber bands or bungee cords, the tension in resistance bands and cords increases as they are stretched; this provides the resistance necessary for strength training. You can combine different levels of resistance to create a customized workout.

Resistance bands and cords are an effective complement or alternative to any strength and power training workout. For example, a boxer can wrap a resistance band around her back or a stable machine, grip the ends of the band in each of her hands, and throw a variety of punches (figure 6.12). This is a great way to build punching power and strength in a manner that isn't possible with other equipment. Resistance bands are also very popular among advanced lifters for targeting the lock-out of lifts such as the squat or bench press. Attaching resistance bands to the ends of the bar and anchoring them to the floor or the bottom of the rack adds resistance at the top of the lift, which allows the lifter to have overload on certain lifts and have a stronger lock-out.

Resistance bands and cords also have the characteristic recoil or "pulling back" effect found in normal rubber bands. This produces the added benefit of exercising agonist muscles while stretching out antagonist muscles (see chapter 1 for a discussion of agonist and antagonist muscles). For example, when performing a biceps curl, the agonist muscles are your biceps and any other muscle aiding in the movement, whereas the triceps are the antagonist (or opposing) muscle. This tendency for the band or cord to

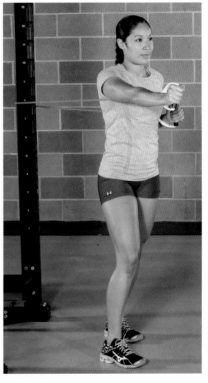

FIGURE 6.12 Performing punches with an elastic band increases the tension throughout the movement.

return to its original shape leads to improvements in overall strength and joint stability.

It is not uncommon to see resistance bands and cords being used in a rehabilitation setting. The light resistance they provide makes them perfect for beginning exercisers as well as people who have limited muscle strength or who are recovering from an injury. Sitting or standing on a smaller elastic band and performing a shoulder press can allow the user a light resistance to help build up strength and assist in shoulder recovery.

Most resistance bands and cords are relatively inexpensive. Like medicine balls, resistance bands and cords offer a convenient and inexpensive form of exercise. Connect one end to a stable stationary object and you are ready to perform a variety of exercises. Also, the compact size of the bands and cords makes them easy to travel with, so you can do a strength training workout almost anywhere. Because these cords and bands stretch, they make it possible to strengthen the corresponding muscle throughout the entire range of motion.

Regrettably, resistance bands and cords do not come without limitations. It can be difficult to find resistance bands or cords in some public gyms. Moreover, very few sporting goods stores carry these items for retail purposes. However, a simple Internet search for a fitness, training, or rehabilitation equipment store can help you get your hands on a set of resistance bands or cords. Another drawback of the bands and cords is that because the resistance gets greater the farther you stretch them, you get only minimal resistance at the beginning of the movement, resulting in minimal gains in strength and power at these early angles. As a result, users may experience uneven gains in muscle strength and power. Fortunately, though, resistance bands and cords are very safe, and using them requires no specific training. Resistance bands and cords can be great additions to your overall exercise plan. Nonetheless, they should not be used as your sole means of gaining strength and power; rather, they should be used to supplement your existing training.

Summary

Some sort of progressive resistance training is necessary to maintain muscle strength and health. However, such training also benefits the strength of bones, tendons, and ligaments and has been shown to increase overall feelings of energy. Having the proper strength and power to perform functional everyday activities is essential to a person's well-being and independence and is very useful when competing in athletic events, either recreationally or professionally. Fortunately, a wide selection of resistance training forms is available to fit almost anyone's needs.

All it takes to begin any strength and power training program is the understanding of what your goals are and what types of exercises you can do to achieve those goals. For instance, if you are rehabilitating a previously injured area, you may choose to perform isometrics. You may look to isokinetics if you want to improve limb movement speed or to plyometrics if you want to increase power and explosiveness. If you simply want to improve general strength and muscle health, you can use isotonics. Whatever your goals or intentions, some type of resistance training exists that will be useful and conveniently fit into your lifestyle.

7

Workout Schedule and Rest

Dustin D. Dunnick, Kylie K. Harmon, and Lee E. Brown

Now that you have learned how to assess your baseline strength (chapter 5) as well as what types of strength and power training are best for achieving different goals (chapter 6), you need to understand the components that go into creating a successful resistance training program. This chapter will familiarize you with the different variables involved in creating a workout schedule. It also introduces some of the language that strength training professionals use in developing and modifying programs. In part IV of this book, you will learn how to take the information presented here and manipulate it to develop a goal-specific strength training program.

The benefits you can get from resistance training are highly dependent on the time and effort you devote to your program. However, busy schedules and hectic workdays should not discourage you from training. Remember that even minimal bouts of exercise may offer a benefit. As you grow accustomed to resistance training, however, you will need to devote more energy to each workout in order to continue to achieve strength gains. Adding a program with proper sets, reps, and rest periods as well as focusing on form and technique will help in achieving your individual goals.

This chapter covers the specific variables you must consider when constructing an effective resistance training program. Through the manipulation of these variables, you can alter the outcome of your training—that is, you can further develop your strength, power, or endurance. Although some of this material may appear to overlap that in previous chapters, the information presented here will help you create a goal-centered resistance training program.

The authors acknowledge the significant contributions of Brian W. Findley, Daniel P. Murray, and Sagir G. Bera to this chapter.

Adjusting Training Variables to Goals

The best way to begin planning your workout schedule is to determine why you want to start a resistance training program. This is where performing a needs analysis is important (see chapter 5). As you learned in chapter 5, strength training has many benefits. Adaptations to resistance training are not limited to increased muscle size and strength. You can also train to improve muscular endurance, power, and athletic performance. The personal goals you establish will greatly affect how you design your program. These goals will influence the workout variables you use in your program design.

You'll recall from chapter 3 that several acute training variables can be adjusted to help you meet your goals. The main seven are as follows:

- **Choice.** Choice is simply the exercise an individual choses for a program or single workout.
- **Order.** The order of exercises chosen for a program or workout (e.g., doing the most taxing exercises first and prioritizing multijoint movements over single-joint movements) can be more important than the exercises themselves.
- **Frequency.** Frequency is the number of training sessions per week for a muscle group.
- **Intensity.** In strength training, intensity refers to the load being lifted compared with the maximum load or 1RM. The closer a load is to maximum, the higher the exercise intensity.
- **Volume.** Volume is determined by sets × repetitions. Volume can be used to describe a single exercise or a complete workout session.
- **Rest interval.** A rest interval is the amount of time spent recovering between each set.
- **Progression.** Progression is an increase in work being completed over time. This usually is represented by an increase in volume or intensity during a training program.

Like training variables, your program design also includes goals. The four main goals are listed in the following sections.

Hypertrophy

One of the most common reasons why people start resistance training is to achieve an increased muscle size, also referred to as *hypertrophy*. If you are new to training, it may take as long as four to eight weeks before you notice differences in muscle size (Moritani and deVries 1979). Keep this in mind so you don't get frustrated with the lack of results in the initial stages of training.

Even in individuals who have previously participated in resistance training, hypertrophy is not maximized unless the program is designed correctly. In general, hypertrophy training is most effective when you use moderate to heavy loads (67-85 percent of 1RM) and large training volumes (3-6 sets of 6-12 repetitions; Kraemer and Ratamess 2005). Hypertrophy protocols require rest periods of between 30 and 90 seconds. This allows sufficient time for some recovery between sets, but it also ensures that the muscle is completely fatigued by the completion of the last set.

Strength

Another common goal of resistance training is to increase maximal strength. As discussed in chapter 3, the greater the overload during resistance training, the greater the adaptations that occur. In keeping with this principle, resistance training carried out with the goal of improving maximal strength is most successful when you use heavy loads or high intensities—loads lifted near the 1RM (>85 percent 1RM) and performed with few repetitions (2-6). A moderate to high number of sets (2-5) with two to five minutes of rest between sets is recommended for maximal strength gains.

The exact load that best produces improvements in maximal strength has been widely debated. It generally is agreed that loads between 85 and 95 percent of 1RM create the muscular overload needed for improvements in maximal strength. A recent analysis of existing research suggests that 85 percent of 1RM may be the best load for producing maximal gains in muscular strength (Peterson et al. 2004).

Maximal strength protocols require the longest rest intervals. When intensity is at its highest, as it is when training for maximal strength, you should take at least three minutes of rest between sets. Many professionals have recommended taking up to five minutes of rest between high-intensity sets, but recent research has revealed that performance is similar on subsequent sets whether rest periods are three or five minutes (Kraemer and Ratamess 2005).

Beginner and novice lifters will experience changes in maximal strength with a wide range of training loads. Therefore, it usually is better for beginners to start out with lower-intensity and higher-volume programs. They can then advance to higher-intensity programs when their progression in strength improvements reaches a plateau.

Power

In physics terms, *power* is the amount of force applied to move an object divided by the time it takes to move that object. In other words, the quicker an object is moved, or the greater the force applied to move the object, the greater the power. The same holds true for muscular power. Because power is a combination of both strength and speed, it often is an important variable for those seeking improvements in athletic performance.

The goal is to move the given load as quickly as possible; this improves explosive strength and the speed with which a given load can be moved. Power training traditionally has been performed with heavy loads, similar to those prescribed for maximal strength training. Heavy loads were believed to be necessary for producing significant muscular overload. Because the goal of training is to lift the heavy load *explosively*, it was thought that doing so in training would create maximal improvements in power.

More recently, it has become apparent that moving lighter loads (30-60 percent of 1RM) with low volumes (few sets and few repetitions) as quickly as possible can be more effective in producing greater power gains (McBride et al. 2002). This load is light enough to move quickly but heavy enough to require some force for it to be moved. Thus, the combination of force production and speed of movement yields peak power.

Although lighter loads allow the lifter to achieve greater movement speeds during training—and thus train the speed component of power—heavier loads train the strength component of power. Either strategy can be effective in improving muscular power, but it appears that training with lighter loads (which allow greater movement speeds) may accomplish this goal more effectively.

The problem with power training with lighter loads, however, is that no consensus exists on the amount of sets and repetitions that should be performed. The research done in this area has been concerned strictly with the comparison of heavy and light loads and not with training volume. Studies of power training with light loads have used volumes ranging from 3 to 6 sets of 3 to 6 repetitions; however, 3 repetitions appears to be the optimal number to avoid fatigue. You should allow for two to five minutes of rest between sets of power exercises; this is similar to the rest periods used for maximal strength training.

Muscular Endurance

Another goal of resistance training can be to improve local muscular endurance. Training for endurance is quite different than training for maximal strength because muscular endurance training aims to improve the ability to perform more submaximal contractions for longer periods of time. As a result, this type of training calls for light loads (generally <65 percent of 1RM) and high volume (2-3 sets of 15-25 repetitions).

Muscular endurance protocols require very little rest time between sets—usually 30 seconds or less. In fact, the purpose of muscular endurance training is to produce a greater duration of muscular work and resistance to fatigue. The short duration of rest time promotes longer durations of muscle activity and helps stave off neuromuscular fatigue.

Muscular endurance training protocols can be very effective for beginners and special populations as well as for athletes training for endurance sports such as mountain climbing and orienteering. People who are unaccustomed to resistance training may be opposed to the amount of work required to lift higher percentages of their 1RM, thus making muscular endurance training a more desirable option. Because new resistance trainers will see benefits with nearly any combination of training volume, a muscular endurance protocol often is a good way to introduce them to the activity.

For intermediate and advanced resistance training, muscular endurance protocols bring variety and balance to a program. Although a desire to increase muscular endurance usually isn't the main reason people start resistance training, the benefits of doing so are widespread and can make it easier to perform activities of daily living, such as gardening or carrying objects. As you will see in later chapters, providing balance and variety in a workout program is essential to maximizing progress.

Athletic Performance

For decades, athletes of all sports have used resistance training as an essential preparatory tool. It is well established that improvements in strength and power enhance athletic performance. To be effective in creating these enhancements, workout programs need to be designed with the specific characteristics of the sport in mind. For example, the exercises and training goals included in the program must fit with the muscle groups and movement patterns used in the sport. A close examination of the sport's requirements reveals not only what muscle groups to train but also whether strength, power, or muscular endurance should be the main focus. For example, basketball requires explosive leg power for jumping as well as muscular strength for the physical contact that can occur under the basket. Therefore, explosive power exercises for the lower body and exercises for overall muscular strength would be important to include for most basketball players.

Exercise Choice and Order

Exercises can be grouped into three categories—power, core, and assistance—based on how they relate to your goals.

- **Power exercises** are explosive movements in which the lifter attempts to move the weight as quickly as possible. Some classic power exercises include the power clean and the push jerk. Power exercises use many muscle groups and require the movement of several joints (as do core exercises; see chapter 11). When performing power exercises, the lifter should be at their freshest in order to minimize fatigue and reduce the risk of injury; therefore, power exercises should be performed first in the workout program. Power exercises are important to include in a well-balanced resistance training program, especially for those seeking to improve athletic performance. Use caution with these exercises, though, because proper form is vital. Instruction and supervision from a qualified exercise professional are always recommended when performing power lifts.

- **Core exercises** use large muscle groups located close to the center of the body. They generally incorporate several muscle groups across multiple joints. These exercises primarily work the muscles of the chest, shoulders, back, and hips and might include the front squat, lunge, and bench press. Because core exercises work multiple muscle groups, you should perform them before assistance exercises.

- **Assistance exercises** work smaller muscle groups in the arms and legs and usually are limited to the movement of one joint. They are used to work specific muscle groups in isolation, and they might include the dumbbell biceps curl, triceps extension, and calf raise. Assistance exercises generally are performed after core exercises so that the individual muscle groups don't get fatigued before they are called upon to execute multijoint movements.

Organizing Workouts

Several factors must be considered as you schedule and organize your training workouts. First, determine how much time you have available for each session—for example, can you spend 30 minutes per session, or do you have a full 2 hours to spend at one time? You also need to determine how many times you can work out each week (i.e., frequency). We discuss more issues related to exercise frequency and how to be efficient in your workouts in the next section.

Next, you must determine what exercise equipment you have at your disposal. Do you have a facility with free weights and machines? Do you have access to things such as plyometric boxes and medicine balls? Answers to these questions will factor into what exercises you choose to include in your workout. We discuss more about choosing exercises and the order in which to do them later in this chapter.

Finally, you need to consider your training background. Are you prepared physically and do you have enough strength training experience to begin an advanced, complex, or difficult workout? Or do you need to start by following a program for beginners? Part IV provides some sample beginner, intermediate, and advanced strength training programs as well as guidelines on how to determine which program is right for you.

Workout Frequency

The first thing to decide when developing a workout schedule is the frequency with which you will train. Workout frequency generally is considered to be the number of workouts completed each week. Typically, an effective workout frequency is two to five times a week.

Frequency is directly related to how much time you have available and are willing to devote to resistance training. You will experience greater results when you are able to hit the gym more often in a given week, but this greater frequency also needs to be balanced with proper rest periods to maximize the gains. Although a greater frequency will result in greater overall gains, you can still achieve positive results with as few as two days per week and should not be discouraged if you cannot train more frequently. Any time spent resistance training is beneficial and helps contribute to a healthy lifestyle.

The total amount of time you spend in the gym is determined by your busy schedule, but you should realize that greater benefits will result from more consistent and regular training. Also, remember that the load you lift and the frequency of the workout should be inversely related. In other words, if you lift relatively heavy or near-maximal loads, then you will need more rest between workouts; therefore, your workouts will be less frequent than those of someone who is lifting relatively lighter loads. (We discuss more about rest periods between workouts later in this chapter.)

To continue making strength gains, you should increase your workout frequency as you become more experienced in the gym as well as incorporate new or different variations of exercises into your training. Again, beginners are able to advance and see strength gains when they undertake any sort of resistance training. Having a lower workout frequency when you are starting out allows your muscles to experience the appropriate rest and recovery between sessions. As you establish consistency in your workouts, gains become more difficult to achieve. Adding more days to your program is one way to achieve greater results.

Several methods can be used to optimize your strength training so that you are working efficiently and achieving the greatest gains possible while allowing enough rest between sessions. These methods include using a split routine (i.e., alternating workouts according to body part or region, muscle group, or type of movement); alternating heavy and light days; and using circuit training, pyramid training, or super or compound sets.

Split Routine

A good way to add days to your workout frequency is to use a split routine in which you complete different exercises on different days of the week. This common approach allows you to work some body parts and rest others on a given day. It also permits you to train on consecutive days; because different muscle groups are trained on different days, you don't have to worry about training fatigued muscles from the day before.

Trying to fit everything you want to accomplish into one workout can be overwhelming. You may want to have a comprehensive program that encompasses all major muscle groups of the body; however, you might not have a block of time large enough to accomplish all that in one workout. Splitting your routine maximizes your time and effort by allowing you to exercise a broad range of muscle groups without spending hours in the gym for each workout.

Split routines also help give your workouts variety. Performing the same set of exercises every time you work out can get boring and stale. Changing things up from day to day and focusing on two or three body parts per session, rather than the entire body, provides more diversity in your program and helps limit tedium.

You can split your routine in a variety of ways. One method is to design body part or muscle group workouts, such as working the upper body and lower body on different days. Another method is to group muscles that produce similar body movements together, such as putting all pushing movements or pulling movements in one workout.

Body Part or Muscle Group Workouts   Probably the most common way that people split their workouts is by body part or muscle group. This type of split allows you to either create a well-balanced generalized program or focus your workout on a single body part that needs attention.

One way to organize your training is by alternating upper-body and lower-body workouts. This provides balance between training the upper- and lower-body muscles and ensures that appropriate recovery takes place between workouts. This method is a good way to introduce beginners to resistance training.

Because each training session is intended to be general in nature (either upper body or lower body), you are able to pick from a wide variety of available exercises. This variety is another reason why beginners favor this kind of workout. Performing the same routine over and over can turn resistance training into a monotonous activity.

For participants who have more experience in resistance training, body part routines can be used to target focus areas. As you become more familiar with working out, you may become aware of certain muscle groups that you would like to focus on more heavily or that you simply enjoy training. Specific body part routines can also center your workouts on muscle groups that are not progressing as well as others. For instance, suppose your bench press workouts have hit a standstill because you are unable to finish the movement on the last few repetitions without help from your spotter. Because the triceps are heavily involved in elbow extension at the end of the bench press motion, you decide to focus your next few upper-body workouts on your triceps. In a few weeks, you see your bench press load increase again because you now have the strength to finish off the movement.

Push–Pull Workouts   You can also split your workout by separating lifts into pushes and pulls and doing each on separate days. Pushes consist of movements in which a load starts close to the body and is moved away. Conversely, pulls involve movements in which the load starts farther away and ends up closer to the body.

Pushes and pulls often use opposing muscle groups to perform the given action. Pushes tend to be dominated by muscles of the chest, shoulders, and posterior arm (triceps), as in the barbell bench press and overhead lifting movements such as the military press or push press. Pulls tend to be dominated by muscles of the back and anterior arm (biceps), as in the lat pull-down and in rowing movements. Muscle groups of the lower extremities are difficult to place in either the push category or the pull category because most tend to be involved in both movements.

The push–pull concept can also be used in a single workout. Beginners may sometimes want to alternate push and pull exercises in a workout when they are working the upper body. This technique allows for appropriate rest of muscle groups between exercises and ensures that training is balanced among major muscle groups.

Alternating Heavy and Light Days

Varying the volume and the main goal (e.g., hypertrophy, strength, or power) of your training is a great way to maximize gains and avoid plateaus. A scheduled cycle of changes in training variables is known as *periodization* of training and is discussed in chapter 3; applications of this kind of training are shown in part IV. Switching the volume of your workout for a few training sessions can enable you to make breakthroughs during times when progress might otherwise have slowed.

Let's illustrate this point with an example. Say you have been training for eight weeks using a hypertrophy program for your upper body. For the past two of those eight weeks, you have been unable to increase the load while trying to maintain the appropriate number of repetitions (8-10). This could be because your maximum strength has not improved to the same extent that your 8 to 10RM has. In this instance, performing the next few workouts with a maximum strength protocol (i.e., increasing load and decreasing reps) may help get you through your plateau.

On the other hand, if your trouble with progression relates to an inability to recover between sets, you may be lacking in muscular endurance. In this case, you may want to perform the next few workouts with lighter loads and increased repetitions. This could improve your muscular endurance enough to recover better between sets when you return to your hypertrophy protocol.

Circuit Training

Circuit training is a unique resistance training method in which single sets of several different exercises (usually 10-12) are completed in succession, with little or no rest between exercises. Typically, one to three circuits of these exercises are performed during a training session. Loads are kept light (generally 40-60 percent of 1RM), and exercises either are performed with a high number of repetitions (12-15) or, more often, are performed for a set time (e.g., 30 seconds) with very short or no rest time between exercises. The purported benefit of this form of training is that it produces improvements in strength and muscular endurance in one workout.

The routine usually works the full body (e.g., leg press, barbell bench press, bent-knee sit-up, leg extension, standing military press, seated leg curl, dumbbell biceps curl, calf raise, lat pull-down, back extension, and cable seated row; see chapters 9-11); all the major muscle groups around each joint are trained every workout. To provide rest for the body, most circuits are sequenced to alternate exercises from lower body to upper body (e.g., leg exercise and then arm exercise). Heart rates during circuit training typically are higher than during most other weight training programs because of the short rest periods.

Because circuit training places higher cardiovascular demands on the body, people often use this type of training to try to improve cardiovascular fitness. Like strength, cardiovascular fitness can improve quickly and with little training in those who are very unfit. Although circuit training likely can improve cardiovascular conditioning in people with lower base levels of fitness, the aerobic effects are much less pronounced in those who are more fit. Even if this type of training does affect cardiovascular fitness to some degree, larger gains will be achieved with actual aerobic endurance training.

Similarly, improvements in basic strength after circuit training are more potent in previously untrained people. The protocols for developing maximal strength and hypertrophy by using heavier loads are much more likely to improve strength and to a greater degree. Circuit training may be a good introductory form of training because it is fast moving and usually shorter in duration than a more traditional resistance training session; however, the low loads limit strength gains.

In fact, one of the most compelling reasons to engage in circuit training is that a workout can be accomplished in a short period of time. Performing three circuits of 10 exercises for 30 seconds each with only seconds between exercises could take as little as half an hour. Circuit training is a great option for those who otherwise would not resistance train because they don't have time.

Undoubtedly, the greatest effect of circuit training is improved local muscular endurance. The combination of light loads, high repetitions, and short rest intervals is perfect for those seeking such gains.

Pyramid Training

Pyramid training refers to a change in the intensity of an exercise from set to set. Pyramids can be ascending, descending, or triangular. Ascending pyramids begin with lighter loads, and each subsequent set is performed with a heavier load. Descending pyramids begin with a heavy load, and each subsequent set is performed using a lighter load. Triangular pyramids ascend and descend, and the heaviest load is lifted in the middle sets. Repetitions vary during pyramid training in order to accommodate the changing loads. An example of this would be performing a 10RM, 8RM, 6RM, 4RM, 2RM, 4RM, 6RM, 8RM, and 10RM with the resistance set to allow only the listed number of repetitions. As mentioned in chapter 3, this type of training is very time intensive, so it often is reserved for only a few exercises in a given workout.

Pyramid training combines several aspects of both maximal strength and hypertrophy protocols. Volume is relatively high because many sets are performed and some sets contain a high number of repetitions. This characteristic of hypertrophy training is coupled with the inclusion of at least one set in which a heavy load is lifted. This high-intensity set is indicative of maximal strength protocols.

Although this method does allow for a variety of muscle stimuli in a single workout, the volume may not be appropriate for all goals. For example, if your goal is maximal strength, this type of routine may lead to an undue amount of muscular fatigue by the time you perform the high-resistance, low-repetition sets (e.g., the 2RM to 4RM sets in the previous example). This fatigue may prevent the neuromuscular adaptations necessary for building maximal strength. However, like circuit training, pyramid training may be used occasionally to break up the monotony that comes with repeating the same workout over and over.

Super Sets and Compound Sets

Using compound sets and super sets is a good way to increase time efficiency during your workouts. The terms *compound set* and *super set* are often used interchangeably, but they refer to two distinct techniques. For the purpose of this discussion, *super sets* are multiple sets of exercise in which a set that uses the agonist muscle group is immediately followed by an exercise that uses the antagonist muscle group (e.g., biceps curls followed by triceps push-downs). *Compound sets*, on the other hand, are sets in which the first set of the second exercise uses the same muscle group as the first exercise and is immediately followed by a third set of the first exercise (e.g., triceps push-downs followed by triceps extensions and then another round of triceps push-downs).

Super sets are useful when you are lifting for maximal strength and need long rest periods between sets. Ordering the exercises so that agonists and antagonists are trained back to back can allow you to move from exercise to exercise with less time spent resting.

Researchers previously thought that performing super sets allowed the antagonist, which is trained second, to produce greater force because the agonist is fatigued and cannot resist the movement of the antagonist. However, recent evidence shows that the opposite is actually true. Because the antagonist is somewhat involved during the contraction of the agonist, the antagonist itself is slightly fatigued during the previous set. This fatigue causes a slight decrease in its ability to produce force.

This effect is better understood using an example. You may expect the quadriceps to perform better immediately after a set of leg curls because the hamstrings are fatigued and less likely to be able to resist (eccentrically) the action of the quadriceps. Instead, the performance of the quadriceps will be slightly hindered because they were somewhat active (i.e., providing a stabilizing cocontraction) during the hamstrings exercise.

Compound sets are done with the purpose of exercising a muscle in a fatigued state. The idea is to completely exhaust the muscle being worked and produce a greater amount of overload.

Rest Between Workouts

You've already learned that the rest you take between sets of a given exercise during a training session is directly related to the intensity with which you are performing the training. In other words, as intensity increases, rest also increases as the body requires more time to recuperate in preparation for the next set (see chapter 3). We discuss earlier in this chapter how this factor affects your training in various ways depending on your goals.

The time taken between workouts can be referred to as the *intertraining-session rest period*. Specific recommendations are not often given for intertraining-session rest periods; rather, these rest periods usually are the by-product of the chosen frequency of training sessions per week. It is widely believed that at least 48 hours of rest is necessary for a muscle to sufficiently recover after a training session.

Regardless of whether we are able to determine the optimal intertraining-session rest time to promote the greatest gains, this variable needs to be guided by your training experience. When you are new to training, keep your frequency at two or three sessions per week. In fact, some research has shown that beginners can improve with as little as one session per week. As your experience mounts, improvements in recovery will allow you to increase the frequency of your training.

Similarly, when progress is slowing or lacking, training frequency or rest should be one of the variables that you examine. When frequency is too low, the muscles are not receiving enough of an overload to incur change. When training frequency is too high, intertraining-session rest is insufficient and the muscles are unable to recover well enough to perform at their best during the next training session. Tinkering with training frequency at the end of training cycles can be another good way to manage your training plateaus.

Summary

Remember that your training goal will dictate to a large degree how you manipulate your training variables. In other words, instead of just doing the same thing each workout, plan to train the correct way for the desired outcome and adjust your plan as needed.

8

Safety, Soreness, and Injury

Kylie K. Harmon, Dustin D. Dunnick, Kavin K.W. Tsang, and Lee E. Brown

This chapter discusses one of the most important topics in the field of resistance training. Although someone may not be interested in reading long-winded explanations about proper form and technique or the importance of following safe training guidelines, learning how to avoid an injury is much better than trying to figure out how to fix one. Practicing preventative techniques goes a long way toward reducing the occurrence and severity of injuries that can cause pain, dysfunction, and a costly loss of training time.

We must emphasize that resistance training prevents and aids in the recovery of far more injuries than it causes. People who avoid working with weights because of the fear of developing or exacerbating an injury are misguided in their thinking. In fact, with qualified instruction and strict adherence to proper technique, the incidence of injuries actually created by resistance training is extremely small. In other words, the positives of resistance training far outweigh the potential negatives.

Throughout this chapter, we discuss the importance of safely engaging in resistance training. We also address the soreness associated with unaccustomed exercise and how this soreness passes in a short time. Finally, we give some information to help you identify and manage injuries.

Lifting Safely

In the weight room, injuries most often occur when individuals do not follow directions or do not use proper form. In addition to properly warming up and

The authors acknowledge the significant contributions of Brian W. Findley, Daniel P. Murray, and Sagir G. Bera to this chapter.

cooling down from your strength training workout, you should always wear appropriate clothing and shoes, and you must learn the proper techniques for each lift.

Warming Up and Cooling Down

Resistance training demands a proper warm-up. Athletes should start every strength training session by performing a general warm-up of 5 to 10 minutes of light aerobic exercise, jogging, or cycling on a cycle ergometer. A dynamic warm-up, consisting of movements that increase body temperature and prepare the muscles for activity, should also be performed. Dynamic warm-up protocols typically consist of full-body movements aimed at warming up the muscles—particularly the muscles that will be involved in the training session—throughout the available range of motion. Movements commonly included are walking knee hugs, cross-knee hugs, skip series, walking lunges, walking hamstrings and quadriceps stretches, inch worms, high knees, and butt kickers performed for a series of 10 to 20 meters. However, this list is by no means exhaustive. The options for what can constitute a dynamic warm-up are endless.

After a thorough dynamic warm-up, a specific warm-up is performed with one or two sets of light loads (around 50 percent of 1RM) to improve blood flow to the muscles that will be exercised. Warm-up sets also improve a muscle's ability to produce force during subsequent training sets. Performing these sets before each exercise takes only a short amount of time, and the first training set can be performed almost immediately after the last warm-up. Warm-up sets should not be counted in your total number of sets for the day. Proper warm-up sets are especially important before high-intensity workouts. Exercising a muscle at or near its maximum intensity without first preparing it physiologically is a dangerous practice.

Cool-down periods after workouts help the body recover. The by-products of muscular contraction (e.g., lactic acid) tend to sit in the muscle after training unless they are cleared back into the blood for processing and waste removal. Cooling down is one way to facilitate this clearance and help the muscle recover more quickly between workouts. Cool-down periods don't have to be excessive in duration. Spending 5 to 10 minutes on a cycle or treadmill (at a low to moderate intensity) after a lower-body workout is sufficient. Similarly, performing 5 to 10 minutes of upper-body aerobic training (e.g., on an upper-body cycle) will help clear waste products after an arm workout.

Stretching

Stretching is another beneficial activity to include in your resistance training program. Muscular flexibility and good range of motion of the joints improve your ability to perform exercises using appropriate form. Improved flexibility, especially of the lower extremities, also seems to help limit lower-back injuries.

Many experts advocate stretching as part of the warm-up process before resistance training, yet recent evidence indicates that this practice is not beneficial. Several studies have shown that static stretching a muscle just before training may decrease its ability to produce force (Cramer et al. 2004); however, this decrement in performance generally lasts no more than two to five minutes (Wolfe et al. 2011). Static stretching programs seem most worthwhile when performed at the end of a workout along with the active cool-down period. The increase in blood flow from training warms the muscle, which allows it to stretch farther and better maintain gains in flexibility.

Several methods of stretching exist, including static, dynamic, ballistic, and proprioceptive neuromuscular facilitation. Static stretching involves slowly stretching a muscle to its end range (i.e., as far as you can stretch it) and holding that stretch for a prescribed duration of time. Intensity of the stretch should be moderate in order to achieve good results without overstretching and causing pain (figure 8.1). The optimal duration for static stretching seems to be 30 seconds with a brief pause between repetitions. Performing two or three repetitions of the stretch is common practice, although better results often are described if the number of repetitions and stretching sessions per day is increased (Malliaropoulos et al. 2004). After any strength training workout athletes should be sure to stretch the entire body, emphasizing the major joints. Dynamic stretching, as described previously, consists of actively moving a muscle through its available range of motion in an attempt to increase flexibility.

Proprioceptive neuromuscular facilitation is a stretching technique that involves relaxing and actively contracting a muscle to ultimately provide a greater stretch. Typically performed with a partner, proprioceptive neuromuscular facilitation

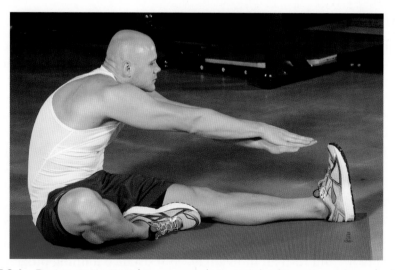

FIGURE 8.1   During static stretching, a muscle is stretched to near-end range of motion and held for up to 30 seconds.

involves the passive stretch of a muscle, followed by an active contraction of the muscle and a final passive stretch of the muscle. The lying hamstrings stretch is an example that is easy to visualize. The person being stretched lies on the floor, and a partner passively stretches the hamstrings by pushing the leg up toward the face as far as possible without creating excessive discomfort. After a brief hold, the person being stretched actively contracts the muscle. After the contraction, the muscle is again relaxed and passively stretched. Due to the inhibition of the Golgi tendon organs, which detect tension in the muscle, the muscle is able to be stretched to a greater depth.

Lifting Attire

Wearing proper attire during resistance training helps regulate body temperature and facilitate lifting movements. Long pants and long sleeves made of heavy, restrictive material may inhibit movement during exercise and may trap heat that the body needs to release. If the body is unable to release enough heat or if the sweat it produces cannot evaporate, the core temperature of the body may increase, leading to dehydration and impaired performance. Wearing comfortable, breathable materials during training sessions helps prevent this. Clothing that allows for optimal mobility is best.

Footwear is also an important consideration in the gym. Open-toed shoes or sandals are not appropriate for resistance training. Comfortable athletic shoes help protect the feet and toes from being stubbed or scraped against heavy equipment, and they offer good support for the feet when lifting heavy weights. Athletic shoes likely won't save you from injury if you drop a heavy plate on your foot, but they can help cushion your feet and prevent minor traumas.

Performing Exercises Correctly

Although injuries directly attributable to resistance training are rare, they do occur from time to time. The vast majority of these injuries stem from the lifter not using proper form. One of the biggest misconceptions about resistance training is that it will lead to injury of the lower back or neck. It is true that these areas are vulnerable to injury when lifting heavy weights, but you can significantly reduce the risk of these injuries by paying attention to proper positioning and avoiding poor technique. It is also critical that a lifting regimen be properly programmed. By having a set program with proper progression (see chapter 3), a lifter is less likely to jump into more advanced lifting techniques when he or she is unaccustomed to high loads and complex movements.

Watch out for the following pitfalls as you strive for proper form:

• Resist the temptation to load up the bar with as much weight as you can possibly lift and turn an individualized resistance training program into a competition among peers. Overloading the bar is never a good idea. It leads to using momentum to perform lifts, which does not optimally isolate the targeted muscles.

- Don't lurch or twist body parts during a lift. A lifter often will compensate with the legs, back, or neck if a load is too great to lift with proper form. Equipment that enables you to lift while sitting and provides a high back support, such as an adjustable bench, can help keep you from overcompensating with accessory muscles or using momentum.

- Avoid performing a partial range of motion to complete a movement. Squatting beyond intended depth or performing biceps curls with a shortened range of motion are common examples. This can be a sign that the load is too great. The length–tension relationship of a muscle tells us that the most difficult segments of muscle action are at the beginning and end of a given range of motion. Some people tend to perform only the easiest (i.e., the middle) portion of the range using a heavier load than is necessary. Although partial range of motion exercises can help strengthen the portion of the muscle being heavily utilized, lifters should avoid training solely in this manner because a muscle needs to be exercised through its entire range of motion. The human body is made to move through the full range of motion of its muscles and joints and should be strengthened in all the areas that are used in daily life. If a lifter trains a muscle throughout only a certain range of motion, the muscles in the weaker portion of the range of motion are not properly trained.

- Don't deviate from proper positioning of the neck during resistance training exercises. Maintaining good form may be a challenge in the beginning, but repeating good form will strengthen the musculature so it becomes progressively easier. A common mistake is to bring the head forward when performing lifts; this places undue stress on the musculature of the back of the neck and strain on the delicate structures of the posterior aspect of the cervical spine. During seated and standing resistance exercises, the head is in the correct position (neutral) when the ears are in line with or slightly in front of the shoulders (see figure 8.2). Proper positioning can be monitored by a spotter or by performing the exercise in front of a mirror.

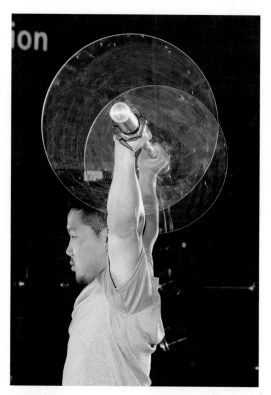

FIGURE 8.2 Aligning your ears evenly with or slightly in front of your shoulders while performing a standing or seated lift will help ensure that your head is properly positioned, thereby keeping your neck and cervical spine free from undue stress and strain.

- Don't compromise proper positioning of the lower back. This can also be a challenge during lifts, especially during core exercises. Overarching of the back is a common compensatory technique when loads are heavier than they need to be or as fatigue progresses. Lifters should identify and eliminate this flawed technique, which may necessitate reducing the load, in order to provide safe lifting for the lower back. Rounding of the lower back often is seen when lifts are performed from the floor, such as in the deadlift. This rounding places the lumbar muscles at a mechanical disadvantage and makes them vulnerable to strain while lifting. Appropriate position entails holding the abdominal muscles tight while maintaining the natural slight arch in the lower back. This ensures that the lumbar spine is held in what is known as the *neutral position* and that undue stress is not placed on either the anterior or posterior aspects.

As an exerciser gains experience and consistently achieves good form, they should progress from machines to free weights.

The use of bad form, which you can observe in almost any gym in the country, has led some exercise professionals to discourage people from performing some highly effective but potentially dangerous exercises. The lat pull-down in which the bar is pulled behind the head and the squat in which the lifter goes below 90 degrees of knee flexion are two exercises that some professionals refer to as bad or dangerous. There is no such thing as a bad exercise; however, some exercises are performed with improper form, and some exercises are contraindicated for certain individuals.

Take the lat pull-down, for example. Some argue that performing this exercise behind the head puts the shoulder in a position where it is vulnerable to injury and causes the lifter to bring the head too far forward. This is true for individuals who lack the appropriate external rotation range of motion in the shoulder to perform the exercise correctly. However, if the appropriate range of motion exists, and if the lifter takes care to pull the bar around and behind the neck instead of pushing the head forward to avoid the bar, then this exercise can be safe and effective. Moreover, the lat pull-down behind the neck may be important to include in training programs for certain athletes, such as wrestlers, who are required to place their shoulders in this position when they participate in their sport.

Part III details the correct form for many strength training exercises. Refer to those descriptions and use a spotter when necessary to ensure that you are using proper form.

Using Straps, Wraps, Belts, and Collars

Lifting straps, wraps, and belts commonly are used by bodybuilding and power-lifting professionals, who often engage in high-intensity training and use heavy loads. Straps are used to help a lifter improve his or her grip on the bar by taking up some of the stress that otherwise would be felt by the hand and forearm. One strap is used for each hand. One end of the strap is wrapped around the wrist, and the other end is wrapped around the bar or dumbbell to be lifted (see figure 8.3). Straps often are used with heavy lifts such as the deadlift.

Wraps can be used around the knees when performing high-intensity exercises for the lower body, such as the squat or leg press. Some people feel that the wraps help support the knees during these heavy lifts and prevent them from incurring undue stress. The wraps should be applied directly around the joint doing the lifting in order to provide greater support for the joint.

Weight belts commonly are used for high-intensity and power lifts.

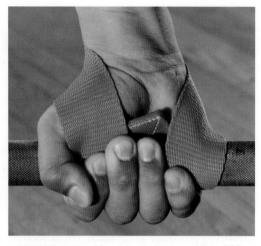

FIGURE 8.3 The closed grip using lifting straps. Notice that the thumb wraps around the bar to prevent slippage.

These belts increase support for the lower back and trunk by increasing intra-abdominal pressure. They may also help cue the lifter to maintain proper lower back positioning during heavy lifting.

The negative aspect of using these pieces of equipment is that the lifter may become dependent on them, which can promote detraining of stabilizer muscles that are also supposed to be working during these lifts. For example, when performing a squat, keeping the back in a slightly arched position and holding the abdominal muscles tight are important parts of correct form. Using a weight belt creates the same stabilizing pressure that the abdominal contraction is supposed to create. When the belt is used, the abdominal muscles and the stabilizer muscles in the lower back can become more relaxed during the lift. This may contribute to their weakness and may therefore be detrimental rather than beneficial. As a result, consider not using a belt, wraps, or straps when lifting less than maximal loads.

Finally, collars are small pieces of equipment that go over the end of the bar in free-weight training. Due to the inherent instability of free weights, collars should always be used to prevent plates from falling off the end of the barbell.

Using Spotters

Exercising with a workout partner or spotter is integral to safe resistance training. This becomes even more important when you are performing high-intensity training or when you are attempting to exercise the muscle to exhaustion. Having a spotter is not a sign of weakness or inexperience. Rather, it is an intelligent decision that shows both a commitment to working your muscles to their limits and a regard for the practice and promotion of proper safety.

A spotter's most obvious contribution to safe resistance training is being there to help you complete a lift in case you are unable to do so on your own.

Therefore, the first things a spotter must know is how much are you lifting and how many reps you intend to perform. Having a spotter allows you to eliminate any fears of being trapped under the bar and lets you work your muscles to a greater state of fatigue. You are able to get the most out of each set because you are lifting the load with maximum effort, volume, or intensity without undue anxiety about safety.

The spotter is also useful for encouragement and motivation. Lifting with a friend or workout partner can make the training session more enjoyable and provide you with motivation to work harder. The encouragement and feedback your spotter gives can also help you press through days when your usual motivation and desire are lacking.

A good workout partner can also coach you to avoid improper form. They may notice that you are not completing full-range repetitions or that you are arching your back with each lift. A well-trained spotter can be key in helping you avoid injuries that might otherwise develop because of bad form. Instructions for spotting on particular exercises are included in part III.

When you are the one acting as a spotter, you must use good spotting form. Getting as close to the weight as possible without disturbing the lift helps ensure proper form. Also, be prepared to offer as much help as needed. In other words, don't underestimate how much you may need to help the person you're spotting. If they need only a little help, it is easy to decrease your contribution to the lift. This is a safer and more effective practice than underestimating the weight at first and then trying to contribute more.

Occasionally, when very heavy loads are being used (e.g., during bar lifts), two spotters are necessary. The appropriate technique is for the spotters to position themselves on both ends of the bar. If the lifter needs help, the spotters must communicate so that they can make equal contributions from both ends.

Injury

An injury occurs when a tissue (e.g., ligament, tendon, muscle, or bone) is subjected to an acute or chronic load that is too great. The damage triggers a response commonly referred to as *inflammation*. Inflammation is misunderstood and often seen as negative, when in actuality inflammation is a bodily response that removes injured tissue and repairs damage. When the body incurs an injury, a cascade of chemical reactions occurs as the body begins to repair the damaged tissue. Inflammation, heat, and redness often are symptoms of this healing process. Therefore, inflammation is the body's way of healing. However, acute inflammation is different from chronic or excessive inflammation, which often is a sign of a larger problem. If inflammation lasts longer than several days or is excessive in severity, you should see your doctor.

The general signs and symptoms of inflammation are redness, heat, pain, swelling, and loss of function. Pain indicates that an injury has occurred, and further stress will cause more damage. Swelling prevents normal function and creates a natural splint that protects the damaged tissue. However, each individual and injury are different, and signs and symptoms may not be present to the same degree. Signs and symptoms typically are more intense at the onset of injury and diminish as the injury begins to heal. Signs are objective indications of injury, whereas symptoms are subjective indications. For example, redness is a sign that a medical professional could see, but pain is a symptom that only the injured party can feel.

It is important to recognize any recurring signs and symptoms when considering a return to activity. Are signs and symptoms increasing, decreasing, or staying the same? If an injury is subjected to too much stress before it heals properly, the body may reinitiate the inflammatory response. No exact timetable for healing exists. Depending on the type of tissue and amount of trauma, signs and symptoms can increase for 48 to 72 hours and may persist for months or even years. Therefore, the old adage of "work through the pain" should be avoided when an injury has occurred.

The PRICE Method of Injury Management

PRICE is an acronym for a commonly accepted injury management protocol: protect, rest, ice, compression, and elevation. The PRICE protocol can be enacted when an injury presents with excessive pain, swelling, or inflammation. Protect the injury from further stress or loading. Although swelling creates a natural splint, the area can be protected further with the application of padding or a brace. Rest the injured area to prevent further trauma and to allow the healing processes to occur. Ice provides pain relief and other anti-inflammatory effects. Compression, generally with an elastic bandage, helps resolve swelling. Elevating the body part above the level of the heart counteracts the effects of gravity and supports the gains of rest and compression.

The practice of PRICE is warranted in the acute management of injury, but modifications may need to occur as healing progresses. For example, active motion helps align healing tissues and should be incorporated as signs and symptoms begin to lessen. Although it is critical that injured tissues are provided an ample amount of rest to heal, active rest can help prepare the body to return to activity as well as prevent excessive loss of muscular gains due to immobilization or decreased loading.

The application of ice or other cold agents has been shown to reduce the temperature of the surrounding tissue, causing vessels to constrict and nerve conduction to decrease. Although this helps attenuate the symptoms of inflammation, constricting vessels can lead to decreased delivery of the substances necessary for healing and may impede the process. No definitive evidence suggests that cold agents are detrimental; at the same time, no evidence shows that they are beneficial in injury management.

Dealing With Muscle Soreness

Unfortunately, muscular soreness is something that often comes with the territory when you begin resistance training. This soreness is the result of the muscle undergoing unfamiliar stress. Although the actual physiological processes involved in producing this soreness are not completely understood, the most likely theory is that unaccustomed exercise actually leads to microscopic tears in the muscle cells. These tears produce swelling, pain, inflammation, and loss of motion in the muscle, leading to decreased or altered function and to stiffness. These symptoms can begin as soon as a few hours after a resistance training session but often will not peak until 48 to 72 hours later. For this reason, the soreness associated with any type of resistance exercise is referred to as *delayed-on-set muscle soreness* (DOMS).

The lack of understanding of the specific processes resulting in DOMS provides us with little ability to treat or prevent it. Rather, we attempt to manage the symptoms of pain and swelling. Ice, heat compresses, stretching, and ibuprofen have been used to treat DOMS. Unfortunately, none of these regimens have resulted in universal success.

One thing we know about DOMS is that it occurs to a lesser and lesser degree as resistance training is repeated. This is known as the *repeated bout effect*. Although you may experience significant discomfort after your first few training sessions, this discomfort is drastically reduced as you continue to train.

DOMS occurs to a greater degree when exercise is intense and is especially evident after intense eccentric training. Therefore, it is recommended that beginners work out with less intensity than intermediate and advanced lifters and minimize eccentric muscle actions in their routines. There is no reason for beginners to start their training with high-intensity workouts when they can accomplish significant gains with lower intensities and, in doing so, reduce the degree of DOMS.

It generally is recommended that lifters wait for the soreness of a prior workout session to fade before lifting again. DOMS acutely reduces strength and diminishes effort, which decreases the quality of a workout and increases the chance of injury. A lifter will be able to return to training without decrements in strength once the soreness is resolved. However, strength and DOMS return to normal levels at different times. Therefore, DOMS is not always a valid indicator of when to return to lifting. Research has shown that although strength may return to normal after 24 to 48 hours, DOMS may persist for 72 hours or longer, especially in beginners.

Identifying and Treating Injuries

As stated earlier, the actual incidence of injury due to resistance training is very low if proper guidelines are followed. Regardless, it is important to be able to distinguish between muscular soreness and injury. Once an injury is identified, you need to know what steps to take to ensure its proper treatment.

Soreness is diffuse and broad, whereas injuries tend to be local, or specific, in nature. Pain that is felt in a localized area—for instance, on one side of the body or in only one muscle or joint—is indicative of injury rather than soreness. Because both sides of the body lift similar loads, soreness tends to present evenly on both sides.

Injuries also last much longer than typical muscular soreness does. If pain does not fade after the 72-hour peak that is often seen with muscular soreness, an injury may be present. If injuries are mismanaged in this early time frame, they can become prolonged and disruptive and may become worse. It is also important to know when to return to activity after sustaining an injury. You should wait for any pain to subside and take note of the movement and function of the injured site. Is the movement pattern altered? Is the limb or joint functioning normally? To prevent further damage, all signs of injury should subside before returning to activity.

Of course, the best recommendation when dealing with an injury is to see a qualified health care professional as soon as possible so that the injury can be taken care of early and appropriately. In the meantime, follow the PRICE principle for treating an injury in its early stages. Practicing these techniques is an effective means of dealing with an acute injury until you can see an appropriate practitioner.

Summary

The most important aspect of any resistance training program is your safety, which can be ensured by following the guidelines in this chapter. Be mindful of the distinction between soreness and injury. Soreness is an expected outcome of almost any new resistance training program. However, injury can result from bad form and technique and usually is associated with unusual or unexpected pain. Injury should always be referred to a qualified physician.

Exercise Technique

This part of the book discusses general technique for strength training exercises. The exercises are grouped into those that target the upper body, lower body, and torso. I also cover explosive lifts.

Before you get started strength training, you should review several safety issues. Although weight training is one of the safest activities, at no time should you compromise safety. Chapter 8 details several precautions you can take to reduce the potential for injury. Please review those precautions before attempting any strength exercise. In addition to those precautions, keep in mind the following safety issues:

- **Medical clearance.** Obtaining medical clearance from a qualified physician before participating in a strength training program is advised. The physician will look for any condition that may compromise your health and safety—things such as coronary risk factors, medications, orthopedic concerns, recent operations, and lifestyle management. This is extremely important information to take into account before you begin training. If any condition exists that has not yet manifested itself, the doctor may detect it during this examination.

- **Grip.** To reduce the likelihood of having a barbell, a dumbbell, or the handle of another piece of equipment slip out of the hands, wrap the thumbs around the bar or handles. This is called a closed grip. It is often tempting to use an open grip in which the thumb is not wrapped around the bar or handle; however, this hand position increases the likelihood that the handle will slip from the hands.

- **Physical space.** Physical space around a lifter can ensure safety as well. The immediate area around a lifter will vary slightly with the exercise, but generally there should be three feet (91.4 cm) of space in any direction around a lifter who is performing a lift. Space is often limited in high-traffic areas and during high-usage times. Be sure to stay away from areas in which the physical space is compromised.

- **Breathing.** Continue to breathe throughout the lift. Generally, you should breathe in during the lowering, or eccentric, phase and breathe out during the lifting, or concentric, phase. The most important thing to remember is that you should never hold your breath while performing resistance training exercises.

- **Lifting technique.** As discussed in chapter 8, lifting technique must never be compromised in an effort to lift more weight or perform more repetitions. Using improper technique results in slower strength gains and can lead to injury. Although everyone uses slightly different technique because of differences in body size and shape, the acceptable range of variance in technique is limited (as you will see in the exercise descriptions in this part of the book). Common lifting errors that compromise technique include swinging the weight to initiate a repetition, moving from the recommended foot position, raising the hips off the bench, not completing the full range of motion, and leaning forward or backward to assist with the movement. Lifting in a controlled manner in both directions is ideal.

- **Proper progression.** Gradually add volume and intensity as the body adapts to training. What may be the ideal training program for one person could be counterproductive for someone else. Therefore, it is best to start with a basic program and add more work over time as the body allows. (The progressive overload principle is discussed in further detail in chapter 3.)

- **Neutral spine.** The spine has three natural curves—cervical, thoracic, and lumbar. The neutral spine position is the position in which the alignment of the vertebrae allows equal distribution of force in all directions. This is the position of the spine typically seen when a healthy person stands erect. A neutral spine position is desirable because it allows for the greatest application of force while also limiting the risk of injury. Injury to the spine can occur if its range of motion is exceeded.

- **Spotting.** The spotter is responsible for the lifter's safety, and by spotting correctly, he or she can further reduce the likelihood of injury. A detailed description of the correct spotting technique is included in the exercise descriptions where appropriate, with specific instructions for lifts such as those in which the weight is supported overhead (pressing movements) or on the trunk (squats). Clear communication between the spotter and lifter is critical. Before any lifting attempts, the spotter should know exactly how the lifter wants to be assisted as well as the number of reps planned; he or she should also be familiar with the lifter's strength levels. The spotter is also accountable for using collars on the weights and ensuring that the bar is loaded evenly on both sides.

9

Upper-Body Exercises

Rob W. Salatto, Vanessa M. Rojo, and Jared W. Coburn

You can perform an infinite number of exercises to strengthen the muscles of the upper body. In this chapter, we focus on proven exercises that strengthen the muscles of the chest, shoulders, upper back, and arms (see figure 9.1, *a* through *c*) as well as some more advanced exercises. The exercises in this chapter serve several purposes. They can help you achieve good general health and fitness, improve athletic performance, and condition your body for "lifting" sports, such as bodybuilding, powerlifting, and weightlifting. In addition, these exercises can help prevent injuries and assist in completing activities of daily living, such as carrying groceries and moving furniture.

As you perform each of these exercises, pay particular attention to exercise technique. Properly executing movements will maximize your strength gains and minimize your chances of injury. Use a spotter when performing heavy lifts in which you support the bar over the head or face. To protect the back, establish a neutral spine position, where the lower back (lumbar spine) maintains its normal lordotic curvature. In addition, it is important that you maintain a stable position when lifting from a bench, either in a lying or a seated position. Specifically, you should utilize a five-point body contact position:

1. Head is placed firmly on the bench or back pad.
2. Shoulders and upper back are placed firmly and evenly on the bench or back pad.
3. Buttocks are placed evenly on the bench or seat.
4. Right foot is flat on the floor.
5. Left foot is flat on the floor.

Some exercises require a spotter to ensure the safety of the lifter. In particular, this is true of exercises in which a barbell or dumbbell is lifted over the head or face. When necessary, the spotter should grasp the barbell, dumbbell, or lifter's wrists (specific guidelines for different exercises are provided in this chapter) and

The authors acknowledge the significant contributions of Michael Barnes and Keith E. Cinea to this chapter.

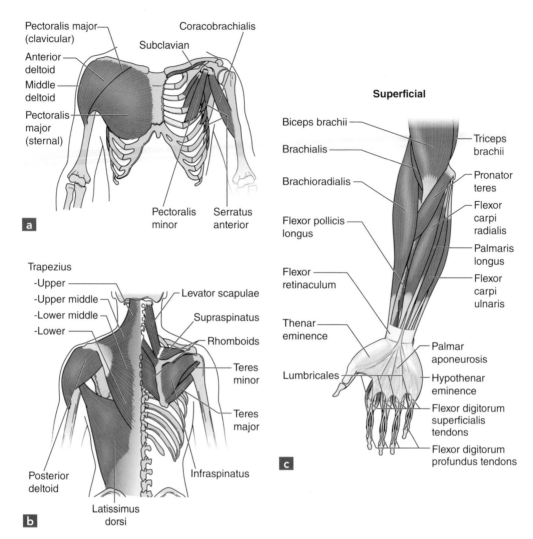

FIGURE 9.1   Major muscles of the (a) chest and anterior shoulders, (b) upper back and posterior shoulders, and (c) lower arm.

provide assistance to complete a repetition, rerack a barbell, or return dumbbells to the floor. Before beginning the exercise, the spotter should also be made aware of how many repetitions the lifter is likely to complete, how much assistance the lifter would like during the exercise, and the timing of the "lift off" for exercises such as the bench press.

To achieve balance in your lifting regimen, combine each pressing exercise with a pulling exercise. For example, if you perform three sets of the bench press, complement your program with three sets of an exercise such as the seated row. This creates balance in both the strength and the size of the muscle groups and ensures joint stability. Most people enjoy training the upper-body muscles because the results are easy to see in the mirror and are easy to quantify on the barbell or machine.

Cable Lateral Raise

Anterior deltoid, medial deltoid

▶ STARTING POSITION

1. Stand erect near the cable column with the exercising shoulder furthest away from the device. Grasp the handle and adjust the cable so that the arm is relaxed against the leg.

2. Select the appropriate resistance on the weight stack.

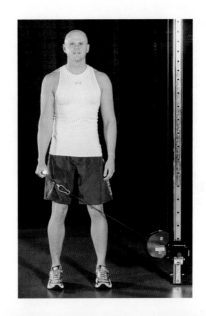

▶ ACTION

3. Maintaining the elbows in an extended position, raise the right arm to the side in a slow, controlled motion until it is approximately parallel to the floor or nearly level with the shoulder. Squeeze the shoulder at the top of the movement.

4. Slowly return to the starting position. Do not let the resistance rest on the weight stack between reps.

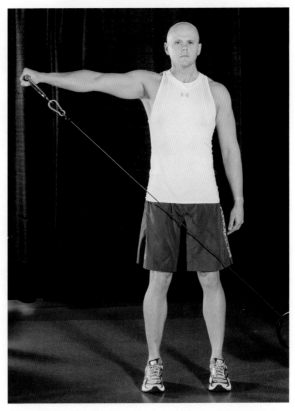

Dumbbell Lateral Raise

Medial deltoid, trapezius

▶ STARTING POSITION

1. Stand with the feet shoulder-width apart. Keep the knees slightly bent. Maintain upright posture throughout the exercise.

2. Hold the dumbbells to the front of the thighs with the palms facing in and the elbows slightly bent.

▼ ACTION

3. Maintaining upright posture and the elbows slightly bent, simultaneously raise both arms to the sides in a smooth, controlled fashion until they are parallel to the floor or nearly level with the shoulders.

4. Lower the dumbbells, following the same path used for the upward movement, while maintaining upright posture and a slight bend in the elbows.

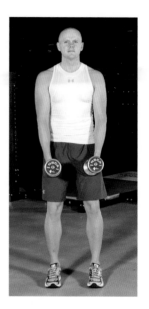

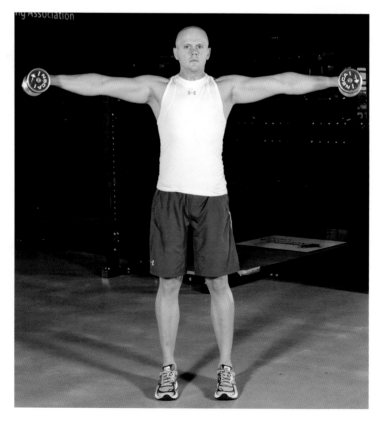

Dumbbell Front Raise

Anterior deltoid, trapezius

▶ STARTING POSITION

1. Stand with the feet shoulder-width apart. Keep the knees slightly bent. Maintain upright posture.
2. Hold the dumbbells in front of the thighs with the palms facing the thighs or facing in.

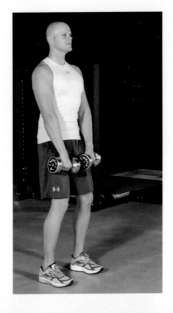

▶ ACTION

3. Maintaining upright posture and a slight bend in the elbows, raise one arm to the front in a smooth, controlled fashion until the dumbbell is at or slightly below shoulder level.
4. Do not jerk the body or use momentum to swing the dumbbell upward.
5. Lower the dumbbell, following the same path used for the upward movement, while maintaining upright posture and a slight bend in the elbows.
6. Repeat this action for the other arm. Alternate arms until the desired number of reps is achieved.

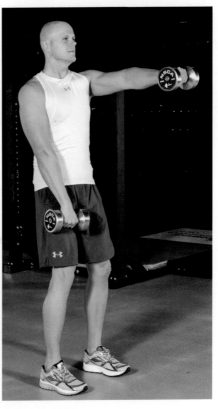

Bent-Over Dumbbell Fly

Posterior deltoid, trapezius

▶ STARTING POSITION

1. Stand with the feet shoulder-width apart and keep the knees slightly bent.
2. Bend at the hips and push the buttocks back until the torso is near horizontal, maintaining a neutral spine position. (The lower back should have a normal lordotic curve.)
3. Hold the dumbbells below the shoulders with the palms facing each other. Keep the arms straight, with a slight bend in the elbows.

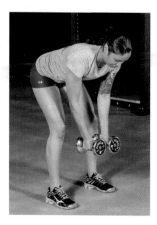

▼ ACTION

4. Maintaining a neutral neck and spine, simultaneously raise both arms to the sides in a smooth, controlled fashion until the dumbbells are at shoulder level. Squeeze the shoulder blades together at the top of the movement.
5. Do not jerk the body or use momentum to swing the dumbbells upward.
6. Lower the dumbbells in a controlled manner following the same path used for the upward movement. Keep the spine in a neutral position.

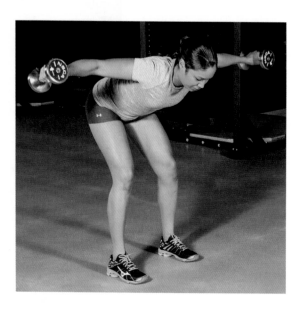

Dumbbell Upright Row

Medial deltoid, upper trapezius

▶ **STARTING POSITION**

1. Stand with the feet shoulder-width apart, maintaining upright posture with the knees slightly bent.

2. Hold the arms in front of the torso with the palms facing toward the thighs and the elbows pointed outward.

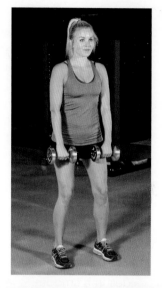

▶ **ACTION**

3. Bend at the elbows to raise the hands to just below shoulder level while simultaneously shrugging the shoulders.

4. Throughout the movement, keep the dumbbells close to the body and the elbows pointed outward.

5. Briefly pause with the hands fully raised while squeezing the shoulders. Begin the descent to the starting position.

6. Do not jerk the body or use momentum to swing the dumbbells upward.

7. Lower the shoulders while simultaneously extending at the elbows to return to the starting position before beginning the next repetition.

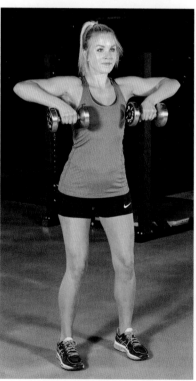

Barbell Upright Row

Medial deltoid, upper trapezius

▶ **STARTING POSITION**

1. Stand with the feet shoulder-width apart, maintaining upright posture with the knees slightly bent.

2. Grip the bar with the hands approximately shoulder-width apart or slightly wider and the palms facing the thighs.

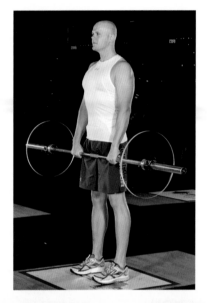

▶ **ACTION**

3. Initiate the movement by bending at the elbows while simultaneously shrugging the shoulders. Raise the hands to shoulder level.

4. Keep the barbell close to the body and the elbows pointed outward.

5. Do not jerk the body or use momentum to swing the barbell upward.

6. Briefly pause with the hands fully raised while squeezing the shoulders. Begin the descent to the starting position. (At the highest position, the elbows should be level with or slightly higher than the shoulders and wrists.)

7. Lower the shoulders while simultaneously extending at the elbows to return to the starting position before beginning the next repetition.

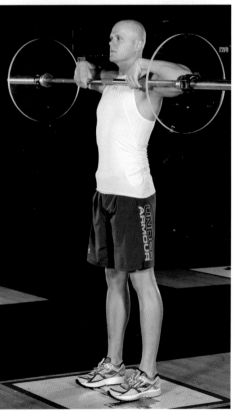

Machine Shoulder Press

Medial deltoid, anterior deltoid, triceps brachii

▶ MACHINE SETUP

1. Adjust the seat height so that the handles are aligned with or slightly above shoulder height.
2. Select the appropriate resistance on the weight stack.
3. Grip either set of handles (with the palms facing forward or toward each other).
4. Position the body with the chest up and the shoulders and head back against the back pad. Keep the feet flat on the ground throughout the movement.

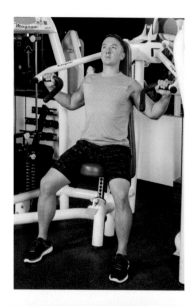

▶ ACTION

5. Press the handles upward in a slow, controlled motion until the elbows are fully extended.
6. Return the handles to the starting position. Do not let the resistance rest on the weight stack between reps.

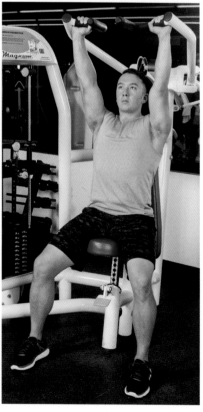

Seated Barbell Military Press

Medial deltoid, anterior deltoid, triceps brachii

▶ **STARTING POSITION: ATHLETE**

1. Sit down on a vertical shoulder press bench and lean back to place the body in the five-point body contact position.
2. Grasp the bar with a closed, pronated grip.
3. Grip should be slightly wider than shoulder-width.
4. Signal the spotter for assistance in moving the bar off the supports.
5. Press the bar over the head until the elbows are fully extended.
6. All repetitions begin from this position.

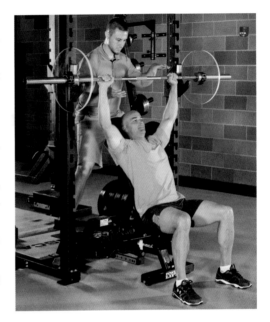

Starting Position: Spotter
- ☐ Stand erect behind the bench with the feet shoulder-width apart and the knees slightly bent.
- ☐ Grasp the bar with a closed alternated grip inside the athlete's hands.
- ☐ Ask the athlete how many repetitions he will attempt to complete.
- ☐ At the athlete's signal, assist with moving the bar off the supports.
- ☐ Guide the bar to a position over the athlete's head.
- ☐ Release the bar smoothly.

Downward Movement: Spotter
- ☐ Keep the hands in the alternated-grip position close to—but not touching—the bar as it descends.
- ☐ Keep the knees slightly bent and the back neutral when following the bar.

▼ DOWNWARD MOVEMENT: ATHLETE

7. With the elbows fully extended over the shoulders, slowly bend the elbows to lower the bar.

8. Extend the neck as necessary to allow the bar to pass in front of the face, and lower the bar until it touches the clavicles and anterior deltoid.

UPWARD MOVEMENT: ATHLETE

9. Push the bar upward until the elbows are fully extended.

10. Extend the neck slightly to allow the bar to pass by the face as it is raised.

11. Do not arch the back or rise off the seat.

12. At the end of the set, signal the spotter for assistance in racking the bar.

13. Keep a grip on the bar until it is racked.

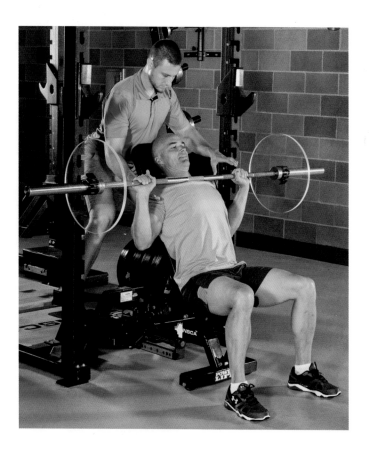

Standing Military Press

Deltoids, triceps brachii

Begin by setting up the barbell on a rack. Many different pieces of equipment can be used for this, such as a squat rack. Use the best, most convenient equipment available.

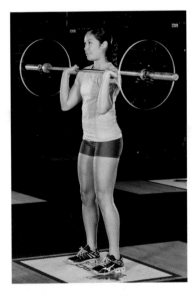

▶ STARTING POSITION

1. Begin with the bar on the top of the shoulders and the feet hip-width apart.
2. Grip the bar one to two inches (2.5-5.1 cm) outside shoulder width with palms facing away from you.
3. Maintain upright posture.

▶ ACTION

4. Push the bar up and over the head until the arms are fully extended over the shoulders. It may be necessary to tilt the head back slightly to avoid hitting the chin or face.
5. Slowly return to the starting position following the same path used for the upward movement.

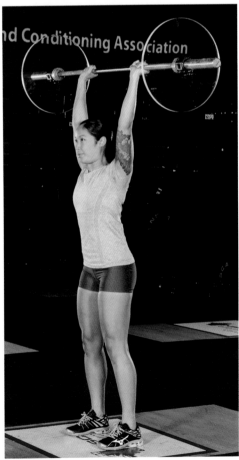

Barbell Shrug

Upper trapezius, levator scapulae

Set up the barbell on a rack. Many different pieces of equipment can be used for this, such as a squat rack or a freestanding shrug platform. Use the best, most convenient equipment available.

▶ STARTING POSITION

1. Position the barbell about mid-thigh, slightly below arm length.
2. With a neutral spine, hold the bar against the thighs and stand with the feet hip-width apart.
3. Position the shoulders back while maintaining upright posture.

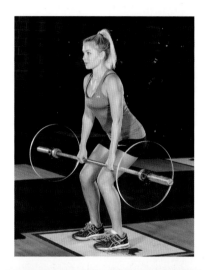

▶ ACTION

4. Elevate the shoulders directly upward as high as possible, ideally three to four inches (7.6-10.2 cm) from the starting point. Pause slightly at the top of the movement, squeezing the shoulders. Keep the arms straight during the entire movement.
5. Return to the starting position along the same path used for the upward movement.

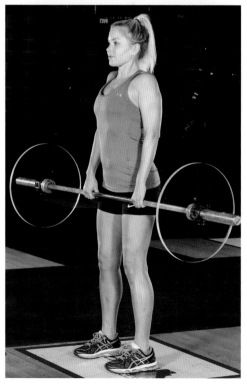

Machine Chest Press

Pectoralis major, anterior deltoid, triceps brachii

▶ MACHINE SETUP

1. Adjust the seat height so that the handles are aligned at nipple height.
2. Adjust the start location for the handles so that they are just in front of the chest.
3. Select the appropriate resistance on the weight stack.
4. Grip the handles with the palms facing forward.
5. Maintain upright posture, with the spine and head against the back pad. (Use the five-point body contact position discussed in the introduction.)

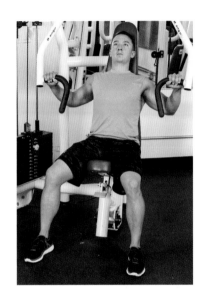

▶ ACTION

6. Maintaining upright posture, extend the handles outward until the elbows are fully extended.
7. Slowly return to the starting position. Do not let the resistance rest on the weight stack between reps.

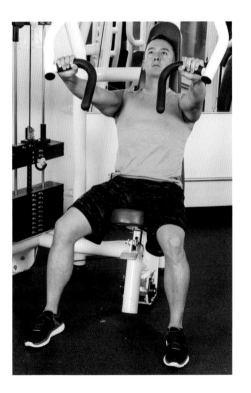

Machine Chest Fly

Pectoralis major, anterior deltoid

The machine used for this exercise is often referred to as the *pec deck*. This exercise uses the machine's vertical handles.

▶ **MACHINE SETUP**

1. Adjust the seat height so that the arms are at shoulder level when holding the vertical handles.
2. Select the appropriate resistance on the weight stack.
3. Keep the elbows slightly bent and grip the vertical handles.
4. Maintain upright posture throughout the exercise.

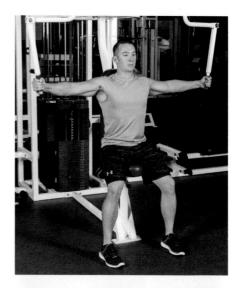

▶ **ACTION**

5. Bring the arms together in a controlled motion until the handles almost touch in front of the body.
6. Slowly return to the starting position. Do not let the resistance rest on the weight stack between reps.

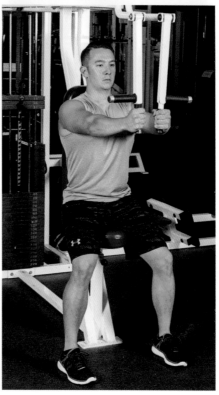

Lying Dumbbell Fly

Pectoralis major, anterior deltoid

▼ STARTING POSITION: ATHLETE

1. After lifting the dumbbells from the floor or rack, sit on the edge of the bench with the dumbbells resting on the thighs near the knee.

2. Grip the dumbbells in each hand with the thumb wrapped around the handle.

3. Lie back onto the bench, bringing the dumbbells to a position next to the shoulders.

4. Be sure to maintain contact with the floor and the bench at five points: both of the feet, the hips, the upper back, and the head.

5. Press the dumbbells in unison to an extended-elbow position above the chest. (Ask the spotter for assistance in moving the dumbbells into the starting position if necessary.)

6. Position the hands directly above the shoulders with the palms facing in and the elbows slightly bent and pointed out to the sides.

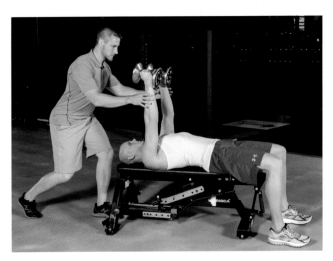

Spotter

☐ Clear the area of any equipment in case the athlete has to drop the weight for any reason.

☐ Ask the athlete how many repetitions he will attempt to complete.

☐ Stand at the head of the bench, prepared to assist the athlete when he lies back on the bench.

☐ With the athlete lying on the bench, place the hands in a ready position under the athlete's forearms toward the wrists. Maintain this position throughout the lift.

▼ ACTION: ATHLETE

7. Maintaining the five points of contact, lower the dumbbells in a controlled and smooth fashion to the sides in a wide arc until they are in a horizontal line with the shoulders.

8. Make sure that the elbows maintain their slightly bent position.

9. Raise the dumbbells following the same path used for the downward movement, performing the full range of motion.

10. Once the set is complete, lower the weight, place the faces of the dumbbells on each thigh, and sit up with the help of the spotter.

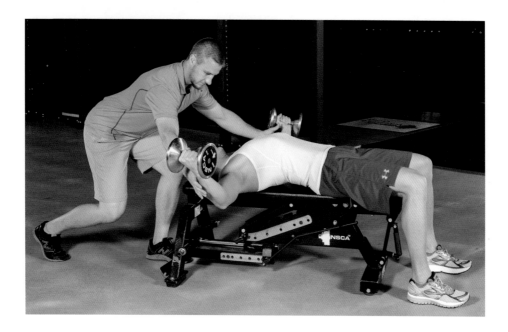

Barbell Bench Press

Pectoralis major, anterior deltoid, triceps brachii

► **STARTING POSITION: ATHLETE**

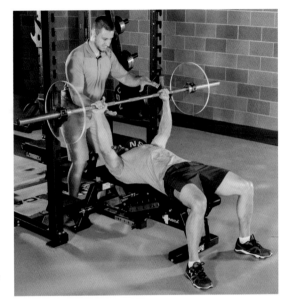

1. Lie on the bench, maintaining contact with the floor and the bench at five points: both of the feet, the hips, the upper back, and the head.

2. Grip the bar with a pronated grip, the hands slightly outside of shoulder width, wrapping the thumbs around the bar.

3. Have the spotter assist with removing the bar from the rack. Support the bar over the chest in line with the nipples.

Spotter

- ☐ Before the athlete starts the exercise, load the bar evenly and use collars.
- ☐ Ask the athlete how many repetitions he will attempt to complete.
- ☐ Stand behind the bar at the head of the athlete and, using an alternated grip inside the athlete's hands, assist with lifting the bar off the rack.
- ☐ Slowly transfer the weight to the athlete when he is in the starting position and has indicated that he is ready.
- ☐ Stand with the knees slightly bent and the hands in a ready position close to the bar. Most athletes need assistance in the upward movement phase of the bench press.
- ☐ Smoothly transfer the barbell back to the rack once the set is completed or if the athlete needs assistance.

▼ ACTION: ATHLETE

4. Maintaining the five points of contact, lower the bar in a controlled motion until it touches the chest at the nipple line. Do not bounce the bar off the chest.

5. While pressing the bar, the upper arms should be at the sides of the body at an angle of approximately 45 degrees from the torso, and the forearms should remain perpendicular to the floor.

6. Press the barbell up to the starting position with the elbows fully extended using the same path used for the downward movement.

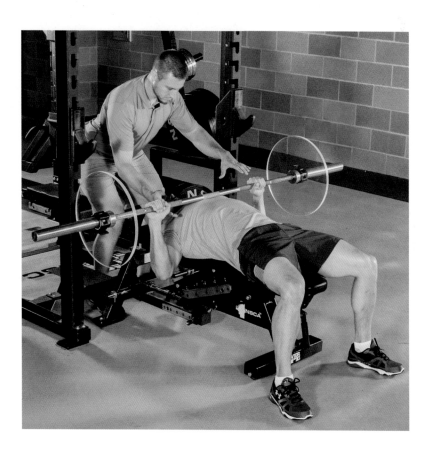

Barbell Incline Bench Press

Pectoralis major, anterior deltoid, triceps brachii

▶ **STARTING POSITION: ATHLETE**

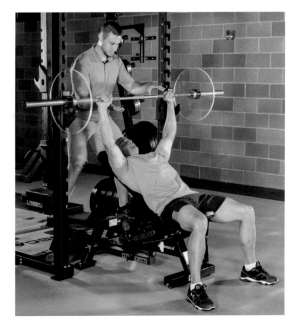

1. Lie on the bench, maintaining contact with the floor and the bench at five points: both of the feet, the hips, the upper back, and the head.

2. Grip the bar approximately two to three inches (5.1-7.6 cm) outside of shoulder width with the palms forward. Wrap the thumbs around the bar.

3. Have the spotter assist with removing the bar from the rack.

Spotter

☐ Before the athlete starts the exercise, load the bar evenly and use collars.

☐ Ask the athlete how many repetitions he will attempt to complete.

☐ Stand behind the bar at the head of the athlete and, using an alternated grip, assist with lifting the bar off the rack.

☐ Slowly transfer the weight to the athlete when he is in the starting position.

☐ Stand with the knees slightly bent and the hands in a ready position close to the bar. Most athletes need assistance in the upward movement phase of the bench press.

☐ Smoothly transfer the barbell back to the rack once the set is completed or if the lifter needs assistance.

▼ ACTION: ATHLETE

4. Maintaining the five points of contact, lower the bar in a controlled and smooth fashion until it lightly touches the upper portion of the chest (between the collar bone and the nipple line). Do not bounce the bar off the chest.

5. While pressing the bar, the upper arms should be at the sides of the body at an angle of approximately 45 degrees from the torso, and the forearms should remain perpendicular to the floor.

6. Press the barbell up to the starting position with the elbows fully extended following the same path used for the downward movement.

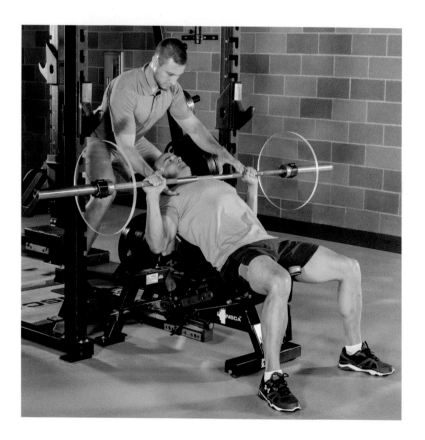

Dumbbell Bench Press

Pectoralis major, anterior deltoid, triceps brachii

▼ STARTING POSITION: ATHLETE

1. Lie on the bench, maintaining contact with the floor and the bench at five points: both of the feet, the hips, the upper back, and the head.
2. Hold the dumbbells in each hand with the thumbs wrapped around the handles.
3. Place the dumbbells slightly to the sides of the chest at nipple level in the down position.

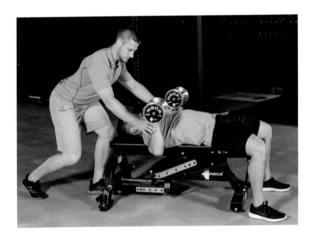

Spotter

- ☐ Clear the area of any equipment in case the athlete has to drop the weight for any reason.
- ☐ Ask the athlete how many repetitions he will attempt to complete.
- ☐ Stand at the head of the bench, feet shoulder-width apart, prepared to assist the athlete when he lies back on the bench.
- ☐ Assist the athlete in getting the dumbbells to the starting position by lifting up on the athlete's forearms near the wrists until the dumbbells are in the up position.
- ☐ Keep the hands in a ready position under the athlete's forearms close to the wrists. Maintain this position throughout the lift.
- ☐ Assist the lifter in sitting up after the set is complete.

▼ **ACTION: ATHLETE**

4. Maintaining the five points of contact, press the dumbbells upward in a controlled and smooth fashion until the arms are extended over the chest.

5. While pressing the dumbbells, the upper arms should be at the sides of the body at an angle of approximately 45 degrees from the torso, and the forearms should remain perpendicular to the floor.

6. Lower the dumbbells using the same path used for the upward movement.

7. Continue pressing and lowering the dumbbells as directed until the desired number of reps is reached.

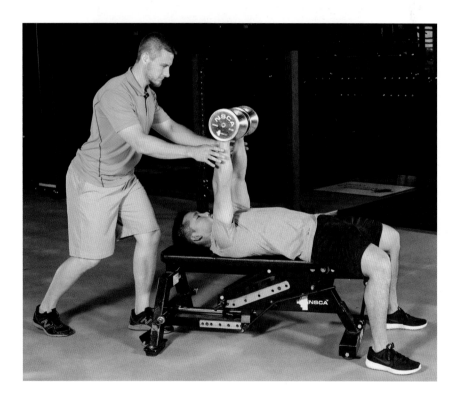

Dumbbell Incline Bench Press

Pectoralis major, anterior deltoid, triceps brachii

▼ STARTING POSITION: ATHLETE

1. Lie on the bench, maintaining contact with the floor and the bench at five points: both of the feet, the hips, the upper back, and the head.
2. Hold the dumbbells in each hand with the thumb wrapped around the handle.
3. Place the dumbbells slightly to the side of the chest at nipple level in the down position.

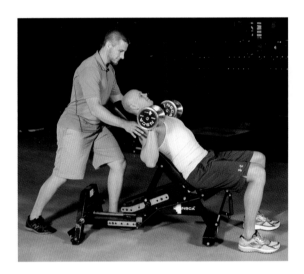

Spotter
- ☐ Clear the area of any equipment in case the athlete has to drop the weight for any reason.
- ☐ Ask the athlete how many repetitions he will attempt to complete.
- ☐ Stand at the head of the incline bench, prepared to assist the athlete when he lies back on the bench.
- ☐ Assist the athlete in getting the dumbbells to the starting position by lifting up on the athlete's forearms near the wrists until the dumbbells are in the up position.
- ☐ Place the hands in a ready position under the athlete's forearms close to the wrists.
- ☐ Assist the athlete in sitting up after the set is complete.

▼ ACTION: ATHLETE

4. Maintaining the five points of contact, press the dumbbells upward in a controlled and smooth fashion until the arms are extended over the chest.

5. While pressing the dumbbells, the upper arms should be at the sides of the body at an angle of approximately 45 degrees from the torso, and the forearms should remain perpendicular to the floor.

6. Lower the dumbbells using the same path used for the upward movement.

7. Continue pressing and lowering the dumbbells as directed until the desired number of reps is reached.

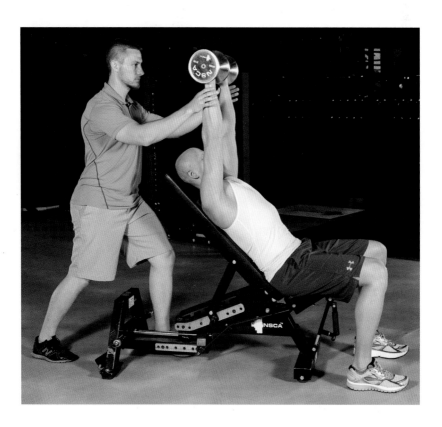

Machine Seated Row

Latissimus dorsi, trapezius, rhomboids, posterior deltoid, biceps brachii

▶ MACHINE SETUP

1. Adjust the seat height to align the mid-chest with the top of the chest pad.

2. Adjust the chest pad to allow for full arm extension.

3. Select the appropriate resistance on the weight stack.

4. Grip the desired handles with the palms facing each other or the palms down.

5. Maintain an upright posture with the chest against the pad.

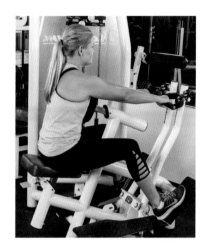

▶ ACTION

6. Pull the shoulders backward in a slow, controlled manner, squeezing the shoulder blades together at the end of the motion.

7. Slowly return to the starting position. Do not let the resistance rest on the weight stack between reps.

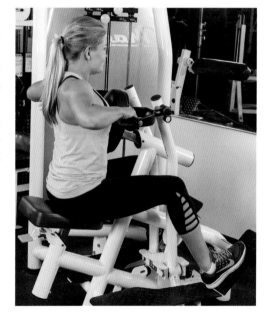

Cable Seated Row

Latissimus dorsi, trapezius, rhomboids, posterior deltoid, biceps brachii

▶ STARTING POSITION

1. Position yourself on a seated cable row apparatus with the knees slightly bent and the feet flat on the supporting platform.
2. Maintain an upright posture.
3. Grip the selected handle with the thumbs wrapped around tightly, and arms extended forward.

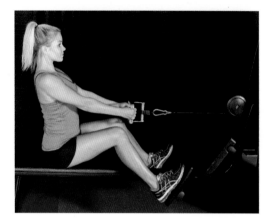

▼ ACTION

4. Pull the handle inward toward the torso, simultaneously flexing the elbows and moving the upper arms backward. Squeeze the shoulder blades together at the end of the action.
5. Slowly extend the arms following the same path used to return to the starting position, performing the full range of motion.

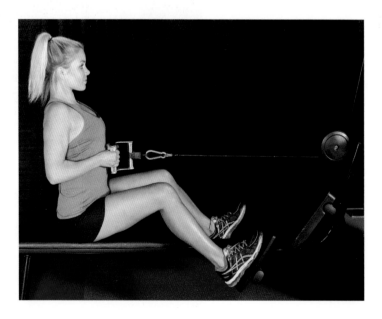

Lat Pull-Down

Latissimus dorsi, biceps brachii

▶ MACHINE SETUP

1. Sit down and adjust the thigh pad so that it rests firmly on the upper legs.

2. Select the appropriate resistance on the weight stack.

3. Stand up and grip the bar wider than shoulder width with the palms facing forward.

4. While gripping the bar firmly, sit down and move the thighs under the pads.

5. Lean back slightly from the hips. Avoid bending the lower back forward or backward.

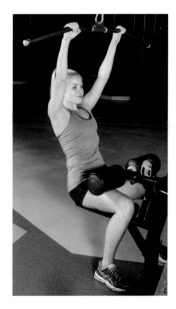

▶ ACTION

6. Pull the bar down to the front of the chest, between the collar bone and the nipple line, in a controlled manner. Simultaneously pull the elbows toward the body.

7. Slowly return the bar to the overhead position to complete the movement.

8. When the desired number of reps has been completed, stand up, gripping the bar firmly, and slowly return the bar to the starting position, controlling the weight on its way down.

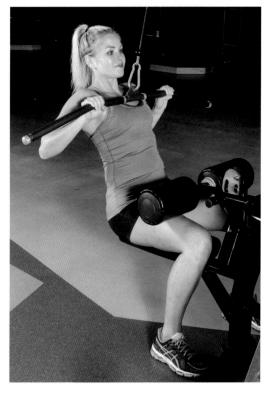

Assisted Pull-Up

Biceps brachii, latissimus dorsi

Assisted pull-up machines can have either a pad to kneel on or a bar to stand on. Apply the directions to whichever machine you encounter.

▶ MACHINE SETUP

1. Select the appropriate resistance on the weight stack.
2. Rotate the lower bar handles outward to make room inside the machine for the body.
3. Lower the foot bar (or knee pad) and lock it into place if assistance is desired.
4. Tightly grip the wider set of handles with the palms facing away from you.
5. Place the feet on the bar (or knees on the pad) while stepping off the supports.

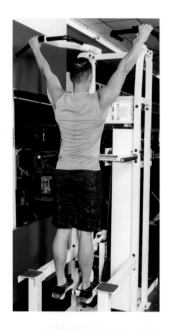

▶ ACTION

6. Pull the body upward by bending the elbows while simultaneously pulling the upper arm toward the body. Continue pulling up until the chin is in line with the hands.
7. Lower the body along the same path used for the upward movement.
8. When finished, remove one foot from the foot bar (or knee from the pad) while it is in the down position and step onto the supports. With the other foot (or knee), control the foot bar (or knee pad) back into its beginning position. When the resistance is completely resting on the stack, step off the machine.

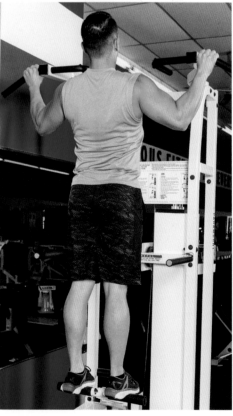

Pull-Up

Latissimus dorsi, rhomboids, biceps brachii

▶ **STARTING POSITION**

1. Grip the bar with the palms facing away from you and the hands wider than shoulder width. Hang from the pull-up bar, maintaining a slight bend in the elbow.

2. The body should hang directly beneath the bar.

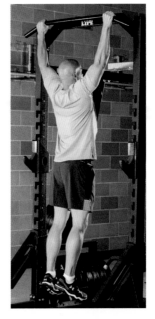

▶ **ACTION**

3. While hanging from the bar and before pulling the body up, squeeze the shoulder blades together. (You should not relax the shoulder blades between reps. Relax them only after the desired number of reps is performed.)

4. Pull the body upward by bending at the elbows while simultaneously pulling the upper arms toward the body. Continue pulling up until the chin is level with the hands.

5. Slowly lower the body along the same path used for the upward movement the starting position to complete the rep.

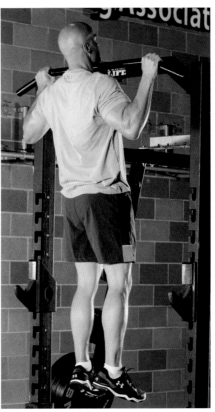

Dumbbell Single-Arm Row

Latissimus dorsi, rhomboids, biceps brachii

▶ STARTING POSITION

1. Place a hand and knee of one side of the body on a bench, with the torso almost parallel to the floor. As you would in a normal standing posture, maintain a neutral spine and avoid bending the lower back up or down.

2. Keep the supporting leg straight but not locked out.

3. With the opposite hand, grip the dumbbell with the thumb wrapped around the handle and the palm facing the bench.

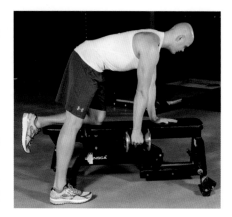

▼ ACTION

4. Simultaneously flex at the elbow and pull the dumbbell upward until it reaches the torso.

5. Slowly lower the dumbbell following the same path used for the upward movement to the starting position to complete the rep.

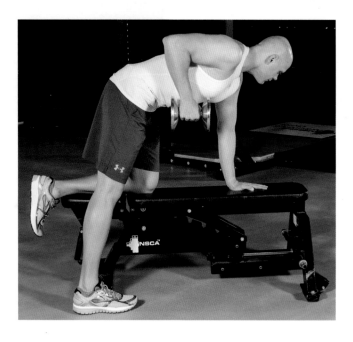

Bent-Over Row

Latissimus dorsi, rhomboids, biceps brachii

▶ STARTING POSITION

1. Stand with the feet shoulder-width apart and slightly bend the knees.
2. Firmly grip the barbell with the palms facing the body, wrapping the thumbs around the bar.
3. Lift the bar from the ground as described for a deadlift in chapter 10.
4. Bend at the hips until the torso is slightly above parallel to the floor and the arms are fully extended. You will maintain this hip-bend position throughout the exercise while rowing the barbell.

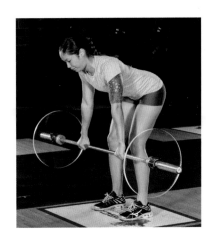

▶ ACTION

5. Maintaining a neutral spine, bend both elbows simultaneously while moving both upper arms backward until the barbell touches mid-torso.
6. Squeeze the shoulder blades together at the top of the movement.
7. Lower the barbell following the same path used for the upward movement, keeping the spine in a neutral position.

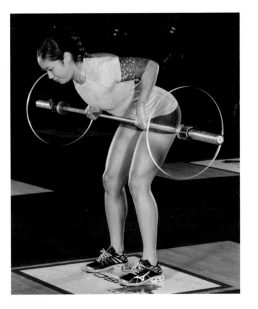

Machine Seated Triceps Push-Down

Triceps brachii

▶ MACHINE SETUP

1. Adjust the seat height so that the arms rest flat on the arm pad, aligning the elbows with the machine's axis of rotation.
2. Select the appropriate resistance on the weight stack.
3. Rotate the handles backward and grip them firmly.
4. Position the back against the back pad.

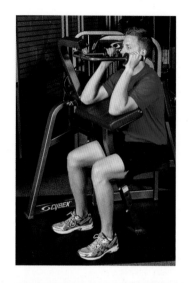

▶ ACTION

5. Extend the elbows to move the handles in a controlled motion until the elbows are fully extended.
6. Slowly return to the starting position. Do not let the resistance rest on the weight stack between reps.

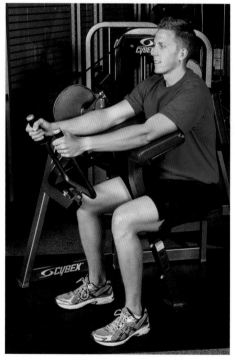

Cable Triceps Extension

Triceps brachii

▶ **STARTING POSITION**

1. Stand in front of the machine with the elbows at the sides of the body and bent to approximately 90 degrees so that the forearms are parallel to the floor.

2. Firmly grip the handle, wrapping the thumbs around it.

3. Keep the elbows directly beneath the shoulders throughout the movement.

4. Maintain an upright posture.

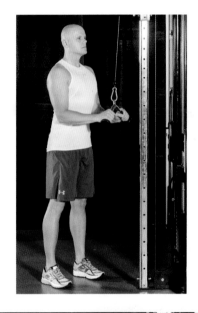

▶ **ACTION**

5. Push down on the handle until the elbows are fully extended. Do not move the upper arm.

6. Slowly return to the starting position following the same path used for the downward movement. Do not let the resistance rest on the weight stack between reps.

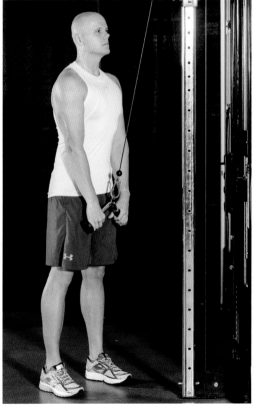

Assisted Dip

Pectoralis major, triceps brachii, anterior deltoid

► **MACHINE SETUP**

1. Select the appropriate resistance on the weight stack.
2. Rotate the lower bar handles inward.
3. Lower the foot bar (or knee pad) and lock it into place if assistance is desired.
4. Tightly grip the handles with the palms facing toward you.
5. Place one foot at a time on the foot bar (or knees on the knee pad) while stepping off the supports.

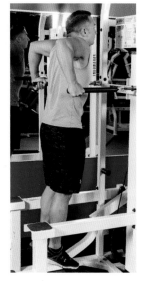

► **ACTION**

6. Bend at the elbows while lowering the body in a controlled and smooth fashion until the upper arms are horizontal to the floor. Maintain upright posture throughout the movement.
7. Press up to return to the starting position following the same path used for the downward movement.
8. When finished, remove one foot from the foot bar (or knee from the knee pad) while it is in the down position and step onto the supports. With the other foot (or knee), control the foot bar (or knee pad) back into its beginning position. When the resistance is completely resting on the stack, step off the machine.

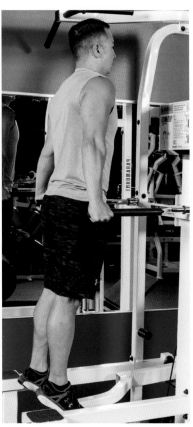

Dip

Pectoralis major, anterior deltoid, triceps brachii

A bench may be used to begin this exercise. Position the bench in front of the dip bars and, after gripping the handles, step off to assume the starting position.

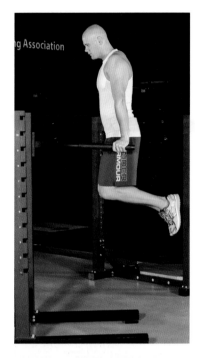

▶ STARTING POSITION

1. Firmly grip the dip bar handles.

2. Maintain upright posture. You may bend the knees if you choose.

▶ ACTION

3. Lower the body in a slow and controlled fashion by bending at the elbows until the upper arms are horizontal to the floor.

4. Pressing upward, return to the starting position.

5. Repeat until the desired number of reps are completed.

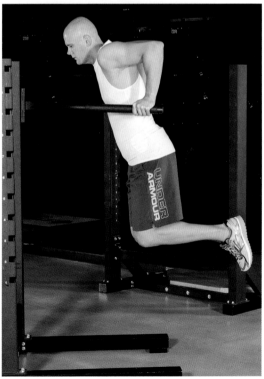

Close-Grip Bench Press

Triceps brachii

▼ STARTING POSITION: ATHLETE

1. Lie on the bench, maintaining contact with the floor and the bench at five points: both of the feet, the hips, the upper back, and the head.
2. Grip the bar with the hands directly shoulder-width apart, wrapping the thumbs around the bar.
3. Have the spotter assist with removing the bar from the rack. Support the bar over the chest in line with the nipples.

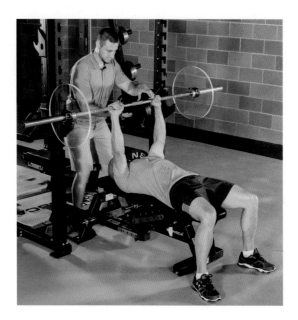

Spotter
- ☐ Before the athlete starts the exercise, load the bar evenly and use collars.
- ☐ Ask the athlete how many repetitions he will attempt to complete.
- ☐ Stand behind the bar at the head of the athlete and, using an alternated grip, assist with lifting the bar off the rack.
- ☐ Slowly transfer the weight to the athlete when he or she is in the starting position.
- ☐ Stand with the knees slightly bent and the hands in a ready position close to the bar. Most athletes need assistance in the upward movement phase.
- ☐ Smoothly transfer the barbell back to the rack once the set is completed or if the athlete needs assistance.

> continued

Close-Grip Bench Press   *> continued*

▼ **ACTION: ATHLETE**

4. Maintaining the five points of contact, lower the bar in a controlled motion until it touches the chest at the nipple line. The upper arms should be close to the sides of the body. Do not bounce the bar off the chest.

5. Press the barbell up to the starting position using the same path used for the downward movement.

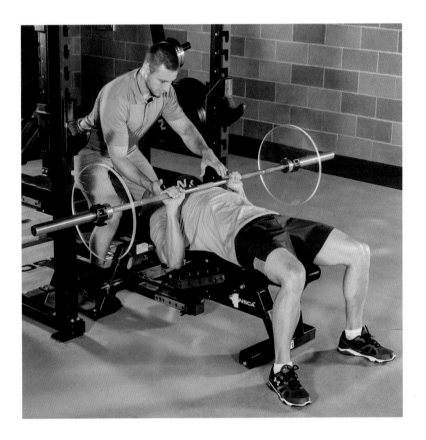

Lying Triceps Extension

Triceps brachii

This movement commonly is referred to as a *skull crusher*.

▼ STARTING POSITION: ATHLETE

1. Lie back on a bench and use an EZ bar to perform the movement.
2. Lie on the bench, making sure that the body makes contact with the floor and the bench at five points: both of the feet, the hips, the upper back, and the head.
3. Hold the bar with the palms facing the feet, wrapping the thumbs around the bar.
4. Have a spotter assist with placing the bar over the chest with the elbows fully extended for the starting position.

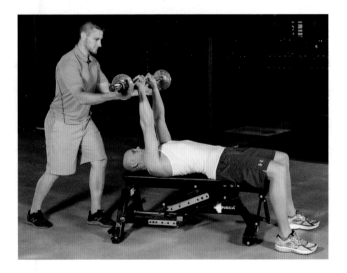

Spotter

- ☐ Before the athlete starts the exercise, load the bar evenly and use collars.
- ☐ Ask the athlete how many repetitions he will attempt to complete.
- ☐ Stand behind the bar at the head of the athlete and, using an alternated grip, transfer the weight to him.
- ☐ Stand with the knees slightly bent and the hands in a ready position close to the bar. Most athletes need assistance in the upward movement phase.
- ☐ Take the bar from the athlete when the set is completed or if the athlete needs assistance.

> continued

▼ ACTION: ATHLETE

5. Maintaining the five points of contact and keeping the upper arms stationary, bend at the elbows to slowly lower the bar toward the forehead. Do not touch the forehead.

6. Keep the movement controlled, with the elbows over the shoulders for the duration of the movement.

7. Press the bar up to the starting position following the same path used for the downward movement.

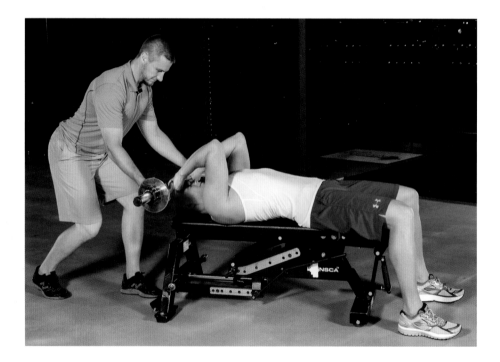

Machine Biceps Curl

Biceps brachii

▶ MACHINE SETUP

1. Adjust the seat height so that the backs of the upper arms rest flat on the arm pad.
2. Align the elbows with the machine's axis of rotation.
3. Select the appropriate resistance on the weight stack.
4. Rotate the handles forward and grip them firmly.
5. Maintain an upright posture, leaning forward slightly if necessary to increase stability.

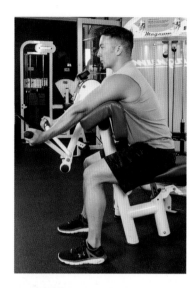

▶ ACTION

6. Bend the elbows in a slow, controlled manner, curling the handles up to the shoulders until the elbows are fully bent.
7. Slowly return the handles to the starting position. Do not let the resistance rest on the weight stack between reps.

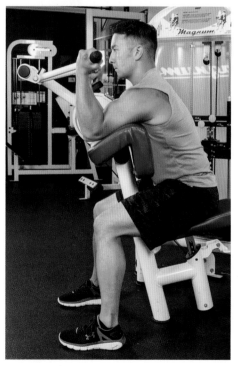

Cable Standing Biceps Curl

Biceps brachii

▶ STARTING POSITION

1. Stand in front of the machine with the elbows fully extended at the sides of the body.
2. Firmly grip the handle, wrapping thumbs around it.
3. Keep the elbows directly beneath the shoulders, where they should remain throughout the movement.
4. Maintain an upright posture.

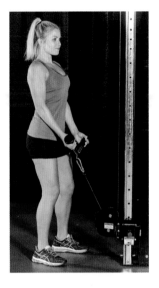

▶ ACTION

5. Pull up on the handle until the elbows are fully bent, squeezing the biceps at the top of the movement. Do not move the upper arms.
6. Slowly return to the starting position following the same path used for the upward movement. Do not let the resistance rest on the weight stack between reps.

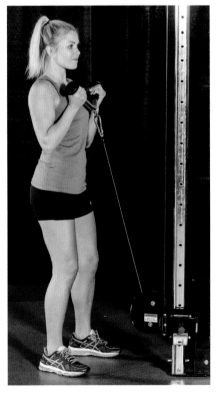

Dumbbell Biceps Curl

Biceps brachii

You may also perform this exercise while standing.

▶ STARTING POSITION

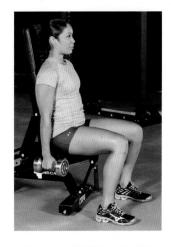

1. Sit with the feet shoulder-width apart. Bend the legs at the knee, and maintain upright posture.
2. Firmly hold the dumbbells next to the seat with the palms facing the thighs, thumbs around the handles.

▶ ACTION

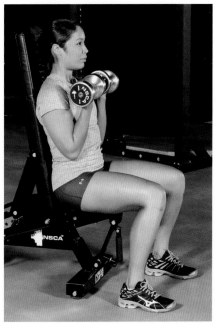

3. Raise the dumbbells in a controlled and smooth fashion by bending at the elbows until they are fully bent. As you bend the elbow, rotate the wrist so that the dumbbell rests with the palm facing the chest at the top of the movement. Squeeze the biceps at the top of the movement.
4. Lower the dumbbells, following the same path used for the upward movement, while returning the palms to their position facing the thighs.
5. Do not use momentum to get the dumbbells moving upward, and do not hyperextend the lower back to complete the lift.

Dumbbell Hammer Curl

Biceps brachii, brachioradialis

You may also perform this exercise while seated.

▶ STARTING POSITION

1. Stand with the feet shoulder-width apart. Keep the legs straight but not locked out, and maintain upright posture.
2. Firmly hold the dumbbells next to the thighs with the palms facing the thighs, thumbs around the handle.

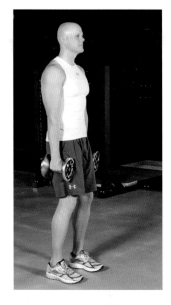

▶ ACTION

3. Raise the dumbbells in a controlled and smooth fashion by bending at the elbows until they are fully bent. Do not rotate the wrists. The palms should remain facing the torso throughout the full range of motion.
4. Lower the dumbbells following the same path used for the upward movement.
5. Do not use momentum to get the dumbbells moving upward, and do not hyperextend the lower back to complete the lift.

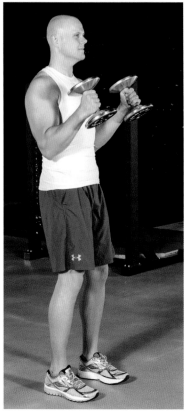

EZ-Bar Curl

Biceps brachii

► **STARTING POSITION**

1. Stand with the feet shoulder-width apart, and keep the legs straight but not locked out. Maintain an upright posture.
2. Hold the EZ bar with the palms facing forward, wrapping the thumbs around the bar and extending the arms fully.

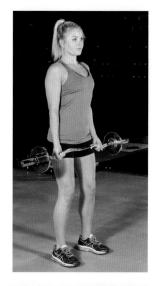

► **ACTION**

3. Raise the EZ bar in a controlled and smooth fashion by bending at the elbows until they are fully bent. Squeeze the biceps at the top of the movement.
4. Lower the EZ bar following the same path used for the upward movement.
5. Do not use momentum to get the bar moving upward, and do not hyperextend the lower back to complete the lift.

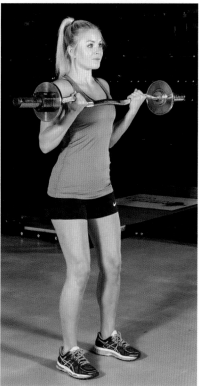

10

Lower-Body Exercises

Katherine E. Bathgate and Andrew J. Galpin

Development of leg strength is essential for both the competitive athlete and the everyday individual. Most activities of daily living require force generated by the muscles of the lower body (see figure 10.1, *a* through *d*); these activities include walking, gardening, hiking, and even standing. Strengthening the muscles of the lower body increases the ability to produce force and perform daily activities more efficiently. The muscles in the lower body not only produce movement; they also protect the skeletal system. This is especially important because the forces that act on an individual in running and jumping activities can cause injury if not controlled properly.

When designing a lower-body exercise program, one should consider the demands placed on the individual. To increase the effectiveness of the program, exercises similar to the movements performed in daily life should be chosen. It is also important to consider any special limitations or injuries and avoid movements that the individual cannot perform safely and pain free.

This chapter consists of a variety of exercises that develop lower-body strength. These exercises differ in the demands they place on the body and therefore cause slightly different adaptations. Each exercise is a tool that can be used to enhance the performance of an individual, whether that performance includes kicking a soccer ball or increasing muscle mass for a bodybuilding competition.

The authors acknowledge the significant contributions of Michael Barnes and Keith E. Cinea to this chapter.

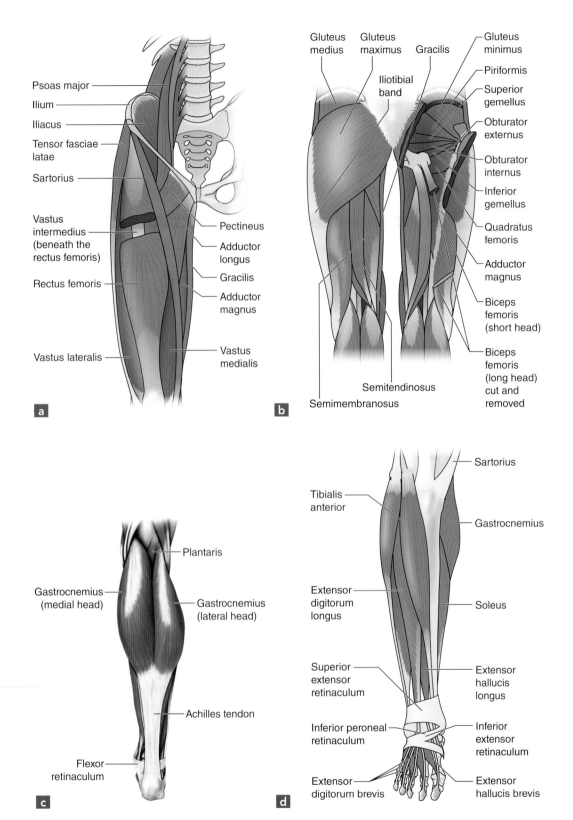

FIGURE 10.1 Muscles of the (a) anterior upper leg, (b) posterior upper leg, (c) posterior lower leg, and (d) anterior lower leg.

Leg Press

Gluteals, quadriceps, hamstrings

▶ MACHINE SETUP

1. Adjust the starting position so that the knees are bent to approximately 90 degrees when placed on the foot plate.

2. Position the feet on the foot plate approximately hip-width apart with the toes straight forward or slightly pointed out.

3. Choose the appropriate resistance on the weight stack.

4. Position the body with the back flat against the back pad; head in a neutral, forward facing position; and hands on the safety handles.

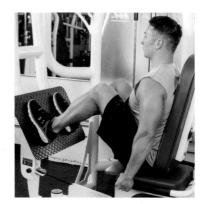

▼ ACTION

5. Push the foot plate away from the body by extending the knees and hips until the knees are almost at full extension. Keep the knees in a path that aligns with the toes and avoid locking out the knees.

6. Return to the starting position in a slow and controlled manner. Do not allow the resistance to rest on the weight stack between reps.

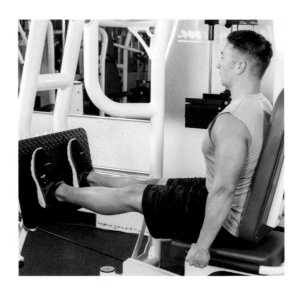

UPPER LEGS AND GLUTEALS

Back Squat

Gluteals, hamstrings, quadriceps

▶ **STARTING POSITION: ATHLETE**

1. Position the rack so that the bar is approximately at shoulder height.
2. Step under the bar to place it on the upper portion of the back and shoulders. The bar should not rest on your vertebrae.
3. Grip the bar at a comfortable position, about a thumb's length from the knurling (the rough part of the bar) or slightly wider than shoulder width.
4. Lift the bar off the rack by extending the hips and knees, then step back, placing the feet about shoulder-width apart and the toes pointed slightly outward. Keep the bar parallel to the floor and the head in a forward facing, neutral position.

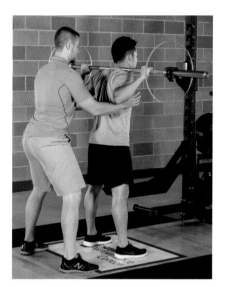

Spotter

- ☐ Ask the athlete if they would like to be spotted from the bar (the spotter's hands are positioned palm-up, under the bar, just outside the athlete's hands), chest (the spotter's arms are positioned under the athlete's armpits with hands facing the athlete's pectorals), or arms (the spotter's arms are positioned under the athlete's armpits with palms facing the toward the athlete's body).
- ☐ Load the bar evenly and use collars to secure the weight.
- ☐ Ask the athlete how many reps they will attempt to complete.
- ☐ Step behind the athlete while the bar is still placed in the rack.
- ☐ As the athlete steps back from the rack, place your arms in a ready position based on their spotting preference. Move as close to the athlete as possible without touching them or disrupting the movement.
- ☐ Squat down in unison with the athlete so that support may be provided throughout the entire movement if needed.
- ☐ Help the athlete back into the rack when the set is completed or when they need assistance.

▼ ACTION: ATHLETE

5. Keeping the feet flat on the floor and weight distributed toward the heels, initiate a backward movement with the hips.

6. Allow the body to descend by bending at the hips and knees, keeping the knees in a path that aligns with the toes.

7. As the body descends, maintain an upright torso and a neutral spine.

8. Descend until the tops of the thighs are parallel to the floor or until thigh–calf contact (if performing a deep squat).

9. Return to the starting position using the same path used for the downward movement.

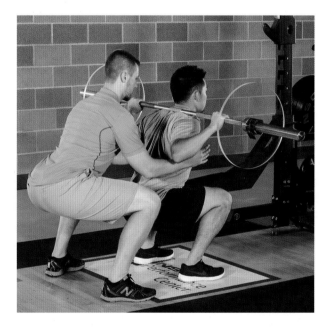

TIPS

- Squat only as deep as you can maintain proper form.
- Avoid excessive forward lean of the torso.

Front Squat

Gluteals, quadriceps, hamstrings

▶ STARTING POSITION: ATHLETE

1. Position the rack so that the bar is approximately at shoulder height.

2. Grip the bar approximately a thumb's length from the knurling (or slightly wider than shoulder width) and rotate the elbows upward from underneath the bar. Using the fingers to help stabilize, allow the bar to rest across the top of the shoulders and clavicle. Fully bend the elbows to position the upper arms parallel to the floor. This is referred to as the front rack position.

3. Lift the bar off the rack by extending the hips and knees. Step back, placing the feet about shoulder-width apart and the toes pointed slightly outward.

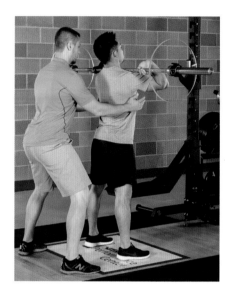

Spotter

☐ Ask the athlete if they would like to be spotted from the bar (the spotter's hands are positioned palm-up, under the bar, just outside the athlete's hands), chest (the spotter's arms are positioned under the athlete's armpits with hands facing the athlete's pectorals), or arms (the spotter's arms are positioned under the athlete's armpits with palms facing the toward the athlete's body).

☐ Load the bar evenly and use collars to secure the weight.

☐ Ask the athlete how many reps they will attempt to complete.

☐ Step behind the athlete while the bar is still placed in the rack.

☐ As the athlete steps back from the rack, position your arms in a ready position based on their spotting preference. Move as close to the athlete as possible without touching them or disrupting the movement.

☐ Squat down in unison with the athlete so that support may be provided throughout the entire movement if needed.

☐ Help the athlete back into the rack when the set is completed or when they need assistance.

▼ ACTION: ATHLETE

4. Keeping the feet flat on the floor, weight distributed toward the heels, and elbows high, initiate a backward movement with the hips.

5. Allow the body to descend by flexing at the hips and knees, keeping the knees in a path that aligns with the toes.

6. As the body descends, keep an upright torso, neutral spine, and the elbows high.

7. Descend until the tops of the thighs are parallel to the floor or until thigh–calf contact (if performing a deep squat).

8. Return to the starting position using the same path used for the downward movement.

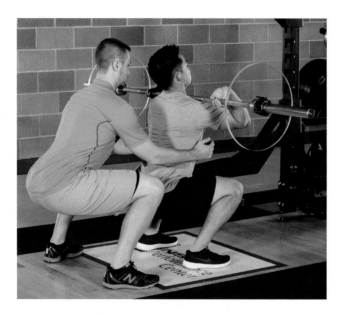

TIPS

- Squat only as deep as you can maintain proper form.
- Avoid excessive forward lean of the torso. The torso should remain in a more upright position compared with the back squat.
- This variation of the squat typically elicits higher quadriceps activation compared with the back squat.

Split Squat

Gluteals, quadriceps, hamstrings

▶ **STARTING POSITION: ATHLETE**

1. Position the rack so that the bar is approximately at shoulder height.
2. Step under the bar to place it on the upper portion of the back and shoulders.
3. Grip the bar at a comfortable position, about a thumb's length from the knurling or slightly wider than shoulder width.
4. Lift the bar off the rack by extending the hips and knees, and then step back. Create a split stance by placing one leg in front of the torso and the other behind the torso. Keep the legs about hip-width apart.

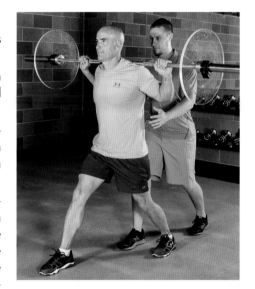

Spotter

☐ Ask the athlete if they would like to be spotted from the bar (the spotter's hands are positioned palm-up, under the bar, just outside the athlete's hands), chest (the spotter's arms are positioned under the athlete's armpits with hands facing the athlete's pectorals), or arms (the spotter's arms are positioned under the athlete's armpits with palms facing the toward the athlete's body).

☐ Load the bar evenly and use collars to secure the weight.

☐ Ask the athlete how many reps they will attempt to complete.

☐ Step behind the athlete while the bar is still placed in the rack.

☐ As the athlete steps back from the rack, position your arms in a ready position based on their spotting preference. Move as close to the athlete as possible without touching them or disrupting the movement.

☐ Position your body in the same split position as the athlete.

☐ Squat down in unison with the athlete so that support may be provided throughout the entire movement if needed.

☐ Help the athlete back into the rack when the set is completed or when they need assistance.

▼ ACTION: ATHLETE

5. Keeping the front foot flat on the floor and the torso in an upright position, allow the body to descend by initiating movement through knee flexion of the rear leg.

6. Descend the body straight down and resist "lunging" forward with the hips. The front leg should be allowed to flex at the knee as the body descends.

7. As the body descends, keep an upright torso and neutral spine.

8. Descend until the top of the thigh of the front leg is about parallel to the ground and the back knee is just above the ground.

9. Return to the starting position using the same path used for the downward movement.

10. Perform the desired number of reps, switch the front and rear legs, and repeat.

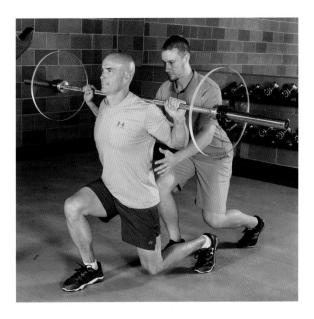

TIPS

- Avoid forward lean of the torso. The shoulders should remain in line with the hips.

- The same exercise can be performed holding dumbbells at the sides in order to limit spinal loading or with the bar in the front rack position to increase activation of the quadriceps. See the front squat for a description of the front rack position.

Step-Up

Gluteals, quadriceps, hamstrings

► **STARTING POSITION: ATHLETE**

1. Choose an appropriate box (typically about knee height) so that the knee joint is at a 90-degree angle when the foot is on the box.

2. Position the rack so that the bar is approximately at shoulder height.

3. Facing the box, step under the bar to place it on the upper portion of the shoulders.

4. Grip the bar at a comfortable position, about a thumb's length from the knurling or slightly wider than shoulder width.

5. Lift the bar off the rack by extending the hips and knees, then step toward the box. Face the box with both feet on the ground.

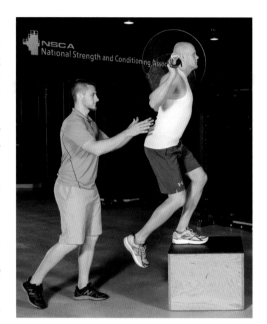

Spotter

☐ Ask the athlete if they would like to be spotted from the bar (the spotter's hands are positioned palm-up, under the bar, just outside the athlete's hands), chest (the spotter's arms are positioned under the athlete's armpits with hands facing the athlete's pectorals), or arms (the spotter's arms are positioned under the athlete's armpits with palms facing the toward the athlete's body).

☐ Load the bar evenly and use collars to secure the weight.

☐ Ask the athlete how many reps they will attempt to complete.

☐ Step behind the athlete while the bar is still placed in the rack.

☐ As the athlete steps toward the box, position your arms in a ready position based on their preference. Move toward the athlete without touching them or disrupting the movement.

☐ Take a small step forward with your lead leg as the athlete steps up on the box.

☐ Bring your back leg next to your lead leg as the athlete reaches the highest position. Be ready to help when cued or needed.

☐ Help guide the athlete back into the rack (after they complete the set or when they need assistance) by stepping backward toward the rack with your arms extended for support or holding the bar if necessary.

▶ ACTION: ATHLETE

6. Place one foot entirely on the box with the knee at about a 90-degree angle. Elevate the body by extending the knee and hip of the front leg. Resist assisting the movement with the rear leg.

7. Elevate the body until the front leg is fully extended and the back leg can be planted firmly on the box. Maintain a neutral spine and avoid excessive forward lean of the torso.

8. Pause before beginning the downward movement. Initiate the downward phase by shifting your weight to the front leg, and then step off the box with the back leg. Step down using the same path used for the upward movement.

9. Perform the desired number of reps, switch the front and rear legs, and repeat.

10. The same exercise can be performed holding dumbbells at the sides in order to limit spinal loading or with the bar in the front rack position, as described in the front squat exercise.

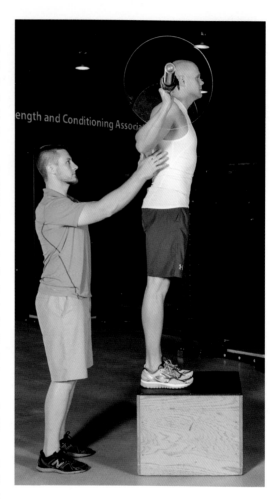

Suspension Trainer Elevated Rear-Foot Split Squat

Gluteals, quadriceps, hamstrings

▶ STARTING POSITION

1. Adjust the suspension trainer so that the handles are about mid-shin height.

2. Facing away from the suspension trainer, place one foot in the lower loop of the suspension trainer. Position the foot so that the loop is around the laces of the shoe and the heel is resting on the hard handle.

3. Step out with the other foot into a split position.

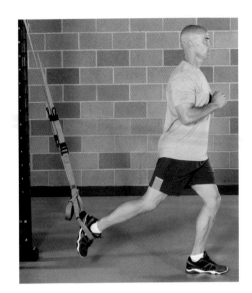

▶ ACTION

4. Descend the body straight down by extending the rear hip back and bending the front leg at the knee joint.

5. As the body descends, maintain an upright torso and a neutral spine.

6. Descend until the top of the thigh is parallel to the floor and the knee is over the toe. Allow the elevated leg to swing back.

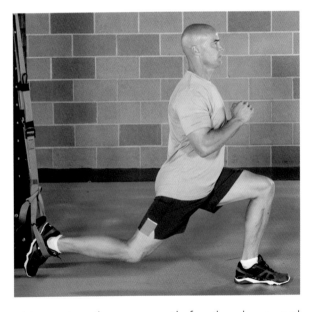

7. Return to the starting position using the same path for the downward movement.

8. Perform the desired number of reps, switch the front and rear legs, and repeat.

9. The intensity of this movement can be increased by adding an explosive hop at the end of the up phase of the movement or by holding a kettlebell at the chest to add resistance.

Leg Extension

Quadriceps

► **MACHINE SETUP**

1. Position the back pad so that the knee joints align with the machine's axis of rotation.
2. Adjust the starting position so that the leg pad rests in a comfortable position just above the ankles and on or directly above the shins when the knees are bent to 90 degrees.
3. Select the appropriate resistance on the weight stack.
4. Sit straight up with the back firmly against the back rest and the head in a neutral position. Grasp the handles at the sides.

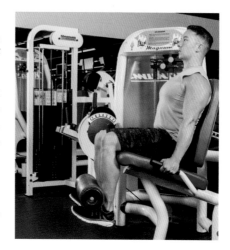

▼ **ACTION**

5. Extend the knees in a smooth and controlled manner until they reach full extension.
6. Return to the starting position in a slow and controlled manner. Do not allow the resistance to rest on the weight stack between reps.

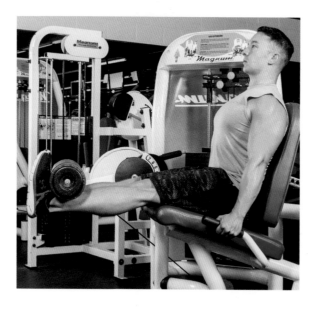

Lateral Lunge

Gluteals, quadriceps, hamstrings

▶ STARTING POSITION

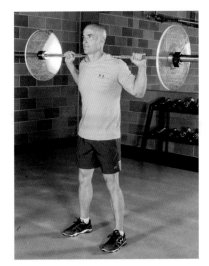

1. Position the rack so that the bar is approximately at shoulder height.

2. Step under the bar to place it on the upper portion of the back and shoulders.

3. Grip the bar at a comfortable position, about a thumb's length from the knurling or slightly wider than shoulder width.

4. Lift the bar off the rack by extending the hips and knees. Step back, keeping the legs about hip-width apart.

▶ ACTION

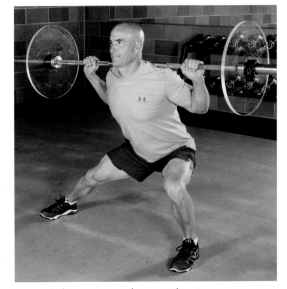

5. With one leg, take a large step laterally out and away from the midline of the body. Place the foot flat and firm against the floor. Keep the toes parallel and pointing forward.

6. Allow the weight of the body to shift horizontally along with the movement of the leg.

7. Descend the body by bending at the hips and knees. The opposite leg should remain straight.

8. As the body descends, keep an upright torso and neutral spine.

9. Return to the starting position by extending the flexed leg and pushing off back toward the other leg.

10. Switch legs and repeat the movement.

TIPS

- Avoid forward lean of the torso. The shoulders should remain in line with the hips.

- The same exercise can be performed holding dumbbells at the sides in order to limit spinal loading.

Lateral Lunge With Slider

Gluteals, quadriceps, hamstrings

▶ **STARTING POSITION**

1. Place a slider on the floor smooth side down and position one foot on top.
2. Position the feet about shoulder-width apart.

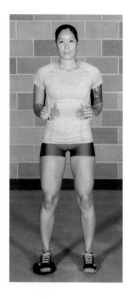

▶ **ACTION**

3. Descend the body, pushing the hips back and sliding the leg (with the slider) away from the midline of the body. Allow the opposite leg to bend at the knee until the top of the thigh is parallel with the floor and the knee is even with the toe.
4. Maintain a neutral spine.
5. Return to the starting position by extending the hip and knee of the leg without the slider and allowing the leg with the slider to return using the same path as the downward movement.
6. Switch legs and repeat the movement.

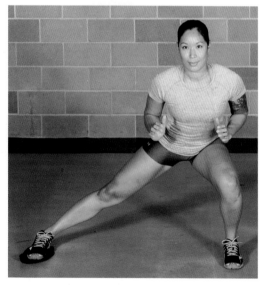

TIP

The intensity of this exercise can be increased by holding a kettlebell at the chest to add resistance.

Deadlift

Gluteals, hamstrings

▼ STARTING POSITION

1. Start with the bar on the floor. Position the feet under the bar so that the bar is over the laces of the shoe and the toes point slightly outward. The legs should be about hip-width to shoulder-width apart.

2. Push the hips backward, lean the torso forward over the bar, and bend at the knees to get into the proper starting position. The shoulders should be over or slightly in front of the bar. Maintain a neutral spine by depressing and retracting the shoulder blades and keeping the chest up.

3. Grip the bar about a thumb's length from the knurling and extend the arms at the elbows.

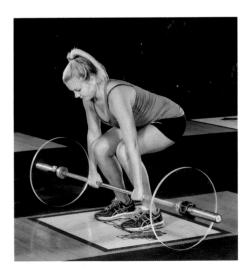

TIPS

- If you are not strong enough to lift standard plates, bumper plates or blocks can be used to maintain the ideal starting position.
- A snatch grip or wide grip can be used to increase activation of the gluteals and quadriceps and to decrease activation of the lower back.

▼ ACTION

4. Keeping the feet flat on the floor and weight distributed toward the heels, begin to pull the bar off the floor.

5. Lift the bar by bringing the hips forward and extending at the knees. Focus on pushing through the ground with the legs, and do not allow the hips to rise before the shoulders. Keep the bar close to the body, the arms straight, and the spine in a neutral position.

6. The shoulders should remain over or slightly ahead of the bar until the bar reaches the knees. Continue the movement until the knees and hips are fully extended.

7. Return to the starting position using the same path used for the downward movement. Keep the spine in a neutral position.

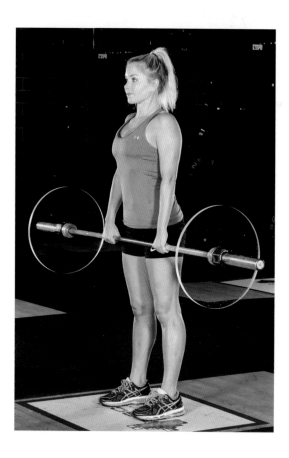

Romanian Deadlift

Gluteals, hamstrings

▼ STARTING POSITION

1. Start with the bar on the floor. Position the feet under the bar so the bar is over the laces of the shoe and the toes point forward. The legs should be about hip-width to shoulder-width apart.

2. Grip the bar approximately a thumb's length from the knurling or slightly wider than shoulder width. Extend the arms at the elbows. Extend the hips and knees to lift the bar off the floor, and step back.

3. Position the feet about shoulder-width apart with the knees slightly bent.

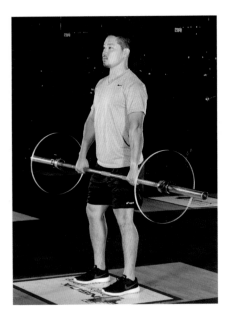

TIPS

- Avoid flexion through the spine and rounding of the back.
- The same exercise can be performed holding dumbbells in front of the body in order to limit spinal loading.

▼ ACTION

4. Keeping the feet flat on the floor and weight distributed toward the heels, lower the bar by bending at the hips (bend and push the hips backwards) to decrease the angle between the torso and thighs. Maintain a neutral spine.

5. Lower the bar until it is in line with the patella tendon or slightly below the knee.

6. Return to the starting position by extending the hips and using the same path used for the downward movement. The knees should remain static and keep the same amount of flexion throughout the entirety of the movement.

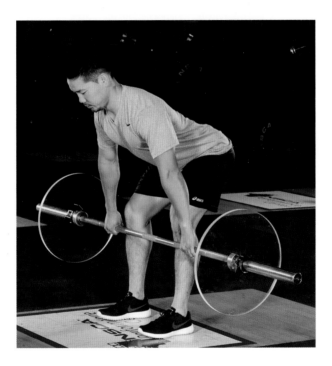

Single-Leg Romanian Deadlift

Gluteals, hamstrings

▼ STARTING POSITION

1. Start with the bar on the floor. Position the feet under the bar so the bar is over the laces of the shoe and the toes point forward. The legs should be about hip-width to shoulder-width apart.

2. Grip the bar approximately a thumb's length from the knurling or slightly wider than shoulder width. Extend the arms at the elbows, lift the bar off the floor by extending the hips and knees, and then step back.

3. Position the feet about hip-width apart with the knees slightly bent.

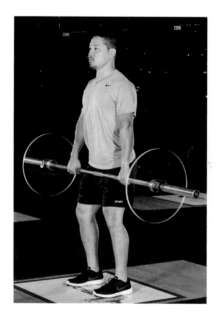

TIPS

- Avoid flexion through the spine and rounding of the back.
- Allow the torso to fall only as far as the back leg can rise. The body should act like a teeter-totter, with the planted leg serving as the fulcrum.
- The same exercise can be performed holding a dumbbell in the hand contralateral to the planted leg to increase activation of the gluteus medius.
- Note: This is an advanced lift and should be attempted only if the deadlift and Romanian deadlift have been fully mastered.

▼ ACTION

4. While maintaining the same knee angle, bend the hips to lower the bar and decrease the angle between the torso and thighs. Simultaneously, allow one leg to rise off the floor, extending it behind the body. Maintain a neutral spine and keep the hips parallel with the floor.

5. Lower the bar until it is in line with the patella or slightly below the knee.

6. Return to the starting position by extending the hips and using the same path used for the downward movement.

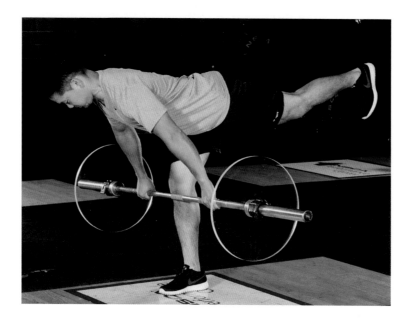

Single-Leg Deadlift

Gluteals, quadriceps, hamstrings

▼ STARTING POSITION

1. Start with the bar on the floor. Position the feet under the bar so the bar is over the laces of the shoe and the toes point forward. The legs should be about hip-width to shoulder-width apart.

2. Grip the bar approximately a thumb's length from the knurling or slightly wider than shoulder width. Extend the arms at the elbows, lift the bar off the floor by extending the hips and knees, and then step back.

3. Position the feet about hip-width apart.

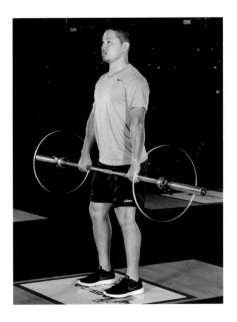

TIPS

- Avoid flexion through the spine and rounding of the back.
- The same exercise can be performed holding a dumbbell in the hand contralateral to the planted leg to increase activation of the gluteus medius.
- This variation elicits higher quadriceps activation compared with the single-leg Romanian deadlift.
- Note: This is an advanced lift and should be attempted only if the deadlift and Romanian deadlift have been fully mastered.

▼ ACTION

4. Initiate downward movement of the bar by bending at the hips and decreasing the angle between the torso and thighs.
5. Lower the bar by bending the hips and bending at the knees. Simultaneously, allow one leg to rise up, extending it behind the body. Maintain a neutral spine and keep the hips parallel with the floor.
6. Lower the bar to the floor.
7. Return to the starting position by extending the hips and using the same path used for the downward movement.

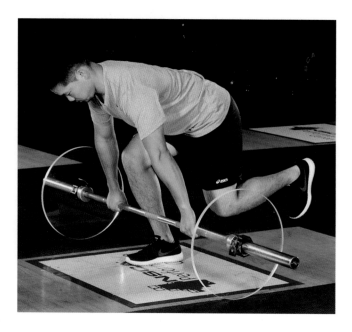

Glute-Ham Raise

Gluteals, hamstrings

► **STARTING POSITION**

1. Position the body in the glute-ham raise device so that the padding ends at the upper thigh. Hook the feet between the pads and place them against the foot plate.

2. Lower the torso so that the legs are extended and the head is pointing toward the ground. Maintain a neutral spine.

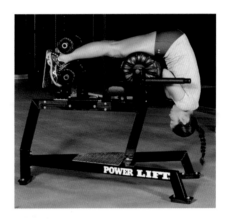

► **ACTION**

3. In a controlled manner, raise the torso by extending the hips until it is parallel with the lower body and the floor. Keep the knees extended until this point.

4. Once the torso is parallel, continue to raise the torso by allowing the knees to flex.

5. Continue to raise the torso until the knees are flexed to about 90 degrees and the torso is perpendicular to the ground.

6. Slowly return to the starting position by extending the knees and using the same path used for the upward movement.

TIPS

• Avoid hyperextension of the spine.

• The intensity of this exercise can be increased by holding a plate or medicine ball at the chest.

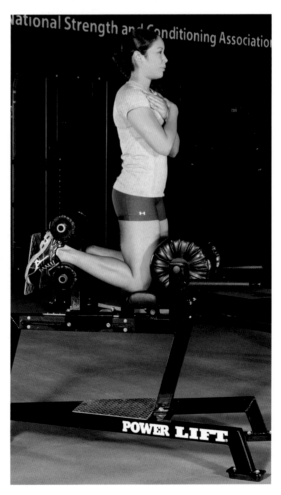

Poor Man's Glute-Ham Raise

Gluteals, hamstrings

▶ STARTING POSITION

1. Loop a long band securely around the top of a squat rack.
2. Pull the band down and grip the band with both hands just below the clavicle.
3. Assume a kneeling position with the knees about hip-width apart.
4. Have a partner support and prevent the rising of the lower legs and feet.

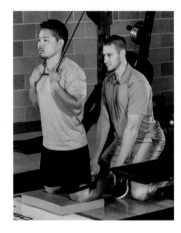

▼ ACTION

5. Initiate the downward movement of the torso by slowly leaning forward.
6. Lower the body as one unit until the body is just off the floor.
7. Return to the starting position by bending at the knees and using the same path used for the downward movement.

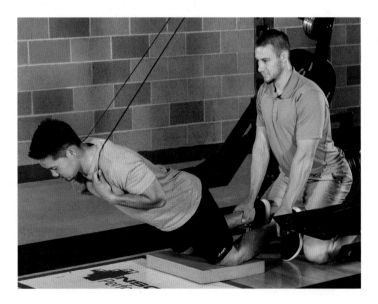

TIPS

- Avoid flexion and extension of the spine.
- The intensity of this exercise can be changed by altering the tension of the band. The more tension in the band, the less intense the exercise. Exceptionally trained athletes may be able to do this exercise without a band.

Hip Thrust

Gluteals, hamstrings

▶ **STARTING POSITION**

1. Place a barbell (with plates or bumpers) on the floor next to of a bench. Sit on the floor with the upper back against a bench and the legs beneath the barbell.

2. Roll the bar up the thigh until it is positioned across the hips (approximately right above the hip crease). A pad may be used for comfort. Grip the bar at the sides of the hips.

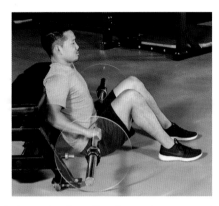

3. Bend the knees to about 90 degrees and place the feet firmly on the ground approximately shoulder-width apart. Then, shift the body back to place the shoulders on top of the bench.

▼ **ACTION**

4. Elevate the body off the floor by fully extending the hips and squeezing the glutes. The feet should remain planted firmly on the floor, and the shoulders should remain planted firmly on top of the bench. Maintain a neutral spine throughout the entire movement.

5. Return to the starting position using the same path used for the upward movement.

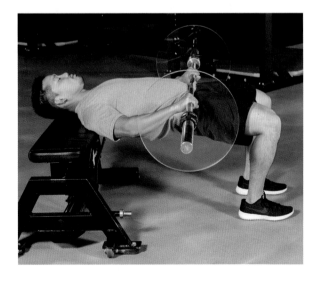

Banded Good Morning

Gluteals, hamstrings

▶ STARTING POSITION

1. Step into a long band with both legs so that the band loops under the soles and around the outer portion of the feet.

2. Pull the band up over the head and position it comfortably around the upper shoulders and trapezius. Loosely grip the band at the chest directly below the clavicle.

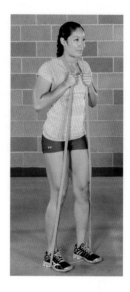

▶ ACTION

3. With the feet planted firmly on the floor about shoulder-width apart, push the hips back to decrease the angle between the torso and thigh.

4. Lower the torso until it is about parallel to the floor or until right before you can no longer maintain good posture. Maintain a neutral spine.

5. Return to the starting position by extending the hips and using the same path used for the downward movement. The knees should remain static and maintain the same amount of flexion throughout the entire movement.

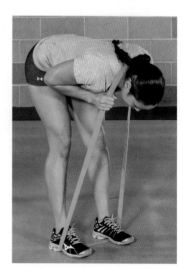

TIP

The intensity of this exercise can be changed by altering the tension of the band. The more tension in the band, the more intense the exercise.

Glute Bridge With Sliders

Gluteals, hamstrings

▶ **STARTING POSITION**

1. Position the body faceup on the floor with the heels resting on the sliders.

2. With the legs approximately shoulder-width apart, bend the knees to about 90 degrees. The sliders should remain between the feet and the floor.

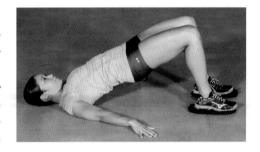

3. Elevate the lower and middle portion of the torso off the floor by fully extending the hips and squeezing the glutes. Maintain a neutral spine.

▼ **ACTION**

4. Fully extend one leg by sliding the slider across the floor. Keep the hips elevated and the opposite leg in starting position.

5. Return to the starting position using the same path used for the outward movement.

6. Repeat this movement with the other leg.

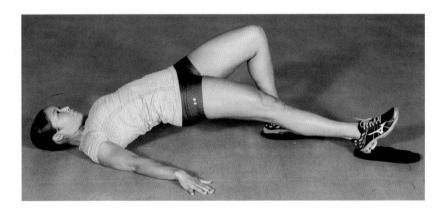

TIPS

- The intensity of this exercise can be increased by extending both legs simultaneously.
- Additionally, two long resistance bands can be used to increase intensity. Loop the resistance bands around a rack and slip each foot into the top of each band. Start the exercise with the bands in a taut state.

Seated Leg Curl

Hamstrings

▶ **MACHINE SETUP**

1. Position the back pad so that the knee joints align with the machine's axis of rotation.

2. Adjust the leg pad so that it is positioned just under the ankles when the knees are extended.

3. Select the appropriate resistance on the weight stack.

4. Sit straight up with the back firmly against the backrest and the head in a neutral position. Grasp the handles at the sides.

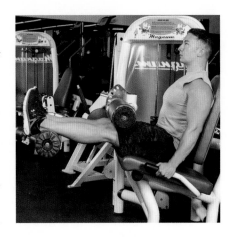

▼ **ACTION**

5. Bend the knees in a controlled motion to move the pad until the heels are beneath the seat and the knees are bent to about 90 degrees.

6. Return to the starting position in a slow and controlled manner. Do not allow the resistance to rest on the weight stack between reps.

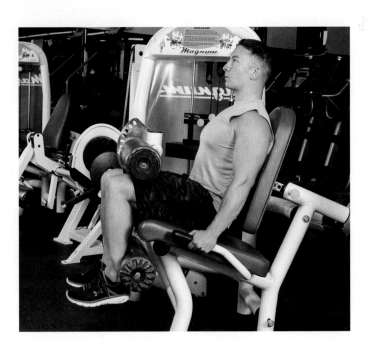

Seated Hip Adduction

Hip adductors

▶ MACHINE SETUP

1. Sit down with the feet on the foot plates and the knees bent 90 degrees.

2. Adjust the starting position so that you feel a slight stretch on the inner thighs.

3. Select the appropriate resistance on the weight stack.

4. Sit straight up with the back firmly against the backrest and the head in a neutral position. Grasp the handles at the sides.

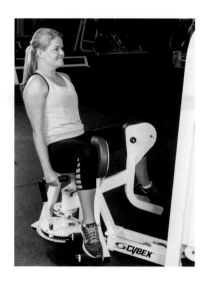

▶ ACTION

5. In a controlled motion, move the pads toward one another by pushing inward at the hips with the inner part of the leg. Keep the knees in line with the shins and ankles.

6. Return to the starting position in a slow and controlled manner. Do not allow the resistance to rest on the weight stack between reps.

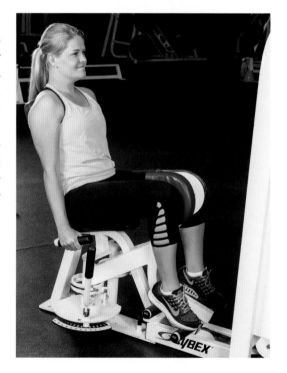

Seated Hip Abduction

Hip abductors

▶ MACHINE SETUP

1. Sit down with the feet on the foot plates and the knees bent 90 degrees.

2. Adjust the starting position so that the feet are close together and the foot plates are touching or almost touching.

3. Select the appropriate resistance on the weight stack.

4. Sit straight up with the back firmly against the backrest and the head in a neutral position. Grasp the handles at the sides.

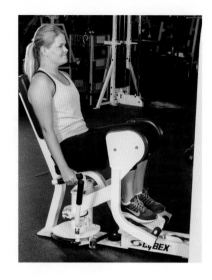

▶ ACTION

5. In a controlled motion, move the pads away from one another by pushing outward at the hips with the outer part of the leg. Keep the knees in line with the shins and ankles.

6. Return to the starting position in a slow and controlled manner. Do not allow the resistance to rest on the weight stack between reps.

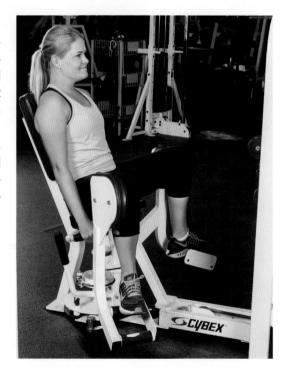

Calf Raise

Gastrocnemius, soleus

▼ STARTING POSITION

1. Position the rack so that the bar is approximately at shoulder height.
2. Step under the bar to place it on the upper portion of the back and shoulders.
3. Grip the bar at a comfortable position, about a thumb's length from the knurling or slightly wider than shoulder width.
4. Lift the bar off the rack and step back, placing the legs about hip-width apart.

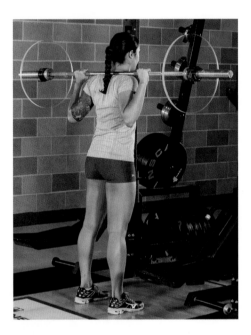

TIPS

- The same exercise can be performed holding dumbbells at the sides of the body in order to limit spinal loading. Additionally, the balls of the feet can be placed on a flat-lying plate to increase the range of motion of the exercise.
- To achieve greater activation of the soleus, the same exercise can also be performed in a seated position with knees at 90 degrees. Position plates or dumbbells on the thighs to add resistance.

▼ ACTION

5. Elevate the body by plantar flexing the ankles and allowing the heels to come off the floor.

6. Fully plantar flex the ankles while remaining on the balls of the feet.

7. Return to the starting position using the same path used for the upward movement.

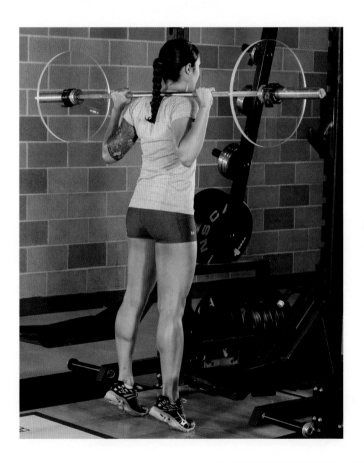

Tib Raise

Tibialis anterior

▶ **STARTING POSITION**

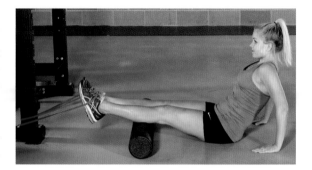

1. Wrap a long band around the side of a squat rack so that both ends are positioned toward the body.

2. While seated on the floor, place a foam roller under the calves. Position the ends of the band around both feet at the laces of the shoe.

3. Scoot the body back so that there is adequate tension in the band.

▼ **ACTION**

4. Dorsiflex the ankle toward the shin using the tension of the band as resistance.

5. Slowly return to the starting position using the same path.

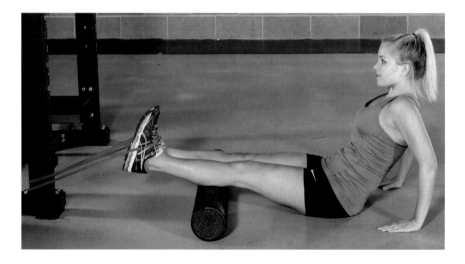

TIP

The same exercise can be performed seated on a bench with a dumbbell positioned between the feet. Place the calves off the bench, parallel to the floor, and perform the same action.

11

Torso Exercises

Andrew J. Galpin and James R. Bagley

Torso (or "core") muscles serve several functions, including stabilizing the spine and pelvis during complex movements (e.g., running, squatting, throwing) and everyday activities (e.g., walking, standing, sitting up).[1] These muscle groups are especially important because they connect lower-body muscles to upper-body muscles, helping transfer forces generated by the legs to the arms and vice versa (figure 11.1, *a* through *c*).

Personal trainers, strength and conditioning specialists, and health care professionals often prescribe torso exercises for both rehabilitation and general strengthening. Abdominal crunches are probably the most popular of these, and although they can be effective, their benefits are limited because they utilize only one muscle group (i.e., rectus abdominis). Therefore, a complete torso training program should include numerous exercises that engage multiple muscle groups (e.g., pelvis, lower back, middle back, sides, rib cage) in a wide range of movements.

This chapter offers many exercises with varying levels of difficulty. We encourage you to explore each exercise and progress at your own pace. It is important to note that performing torso exercises improperly may agitate—or even cause—lower-back injuries. Therefore, maintain proper position of the head, spine, and hips at all times; they should be in the neutral position, not in exaggerated flexion or extension. Quality is more important than quantity!

The authors acknowledge the significant contributions of Michael Barnes and Keith E. Cinea to this chapter.

[1]*Core muscles* should not be confused with *core lifts,* such as the squat, deadlift, and other compound exercises that use large muscle groups.

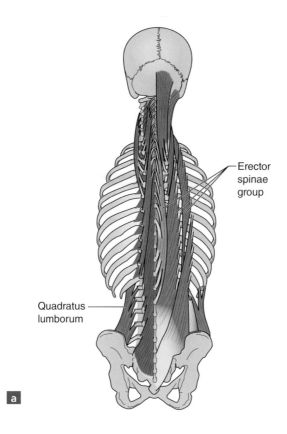

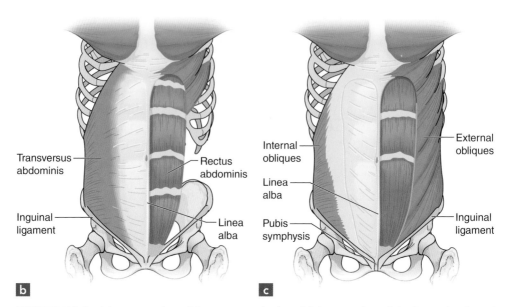

FIGURE 11.1 Major muscles of the torso, including (a) the muscles of the lower back and (b and c) the abdominal muscles.

Bent-Knee Sit-Up

Rectus abdominis

▼ STARTING POSITION

1. Lie faceup on the floor with the fingertips lightly touching each side of the head.
2. Bend the knees to place the feet flat on the floor, and lift the head off the floor.

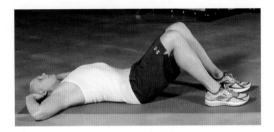

▼ ACTION

3. Keeping the feet flat on the floor, curl the torso off the floor, moving the head and shoulders toward the thighs until the upper back is off the floor.
4. Return to the starting position following the same path used for the upward movement.

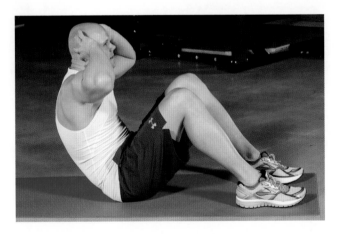

TIPS

- Curl all the way up until the upper back is off the floor.
- Keep the feet flat on the floor throughout the movement.
- Do not jerk the torso or arms to provide momentum to assist the movement.

Abdominal Crunch

Rectus abdominis

▶ **STARTING POSITION**

1. Lie faceup on the floor with the feet on a bench to allow for a 90-degree bend at the knees and hips.
2. With the fingertips at each side of the head, lift the head off the floor.

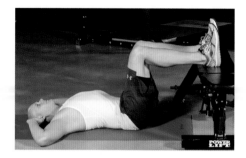

▼ **ACTION**

3. Keeping the feet in position on the bench, curl the torso off the floor, moving the head and shoulders toward the thighs until the upper back is off the floor.
4. Return to the starting position following the same path used for the upward movement.

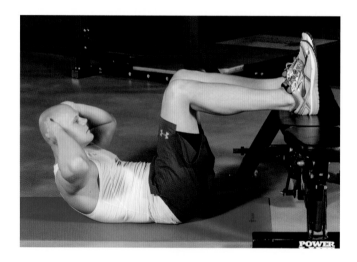

TIPS

- Curl all the way up until the upper back is off the floor.
- Keep the feet on the bench throughout the movement.
- Do not jerk the torso or arms to provide momentum to assist the movement.

Ankle Touch

Rectus abdominis

▼ STARTING POSITION

1. Lie faceup on the floor and bend the knees to place the feet flat on the floor.
2. Place the arms to the sides, and lift the head off the floor.

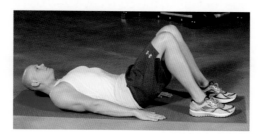

▼ ACTION

3. Keeping the feet flat on the floor, curl the torso off the floor, moving the hands until they touch the ankles or you are not able to reach any further.
4. Return to the starting position following the same path used for the upward movement.

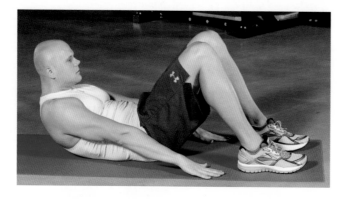

TIPS

- Curl until you touch the ankles or until you cannot move any farther.
- Keep the feet flat on the floor throughout the movement.
- Do not jerk the torso or arms to provide momentum to assist the movement.

Stability Ball Crunch

Rectus abdominis

When using a stability ball, select one that is the proper size for your body. When you are seated on the ball, both your hips and knees should be at about 90-degree angles. Also, be certain that the stability ball is inflated to the proper size before using it. If the ball is under- or overinflated, serious injuries could result. Table 11.1 provides a general guide for finding the correctly-sized ball based on your height.

Table 11.1 Stability Ball Sizing Guidelines

If your body height is	You need a ball this size
Up to 4 ft 10 in. (147 cm)	Small: 45 cm
4 ft 10 in. to 5 ft 5 in. (147-165 cm)	Medium: 55 cm
5 ft 5 in. to 6 ft 0 in. (165-183 cm)	Large: 65 cm
6 ft 0 in. to 6 ft 5 in. (183-196 cm)	X large: 75 cm
More than 6 ft 5 in. (196 cm)	XX large: 85 cm

▼ **STARTING POSITION**

1. Start in a seated position on the ball and roll forward until the middle of the back is supported on the ball, and the torso is approximately parallel to the floor.
2. Keep the feet flat on the floor and place the fingertips at each side of the head.

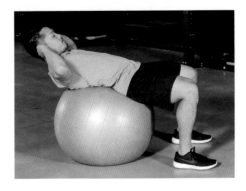

▼ ACTION

3. Keeping the feet flat on the floor, curl the torso upward by moving the head and shoulders until the upper back is off and the lower back remains on the ball.

4. Return to the starting position following the same path used for the upward movement.

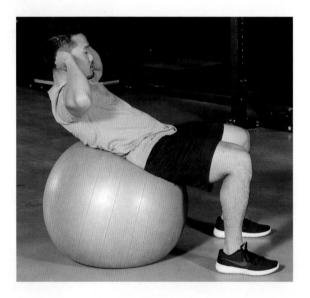

TIPS

- Avoid rolling on the ball.
- Keep the feet flat on the floor throughout the movement.
- Do not jerk the torso or arms to provide momentum to assist the movement.
- You can work the obliques by performing this same movement while lying with the side of the torso on the ball and then curling the torso upward.

Roll-Out

Rectus abdominis

▶ STARTING POSITION

1. Kneel on the floor and place the hands on the stability ball directly in front of the body.
2. Position the feet and knees slightly wider than shoulder width.

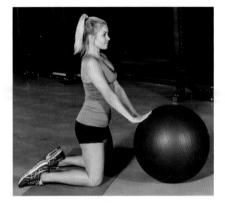

▼ ACTION

3. Reach forward and roll out on the forearms until the movement becomes too difficult for you to go any farther forward or until the body is fully extended. Do not let the hips sag or do not hyperextend the low back. Shoulders, hips, and knees should remain in line when fully extended.
4. Return to the starting position following the same path used for the outward movement.

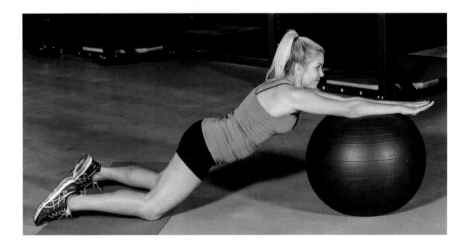

TIPS

- Maintain a neutral spine position.
- Keep the abdominal muscles tight.

Jackknife

Rectus abdominis

▶ STARTING POSITION

1. Lie facedown and support the body in a plank or push-up position, with the hands placed on the floor slightly wider than shoulder width.
2. Place one leg at a time on top of the stability ball until both upper shins are in contact with the ball.

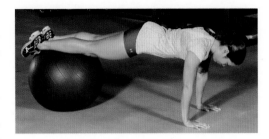

▼ ACTION

3. Keeping the feet together, slowly pull the feet and knees in toward the torso until they are fully drawn in. Flex the knees and hips to roll the ball toward the chest. Shoulders remain over the hands with the head in neutral position for the entire movement. Hips must raise slightly to allow hip and knee flexion to roll the ball forward.
4. Slowly return to the starting position following the same path used for the inward movement.

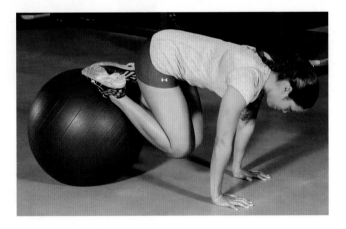

TIPS

- Maintain a neutral spine position.
- Avoid letting the ball move to the side of the legs or letting the hips drop.
- Keep the abdominal muscles tight.

Medicine Ball Overhead Reach

Rectus abdominis

▶ STARTING POSITION

1. Sit slightly to the front of the top of a stability ball, with the torso at about a 45-degree angle.

2. Hold a medicine ball directly in front of the torso with the arms straight.

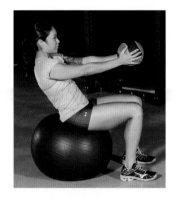

▶ ACTION

3. Keeping the arms straight and the spine neutral, slowly raise the medicine ball upward until it is directly overhead or until it reaches a level just before the torso position cannot be maintained.

4. Slowly return to the starting position following the same path used for the upward movement.

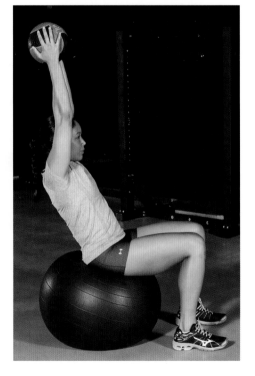

TIPS

- Avoid using a medicine ball that is too heavy.
- Keep the abdominal muscles tight.
- Although this movement actively uses the shoulders, the muscles of the torso are extremely involved in an effort to stabilize the body and control the movement.

Hanging Leg Raise

Rectus abdominis

▶ STARTING POSITION

1. Grip a pull-up bar with the hands shoulder-width apart and facing forward. Allow the body to hang. Arms should be fully extended.

2. If your grip strength is not sufficient, this exercise can be modified by using hanging ab straps that attach to the bar. Place the arms in the ab straps with the elbows bent 90 degrees.

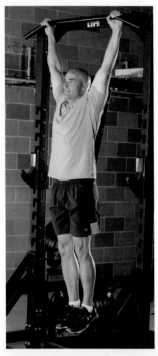

▶ ACTION

3. Contract the abdominal muscles to raise the legs up while bending the knees to a 90-degree angle. To make this exercise more difficult, keep the legs straight at the knee joint throughout the entire range of motion.

4. Lower the legs to the hanging position and repeat.

TIP

Control the body to reduce swinging during the leg-raising motion.

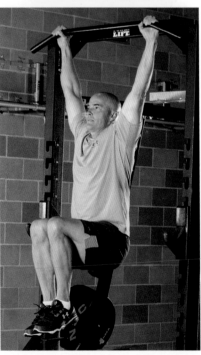

Cable Crunch

Rectus abdominis

MACHINE SETUP

1. Attach a triceps rope to a cable machine and move the cable to the top position.
2. Choose a weight that is challenging but that still allows for perfect technique. Start with a light weight to practice technique.

▶ STARTING POSITION

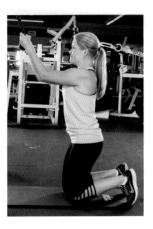

3. Kneel down below the cable with the knees shoulder-width apart. Grip the triceps rope with the palms facing each other. Arms are bent to approximately 90 degrees.

▼ ACTION

4. Keep the head and spine in a neutral position while bending at the hips until the head is just above the ground.
5. Keep the core tight, even when returning to the starting position.

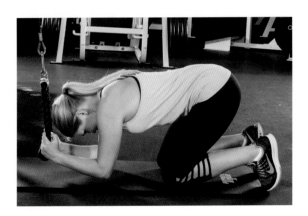

Alternate-Touch Crunch

Rectus abdominis, internal obliques, external obliques

▶ STARTING POSITION

1. Lie faceup on the floor with the feet on a bench to allow for a 90-degree bend at the knees and hips.
2. With the fingertips placed lightly behind the head, lift the head off the floor.

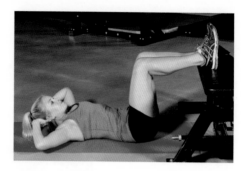

▼ ACTION

3. Keeping the feet on the bench, twist the torso by leading with the shoulder toward the opposite knee until the upper back is off the floor.
4. Return to the starting position following the same path used for the upward movement.
5. Alternate from one side to the other with each repetition.

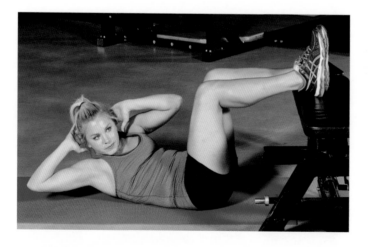

TIPS

- Rotate until the upper back is off the floor.
- Keep the feet on the bench throughout the movement.

Russian Twist

Rectus abdominis, internal obliques, external obliques

▼ STARTING POSITION

1. Lie faceup on the floor. Bend the knees to place the feet flat on the floor, and lift the head off the floor.
2. Keep the spine neutral, with the torso off the floor at a 45-degree angle.
3. Hold the arms straight away from the body with the hands locked together. You can also hold a dumbbell or kettlebell to increase difficulty.

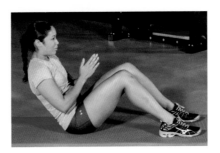

▼ ACTION

4. Rotate the arms from one side to another in a controlled twisting motion without stopping between repetitions.

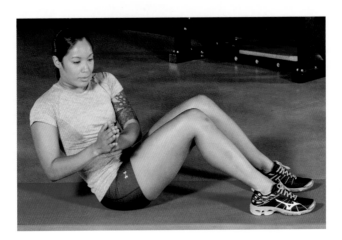

TIPS

- Keep the feet flat on the floor and make sure to continue breathing throughout the movement.
- Slow down the action of the twists to increase difficulty.

Outside Calf Touch

Rectus abdominis, internal obliques, external obliques

▼ STARTING POSITION

1. Lie faceup on the floor and bend the knees so that the feet are flat on the floor.
2. Place the hands on top of one another, reaching toward the knees.
3. Lift the head off the floor.

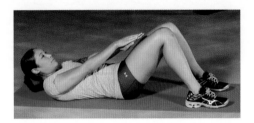

▼ ACTION

4. Keeping the feet flat on the floor, curl and rotate the torso off the floor, moving the hands toward the outside of one calf until they touch it.
5. Return to the starting position following the same path used for the upward movement.
6. Alternate from one side to the other with each repetition.

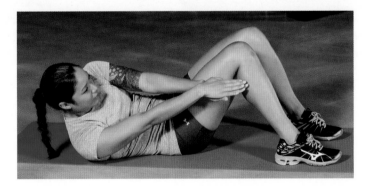

TIPS

- Curl upward until the hands touch the outside of the calf.
- Keep the feet on the floor throughout the movement.

Prone Plank

Rectus abdominis, internal obliques, external obliques

▼ STARTING POSITION

1. Lie facedown with the feet hip-width apart.

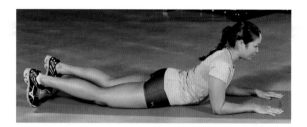

▼ ACTION

2. Bend the elbows to about 90 degrees directly under the shoulders, place the palms flat on the floor, and push off the floor.
3. Keep the spine and head neutral and aligned with the torso so that the ankles, knees, hips, shoulders, and head are in a straight line.
4. Hold the position until failure or for the desired duration.

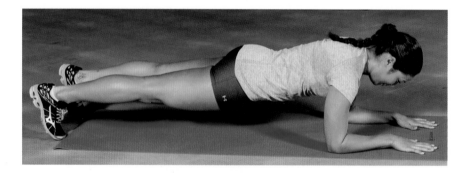

TIPS

- Keep the spine and head neutral by activating the abdominal muscles.
- Focus on the lower portion of the abdominal muscles.

Side Plank

Internal obliques, external obliques

▼ STARTING POSITION

1. Lie on your side with the feet stacked on top of each other. Bend one elbow to about 90 degrees and place it under the shoulder.

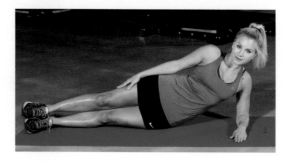

▼ ACTION

2. Keeping the spine and head neutral and in line with the torso, raise your hips off the floor until the bottom ankle, knee, hip, and shoulder are in a straight line.
3. Hold the position until failure or for the desired duration.
4. Switch and repeat with the other side.

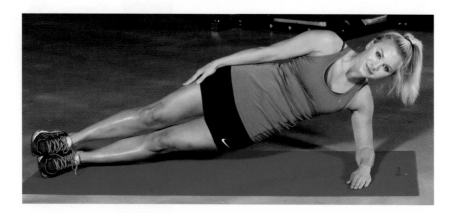

TIP

Keep the spine and head neutral by contracting the internal and external obliques.

Side Bend

Internal obliques, external obliques

▶ STARTING POSITION

1. Stand with feet shoulder-width apart. Hold a weight (kettlebell, dumbbell, or weight plate) in one hand at the side.

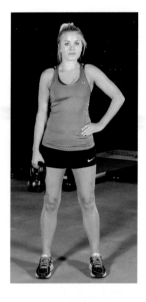

▶ ACTION

2. Bend the upper body to the weighted side without leaning forward or backward. Keep the thoracic spine and neck neutral while bending at the lumbar spine to the point of oblique stretch but not discomfort.

3. Contract the oblique, raising the weight and returning your back to your neutral position.

4. After completing the desired number of repetitions, switch the weight to the opposite side and repeat.

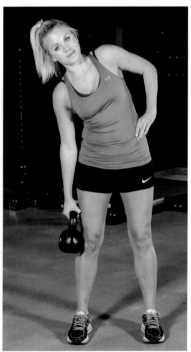

TIP

Choose a weight that is challenging but that still allows for perfect technique. Start with a light weight to practice technique.

Stability Ball Shoulder Roll

Erector spinae, internal obliques, external obliques

▶ STARTING POSITION

1. Sit on the ball and roll forward until the upper back is supported on the ball and the knees are bent to 90 degrees.
2. Place the feet flat on the floor slightly wider than shoulder width.
3. Cross the arms over the chest.

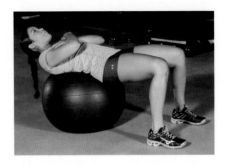

▼ ACTION

4. Keeping the feet flat on the floor, rotate the torso by rolling up on the ball with one shoulder until the upper back is off the ball.
5. Return to the starting position following the same path used for the upward movement.
6. Alternate from one side to the other.

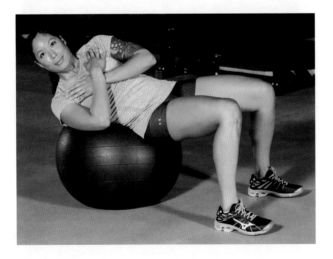

TIPS

- Curl all the way up until the upper back is off the ball.
- Keep the feet flat on the floor throughout the movement.

Back Extension

Erector spinae, gluteals, hamstrings

▶ MACHINE SETUP

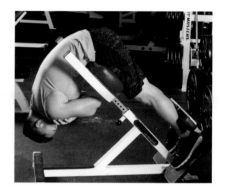

1. Adjust the foot pad so the upper thighs rest on the hips and upper thighs.
2. Position yourself in the machine so that the legs are nearly straight and the torso is approximately 90 degrees from the legs. Keep the neck and spine neutral.
3. Cross the arms over the chest.

▼ ACTION

4. Extend at the hips, raising the torso in a controlled and smooth motion until it forms a straight line with the legs.
5. Return to the starting position following the same path used for the upward movement.

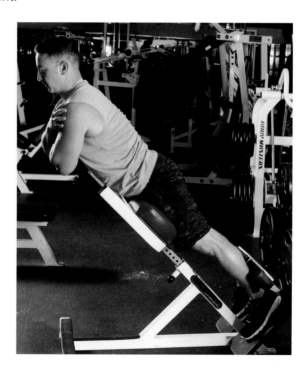

TIPS

- Avoid exaggerating the range of motion and rounding the back and shoulders during the movement.
- Maintain a neutral spine throughout the movement.

Quadruped Walking

Rectus abdominis, erector spinae, internal obliques, external obliques, rhomboid major, rhomboid minor

▶ **STARTING POSITION**

1. Get on your hands and the balls of your feet, with your fingers and toes pointed forward.
2. Fully extend the arms and make sure the knees are in line with the feet.
3. Keep the spine neutral from the hips to the head. The neck should not be extended, the shoulders should not be rounded, and the low back should not have an extended arch or dip.

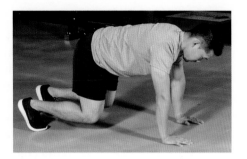

▼ **ACTION**

4. Walk by moving the hand and foot on the same side of the body. Repeat with the opposite hand and foot, as shown in photo.
5. Walk in all directions (i.e., forward, backward, both sides, and even at angles).

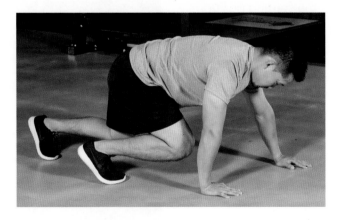

TIP

Maintain the neutral positions of the head, shoulders, back, and hips while moving the legs and arms.

Perpendicular Band Press

Rectus abdominis, erector spinae, internal obliques, external obliques, rhomboid major, rhomboid minor

▶ **STARTING POSITION**

1. Hold an elastic band or the machine cable perpendicular to the machine with both hands at the center of the chest and assume a standing, half-kneeling, or kneeling position. Both hands should be holding the band or cable close to the chest. Both arms are flexed.

2. Keep the neck and spine neutral at all times.

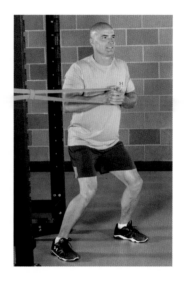

▶ **ACTION**

3. Slowly extend the elbows until they are fully extended, and then return to the starting position.

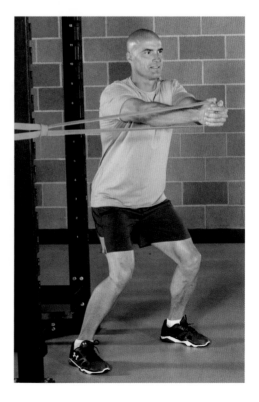

Hollow Position

Rectus abdominis, internal obliques, external obliques, gluteals

▼ STARTING POSITION

1. Lie faceup on the floor. Point the toes toward the ceiling and extend the arms above the head.
2. Keep the lower back pressed to the floor in a neutral position.

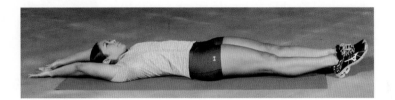

▼ ACTION

3. Keeping the spine neutral, contract the gluteal and torso muscles to slightly lift the feet, arms, neck, and upper back off the floor. Keep the arms and legs extended throughout the entire movement.
4. Hold the position for the desired duration.

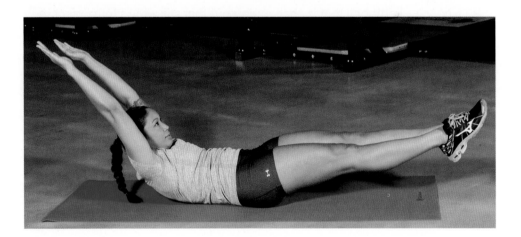

TIP
Keeping the glutes squeezed and pulling the belly button to the floor helps minimize any excessive arching of the lower back.

Kettlebell Swing

Rectus abdominis, erector spinae, gluteals, latissimus dorsi, deltoids, quadriceps, hamstrings

▶ **STARTING POSITION**

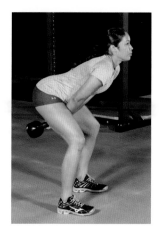

1. Stand over the kettlebell with the feet flat and shoulder-width apart, the toes facing forward or slightly outward, the chest up, and the shoulders back.

2. With a neutral spine, squat down and grip the kettlebell with both hands, palms facing back, with the thumbs wrapped around the handles and the index fingers touching or close together.

3. Grip the kettlebell and stand up, maintaining a neutral spine. Keep the elbows fully extended and the shoulders back, engaging the torso muscles.

4. Shift your body weight toward the heels and soften the knees and hips to a quarter-squat position, with the kettlebell hanging between the thighs.

TIPS

- Choose a kettlebell that is challenging but that still allows for perfect technique. Start with a light kettlebell to practice technique.
- Allow the kettlebell to swing back between the legs and continue.
- Drive through the heels, gluteals, and hips as the kettlebell swings from back to front.

▼ ACTION

5. Flex at the hips to allow the kettlebell to swing backward between the legs. Keep the knees in the same starting flexed position, with the back neutral and the arms extended.

6. Allow the kettlebell to swing backward until the torso is nearly parallel to the floor. The kettlebell should be past the vertical line of the body.

7. Push through the heels, contract the gluteal muscles, and extend the hips and knees to swing the kettlebell upward. Allow momentum to swing the kettlebell up to eye height, keeping the arms extended. At the top of the movement, engage the torso muscles.

8. Control the weight during the descent, and flex at the hips.

9. Prepare the body for the next swing by shifting the weight back toward the heels while bending at the hips, loading the hamstrings and glutes.

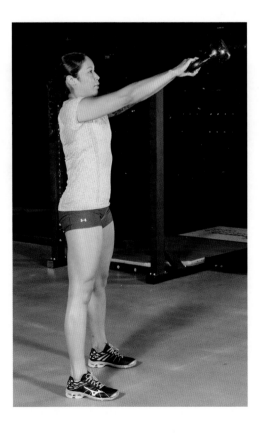

Modified Superman

Erector spinae, internal obliques, external obliques, rhomboid major, rhomboid minor, gluteus maximus

▶ STARTING POSITION

1. Lie facedown perpendicularly across a flat bench.
2. Raise the arms straight in front of the body while elevating the legs so that only the torso is touching the bench. Contract the back muscles to hold up the arms and legs.

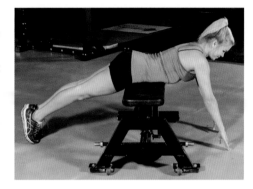

▼ ACTION

3. Align the head (do not lift the neck by looking up), torso, and feet so that all are approximately the same distance from the floor. Keep the spine neutral (not overextended).
4. Hold the plank-like position until failure or for the desired duration.

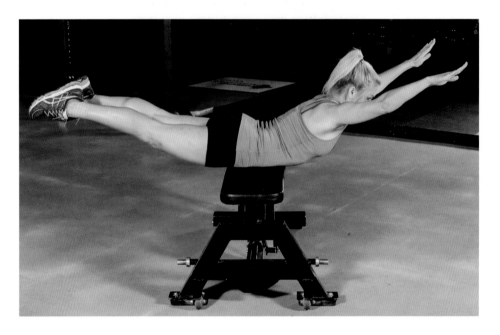

TIPS

- Keep the spine neutral by drawing the belly button in and activating the lower-back, gluteal, and shoulder blade muscles.
- Make sure to continue breathing while holding the position.

12

Explosive Movements

Andrew J. Galpin and J. Albert Bartolini

Explosive strength training benefits all lifters. Performing explosive exercises increases the lifter's ability to rapidly produce and absorb force. These improved abilities benefit athletes in particular because nearly all sports require forceful movements at high speeds. For example, athletes need to accelerate, decelerate, stop, jump, land, and change direction. By performing the exercises included in this chapter, lifters will increase their ability to produce explosive movements. The increased ability to produce explosive power also has implications in day-to-day life because speed is needed to avoid tripping and falling, lift a child, or load equipment onto a truck.

Ground-based explosive movements help develop power through the improved coordination of a particular movement sequence called *triple extension* (i.e., extension of the ankles, knees, and hips), which is fundamental to human locomotion. Improving the coordination of the triple extension enhances an athlete's ability to produce ground forces, which inevitably increases athletic performance.

Many explosive resistance exercises exist, and each varies in complexity. The exercises included in this chapter are some of the most fundamental and frequently used. Although intended to produce force rapidly, the exercises can be executed safely because they can be scaled to the ability of the lifter. It is common for these exercises to be introduced and taught by using unloaded bars and dowels. When properly used, explosive exercises are safe and likely to reduce the risk of injury during sport and day-to-day activities. However, explosive movements are some of the most complex and physically difficult exercises a lifter can perform; highly skilled and qualified strength and conditioning specialists should be consulted when implementing them. Strict adherence to technique is strongly encouraged.

The authors acknowledge the significant contributions of Michael Barnes and Keith E. Cinea to this chapter.

Power Clean

Gluteals, hamstrings, quadriceps, gastrocnemius,
soleus, deltoids, trapezius

▼ STARTING POSITION

1. Approach the barbell on the floor and take a pronated grip on the bar slightly wider than shoulder width. Your arms should be outside your knees.
2. Keep the arms straight, the wrists slightly flexed, and the elbows locked and rotated outward.
3. Stand with the feet flat and hip- to shoulder-width apart. Hold the barbell approximately one inch (2.5 cm) in front of the shins.
4. Pull the shoulders back, elevate the chest, and keep the eyes looking forward with a neutral spine and head.
5. Keep the shoulders over or slightly in front of the barbell and your body weight on the forward half of the feet.

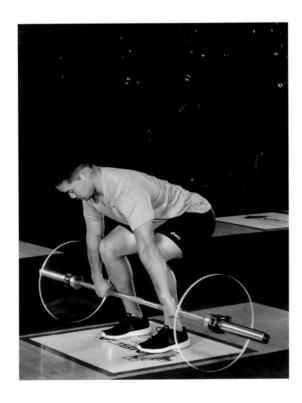

▼ FIRST PULL

6. Keeping the back neutral and the arms straight, extend the hips and knees to lift the barbell off the ground to the mid-thigh in a controlled manner. Avoid jerking the bar off the ground and rounding the back. Also avoid locking out the knees when moving the barbell from below the knees to mid-thigh height.

7. Look straight ahead and raise the shoulders and hips at the same speed.

8. Keep the bar as close to the shins as possible.

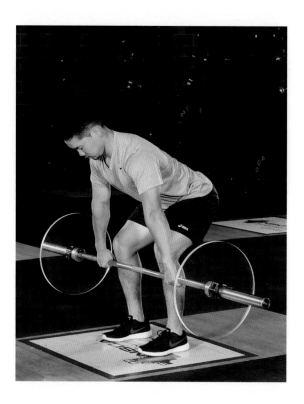

> continued

▼ TRANSITION

9. As the bar rises to just above the knees, thrust the hips forward and slightly bend the knees to move the thighs against and the knees under the bar. Note: The transition phase is similar to the Romanian deadlift; in fact, weightlifters often use the Romanian deadlift to strengthen this movement pattern.

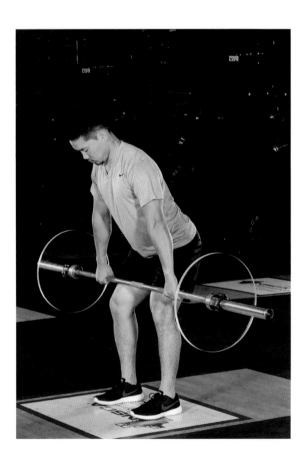

▼ SECOND PULL

10. Keeping the arms straight and the wrists slightly flexed with the bar at mid-thigh level, rapidly extend the hips, knees, and ankles (triple extension) to rise up on the toes.

11. As the legs complete triple extension, elevate the shoulders explosively.

12. Continue looking straight ahead as you elevate the barbell to around chest height without using the muscles in the arms.

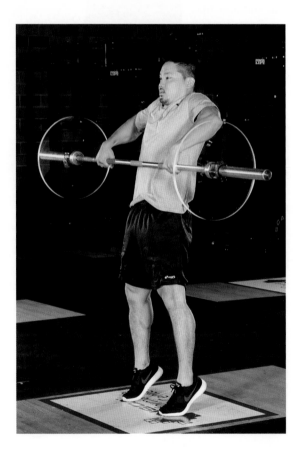

> continued

Power Clean *> continued*

▶ CATCH POSITION

13. When the bar has reached its maximum height, bend the elbows, rotating the arms around and under the bar, and drop under the bar into a quarter squat.

14. Once under the bar, immediately lift the elbows up so that the arms are parallel to the ground. If this is done properly, the bar will be received on the front of the shoulders at the same time that you reach the quarter squat. The shoulders should not slump forward.

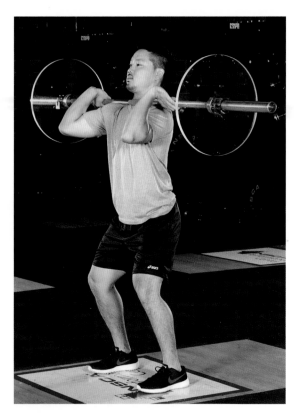

ENDING POSITION

15. Keeping the elbows high and the chest elevated, stand straight up.

16. If the movement is being performed on a proper lifting surface (e.g., platform) and with rubber weight plates (i.e., bumper plates), the bar can be unracked from the ending position by letting it drop to the floor. Carefully guide the bar to the floor with the hands.

17. If either a platform or bumpers are unavailable, the bar should be lowered carefully to the thighs while keeping the spine neutral. Gradually reduce the tension of the arms and slightly bend the knees and hips to cushion the impact. The bar can then be lowered to the floor while keeping the spine and neck neutral, or it can be placed on the rack supports.

High Pull

Gluteals, hamstrings, quadriceps, gastrocnemius, soleus, deltoids, trapezius

Similar to the power clean, the high pull is a variation of the clean. In fact, the power clean and the high pull share identical instructions for the starting position, first pull, transition, and second pull. However, in the high pull variation, the weight is not caught with bent elbows but rather is pulled explosively and allowed to return to the thigh position. Removing the catch phase may ease the burden on the elbow, wrist, and knee joints because it eliminates the eccentric loading that occurs during this action. Thus, although both exercises are similar, significant differences exist.

▼ STARTING POSITION

1. Approach the barbell on the floor and take a pronated grip on the bar slightly wider than shoulder width. Your arms should be outside your knees.
2. Keep the arms straight, the wrists slightly flexed, and the elbows locked and rotated outward.
3. Stand with the feet flat and hip- to shoulder-width apart. Hold the barbell approximately one inch (2.5 cm) in front of the shins.
4. Pull the shoulders back, elevate the chest, and keep the eyes looking forward with a neutral spine and head.
5. Keep the shoulders over or slightly in front of the barbell and your body weight on the forward half of the feet.

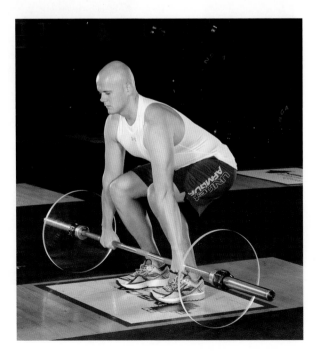

> continued

273

▼ FIRST PULL

6. Keeping the back neutral and the arms straight, extend the hips and knees to lift the barbell off the floor to mid-thigh in a controlled manner. Avoid jerking the bar off the floor and rounding the back. Also avoid locking out the knees when moving the barbell from below the knees to mid-thigh height.

7. Look straight ahead and raise the shoulders and hips at the same speed.

8. Keep the bar as close to the shins as possible.

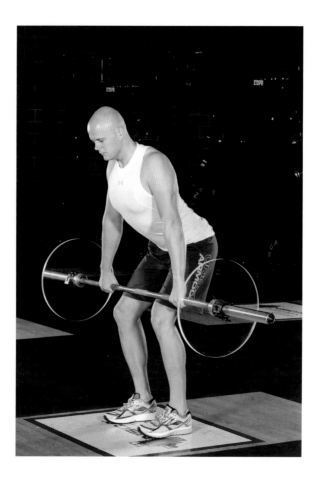

▼ TRANSITION

9. As the bar rises just above the knees, thrust the hips forward and slightly bend the knees to move the thighs against and the knees under the bar. Note: The transition phase is similar to the Romanian deadlift; in fact, weightlifters often use the Russian deadlift to strengthen this movement pattern.

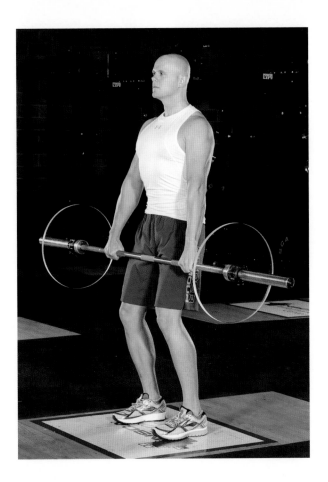

> *continued*

▼ SECOND PULL

10. Keeping the arms straight and the wrists slightly flexed with the bar at mid-thigh height, rapidly extend the hips, knees, and ankles (triple extension) to rise up on the toes.

11. As the legs complete triple extension, elevate the shoulders explosively.

12. Continue looking straight ahead as you elevate the barbell to about chest height without using the muscles of the arms.

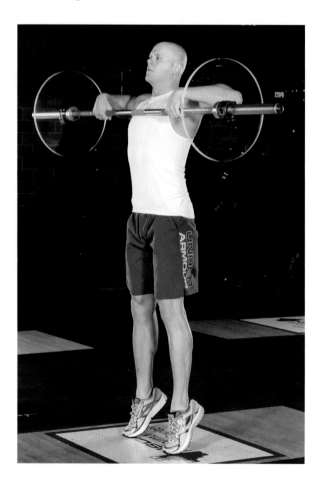

ENDING POSITION

13. When the bar has reached its maximum height around the level of the chest, let the bar return to a resting position on the thighs.

14. Once the bar is on the thighs, return it to the floor by squatting down. Keep the spine in the neutral position.

Hang Power Clean

Gluteals, hamstrings, quadriceps, gastrocnemius, soleus, deltoids, trapezius

Similar to the power clean, the hang power clean is a variation of the clean. In fact, the power clean and the hang power clean share identical instructions for the transition, second pull, catch, and ending position. However, in the hang power clean, the movement starts with the bar in the "hang" position (i.e., just above the knee) instead of on the floor. Removing the portion of the movement in which the bar gets from the floor to the thighs eases the burden on the low back. It also removes one of the more technically challenging phases of the lift, making the hang power clean a viable option for less experienced lifters. Thus, although both exercises are similar and beneficial, significant differences exist.

▶ STARTING POSITION

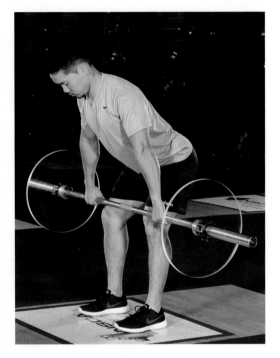

1. Approach the barbell on the floor and take a pronated grip on the bar slightly wider than shoulder width. Your arms should be outside your knees.

2. Keep the arms straight, the wrists slightly flexed, and the elbows locked and rotated outward.

3. Stand with the feet flat and hip- to shoulder-width apart. Hold the barbell approximately one inch (2.5 cm) in front of the shins.

4. Pull the shoulders back, elevate the chest, and keep the eyes looking forward with a neutral spine and head with weight distributed on the middle of both feet.

5. Squat down. Keeping the arms straight, spine neutral, and shoulders above or slightly in front of the bar, pull the bar from the ground to just above the knees in a controlled manner. This is the hang position.

> continued

▼ FIRST PULL

6. Keeping the back neutral, arms straight, and wrists slightly flexed, rapidly extend the hips and knees, lifting the bar to mid-thigh. Avoid jerking the bar, which will cause the back to round. Avoid locking out the knees.

7. Look straight ahead and raise the shoulders and hips at the same speed.

8. Pull the barbell without using the muscles in the arms, and keep the bar close to the body so that it is easier to control and balance.

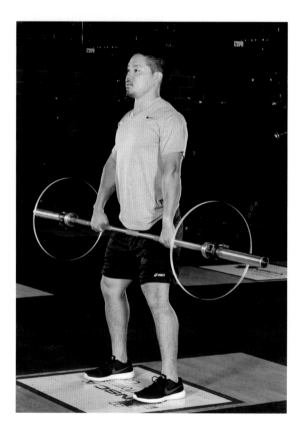

TRANSITION

9. As the bar rises just above the knees, thrust the hips forward and slightly bend the knees to move the thighs against and the knees under the bar. Note: The transition phase is similar to the Romanian deadlift; in fact, weightlifters use the Romanian deadlift to strengthen this movement pattern.

▼ SECOND PULL

10. Keeping the arms straight and the wrists slightly flexed with the bar at mid-thigh height, rapidly extend the hips, knees, and ankles (triple extension) to rise up on the toes.

11. As the legs complete triple extension, elevate the shoulders explosively.

12. Continue looking straight ahead as you elevate the barbell to about chest height without using the muscles in the arms.

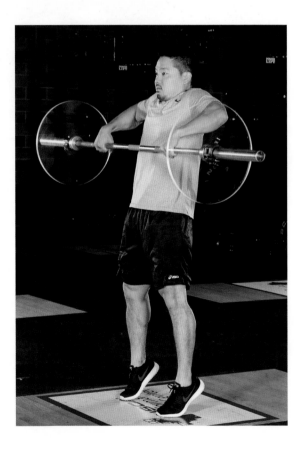

> continued

▶ CATCH POSITION

13. When the bar has reached its maximum height (around the level of the chest), bend the elbows, rotating the arms around and under the bar, and drop under the bar into a quarter squat.

14. Once under the bar, immediately lift the elbows up so that the arms are parallel to the floor. If this is done properly, the bar will be received on the front of the shoulders at the same time that you reach the quarter squat. Do not allow the shoulders to slump forward; this will make it more difficult to control the bar and could place more strain on the lower back.

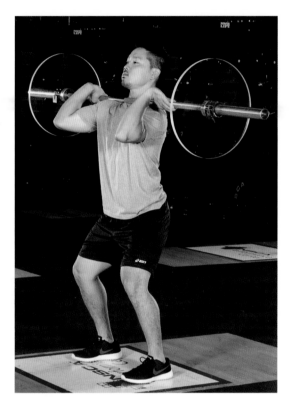

ENDING POSITION

15. Keeping the elbows high and the chest elevated, stand straight up.

16. If the movement is being performed on a proper lifting surface (e.g., platform) and with rubber weight plates (i.e., bumper plates), the bar can be unracked from the ending position by letting it drop to the floor. Carefully guide the bar to the floor with the hands.

17. If either a platform or bumpers are unavailable, the bar should be lowered carefully to the thighs while keeping the spine neutral. Gradually reduce the tension of the arms and slightly bend the knees and hips to cushion the impact. The bar can then be lowered to the floor while keeping the spine and neck neutral, or it can be placed on the rack supports.

Push Press

Gluteals, hamstrings, quadriceps, gastrocnemius, soleus, deltoids

▼ STARTING POSITION

1. Hold the bar on top of the clavicles and front of the shoulders with a grip that is slightly wider than shoulder width, palms facing up.
2. Stand with the spine neutral, the feet hip- to shoulder-width apart, and the eyes looking straight ahead.
3. Pull the shoulders back and elevate the chest.
4. Extend the hips and knees to lift the bar off the supports.
5. Step back, ensuring that the bar adequately clears the supports, and assume a position in which the feet are hip- to shoulder-width apart and even.

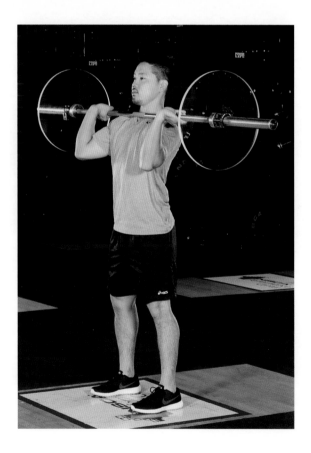

> continued

▼ THE DIP

6. Keeping your body weight toward the heels and the barbell on the shoulders, move into less than a quarter squat by pushing the hips back, bending the knees, and keeping the chest up.

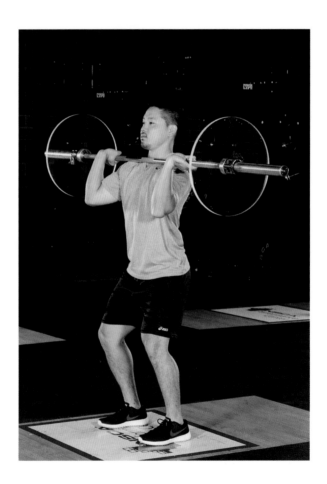

▼ THE DRIVE

7. Without pausing at the bottom of the dip, push upward with the legs by extending the hips, knees, and ankles and then extending the elbows. The act of driving upward will force the bar up off the shoulders.

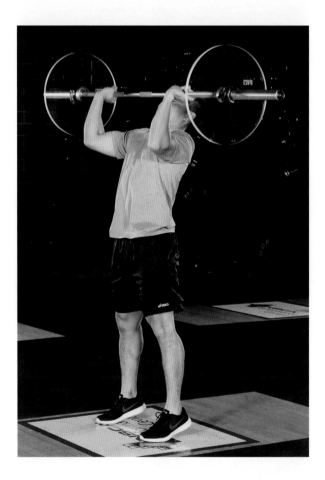

> continued

▼ CATCH POSITION

8. When the bar has reached its greatest height from the drive, continue to press until the arms are fully extended and the barbell is slightly over or behind the ears. The feet are flat during the catch.

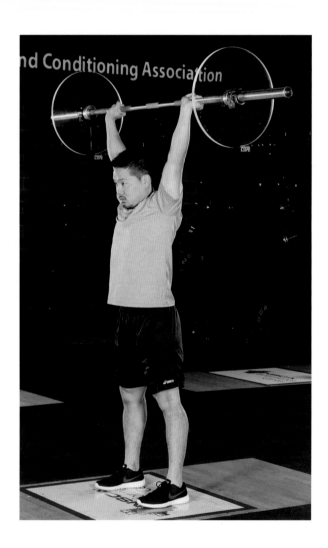

Push Jerk

Gluteals, hamstrings, quadriceps, gastrocnemius, soleus, deltoids

The push jerk and push press are another set of similar yet significantly different exercises. The push press combines leg drive and shoulder pressing, whereas the push jerk focuses almost entirely on the leg drive. During the push press, the shoulders and arms drive the bar up (concentric contraction), hold it overhead (isometric contraction), and lower it back down (eccentric contraction). However, the push jerk emphasizes using the legs almost exclusively to move the bar overhead; the shoulders and arms are used only to catch the bar at the top (eccentric contraction), hold it (isometric contraction), and lower it back down (eccentric contraction). The concentric actions of the shoulders and arms during the push jerk exist but are minimal compared with the forces generated from the legs or from the shoulders and arms during the push press.

▶ STARTING POSITION

1. Stand straight with the feet hip- to shoulder-width apart. Place the bar on top of the clavicles and the front of the shoulders.

2. Take a grip on the bar that is slightly wider than shoulder width, with the palms facing up.

3. Elevate the chest, pull the shoulders back, and tuck the chin.

4. Extend the hips and knees to lift the bar off the supports.

5. Step back, ensuring that the bar adequately clears the supports, and assume a position in which the feet are hip- to shoulder-width apart and even.

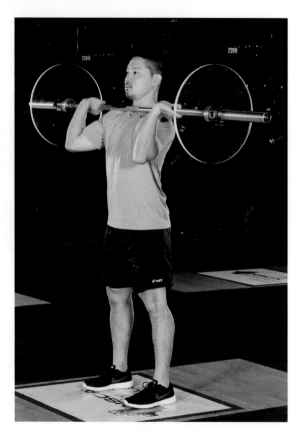

> continued

▼ THE DIP

6. Keeping your body weight on the heels, the barbell on the shoulders, and the chest up, quickly move into less than a quarter squat by pushing the hips back and bending the knees.

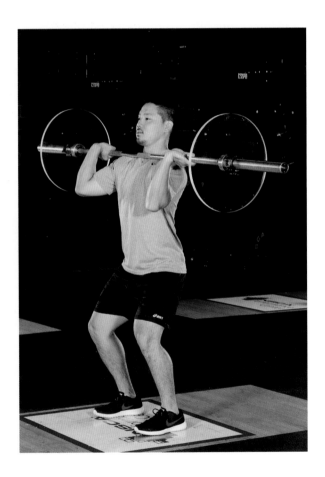

▼ THE DRIVE

7. Without pausing at the bottom of the dip, explosively reverse directions, driving straight up with the legs by extending the hips, knees, and ankles (triple extension) until rising up onto the toes, and then extend the elbows. The act of driving up will force the bar up off the shoulders.

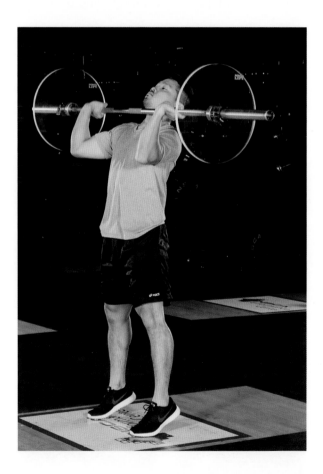

> continued

▼ CATCH POSITION

8. When the bar has reached its greatest height from the drive, quickly flex the hips and knees to a dipped position. Simultaneously continue to press the bar until the arms are extended and the barbell is received overhead at the same moment that the bar reaches its highest position.

9. Catch the bar with the torso erect, the head in a neutral position, feet flat on the floor with knees and hips to a quarter-squat position, and the bar slightly behind the head, forming a straight line through the body.

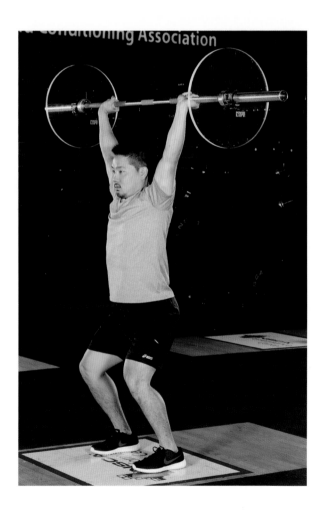

Medicine Ball Slam

Gluteals, hamstrings, quadriceps, gastrocnemius, soleus, deltoids, triceps, rectus abdominis

▶ STARTING POSITION

1. Stand with the feet slightly wider than shoulder-width apart. Hold a medicine ball with both hands directly in front of the chest, palms facing each other. The elbows should be bent and pointing toward the floor.

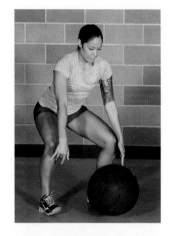

▶ ACTION

2. Lift the medicine ball above the head by fully extending the ankles, knees, hips, torso, and arms while standing on the balls of the feet.

3. Initiate the movement by using the lats and triceps to pull the arms down while simultaneously contracting the torso.

4. Slam the ball onto the floor as hard as possible at an angle slightly away from the body.

ENDING POSITION

5. Catch the ball with both hands on the bounce. Do not let the ball hit other exercisers. Do not let the ball strike your chest, head, or face. In the end position you are leaning over the top of the ball path, and the ball tends to bounce straight up or at a slight angle back to the thrower.

6. Return to the standing position and repeat the desired number of reps.

TIP

A major concern with this exercise is the ball striking the athlete on the rebound. Thus, use a medicine ball that is rubberized or otherwise not bouncy to reduce the risk of injury.

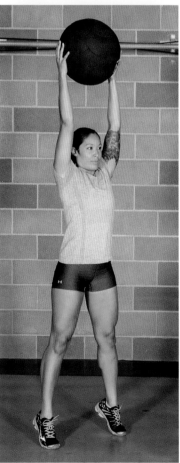

Medicine Ball Put

Pectoralis, anterior deltoid, triceps brachii

This exercise should be performed only in a safe environment, meaning a space free of equipment, other exercisers, and mirrors. The room should also offer a place for the medicine ball to land. A supported concrete wall designed for this purpose is ideal. Do not throw the ball against a wall made of drywall.

▶ STARTING POSITION

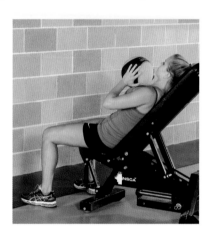

1. Sit comfortably on a 45-degree incline bench with the feet flat on the floor.
2. Grasp the medicine ball with both hands—one on each side.
3. Position the medicine ball against the chest with the elbows tucked in toward the body.

▶ ACTION

4. Without making additional body movement (e.g., trunk or neck flexion), propel ("put") the medicine ball for maximal horizontal distance by fully extending the arms.

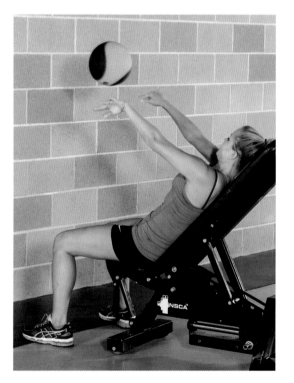

Medicine Ball Rotational Throw

Rectus abdominis, internal oblique, external oblique

▶ STARTING POSITION

1. Stand perpendicular to a wall or partner.
2. Hold the medicine ball over the left hip and bend the arms near the torso.

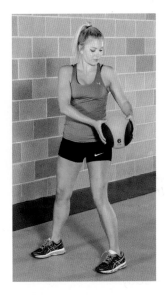

▶ ACTION

3. Shift the weight to the back leg (i.e., the leg farthest from the wall).
4. Push hard off the back leg while simultaneously turning the hips and shoulders toward the wall or partner.
5. Block (i.e., stiffen) the front leg while releasing the medicine ball. The back heel should come off of the ground while pivoting on the ball of the foot. The arms should be fully extended at the time the ball is released.

ENDING POSITION

6. Finish with the hips and shoulders facing the wall or partner.

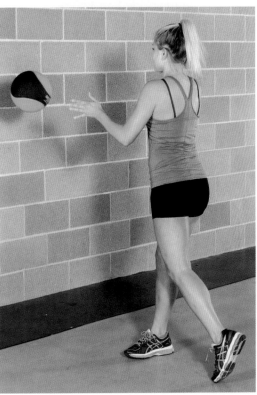

Clapping Push-Up

Pectoralis, anterior deltoid, triceps brachii

▼ STARTING POSITION

1. Assume a standard push-up position with the spine and head neutral, the feet close together, and the arms under the shoulders.

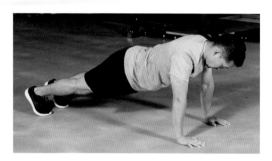

▼ ACTION

2. Lower the body, keeping the elbows close to the torso. Once in the bottom position, immediately accelerate the body upward by extending the elbows as rapidly as possible while maintaining a rigid posture through the knees, ships, and shoulders.

3. Once the upper body is in the air, clap the hands together. Return the hands to catch the upper body, and return to the standard push-up position.

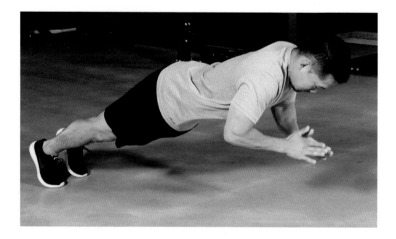

Countermovement Squat Jump

Gluteals, hamstrings, quadriceps, gastrocnemius, soleus

▶ STARTING POSITION

1. Assume a relaxed upright position with the spine neutral, the feet about shoulder-width apart, and the upper arms at the sides. Bend the elbows approximately 90 degrees.

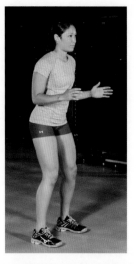

▶ ACTION

2. Begin by dipping to a quarter squat by flexing the hips and knees while moving the arms back.

3. Once the quarter squat is reached, immediately explode upward by extending the hips, knees, and ankles (triple extension) while simultaneously propelling the arms upward to help generate momentum.

ENDING POSITION

4. Land with slight flexion of the ankles, knees, and hips. Transition to flat feet while returning the arms to the starting position.

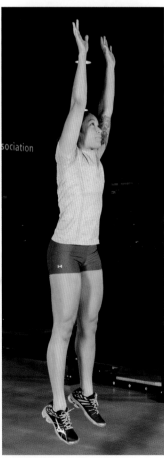

293

Split Jump

Gluteals, hamstrings, quadriceps, gastrocnemius, soleus

▶ **STARTING POSITION**

1. Assume a split stance: Extend one leg forward with the knee over the midpoint of the foot (i.e., bent approximately 90 degrees), and extend the other leg back with the knee bent (90 degrees) and under the hips and shoulders. The hip angle for the front leg should be approximately 90 degrees or slightly less. The hip angle for the back leg should be approximately 180 degrees or slightly less. Feet should be hip-width apart.

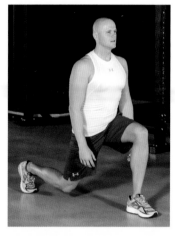

▶ **ACTION**

2. Jump as high as possible from this split stance while propelling the arms upward to generate momentum. Focus on exploding straight up without further flexing the hips or knees.

ENDING POSITION

3. As you land, return to the starting position by flexing the ankles, knees, and hips. After the desired number of repetitions are completed, switch the position of the legs.

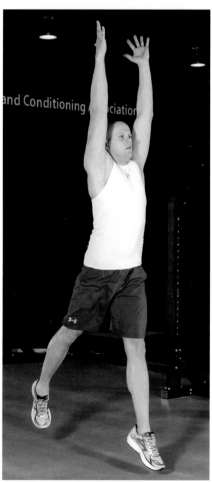

Suspension Trainer Sprinter's Start

Gluteals, hamstrings, quadriceps, gastrocnemius, soleus

▶ STARTING POSITION

1. Stand facing away from the suspension trainer with a neutral grip on the handles.

2. Position the arms over the straps between the arms and the torso, bend the elbows, and tuck the hands close to the body.

3. Stagger the feet, one stride length in front of the other, approximately hip-width apart.

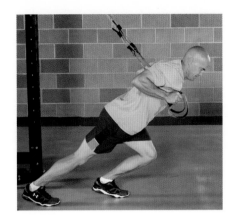

▶ ACTION

4. Slightly bend the ankles, knees, and hips.

5. Rapidly extend the ankle, knee, and hip of the forward leg while forcefully driving the rear knee upward and bending the ankle and hip of the rear foot. When the ankle, knee, and hip are fully extended, there should be able to be a line drawn through the ankle, knee, hip, and shoulder.

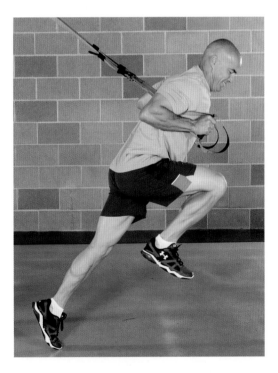

ENDING POSITION

6. Land with slight flexion of the ankles, knees, and hips. Transition to flat feet while returning to the starting position.

7. Do the desired number of repetitions, and then switch foot position.

PART IV

Sample Programs

Regular participation in a strength training program offers numerous health and fitness rewards for most adults. Once thought of as a method of conditioning reserved for elite athletes, strength training is now recommended by professional health and fitness organizations and researchers as an effective means for adults of any age to enhance and maintain musculoskeletal health, functional ability, and quality of life. Strength training has become a popular mode of exercise that can be performed in health clubs, recreation centers, and homes. The key to safe and effective strength training is a well-designed program that involves the correct exercise technique (described in chapters 9 through 12), proper prescription of program variables (described in chapter 3), and a sensible progression to keep the workout effective and enjoyable (see chapter 7).

For a long time, coaches and trainers searched for the optimal combination of sets, repetitions, and exercises that would maximize gains in strength and muscle size. But now we know that a training program that works for one individual may not be effective for another. Thus, strength training programs need to be based on individual needs, goals, and abilities in order to maximize training outcomes, minimize the risk of injury, and increase the likelihood that strength training becomes a lifelong activity. The first step is to identify "at-risk" adults with medical ailments such as high blood pressure, heart disease, or diabetes who should obtain medical clearance before they begin a strength training program (see chapter 8).This important first step will ensure that participation in strength-building activities will be beneficial rather than harmful to those adults who are managing injuries or illnesses. Once an adult is cleared for participation by his or her health care provider, a personalized strength training program can be developed.

The second step is to identify realistic goals and a sensible starting point for each individual. Too often, adults begin strength training at a level that exceeds their current fitness level. Not only can this approach lead to excessive muscle soreness and nonadherence to the program, but it can also result in injury. Moreover, beginners often make dramatic improvements in muscle strength during the first few weeks of strength training; it doesn't make sense for beginners to participate in more advanced training programs, because strength gains will not be any greater and the likelihood of injury will increase. Since strength training programs should be both effective and realistic, the best approach is to design a training program that is consistent with a person's current fitness status and individualized goals.

In addition, when planning your training program, think about the time you have available for training, the equipment that is available to you, your strength training experience, and your health history. Consider the following questions before beginning a strength training program:

- Are there medical concerns that may limit or prevent your participation in a strength training program? Individuals with medical conditions such as heart disease, high blood pressure, diabetes, and arthritis should check with their physician or health care provider before they begin strength training.

- Do you currently participate in a strength training program? While individuals with no experience strength training should start with the beginner program, individuals who have been strength training regularly for more than two or three months may want to start at a higher level of training depending on their training experience and fitness goals.

- What type of strength training equipment is available at home or at your gym? There are advantages and disadvantages to using free weights (barbells), weight machines, and body weight exercises, but all modes of strength training can be effective provided that appropriate training guidelines are followed. The key is to choose a mode of training that is consistent with your needs, goals, and abilities.

- How much time do you have available for strength training during the week? A well-designed strength training program for a beginner can be completed in less than 30 minutes, whereas an advanced program may take longer than 60 minutes to finish. Strength training programs can be tailored to meet specific time requirements.

- What are your specific training goals? A strength training program for a beginner who wants to increase muscle strength is quite different from a program for an athlete who needs to enhance sport performance (see chapter 7). Since there is not one combination of sets and repetitions that will optimize gains for everyone, each individual must prioritize his or her training goals and then follow a program that is specifically designed to achieve those goals.

- Would individualized instruction from a qualified fitness professional be beneficial for you? It is a lot easier to develop good habits from the start than to try to break bad habits once they develop. Qualified fitness professionals can provide motivation, guidance, and instruction on safe exercise technique.

Once these questions are answered, you can design a safe, effective, and enjoyable strength training program that is consistent with personalized goals. As discussed in chapter 7, while there are many different program goals (e.g., to increase muscle strength, to reduce body fat, and to reduce stress), most beginner programs are designed to improve general fitness, strengthen connective tissue (tendons and ligaments), and build a foundation for more advanced workouts. These programs should be distinguished from more advanced training programs, which are typically designed to maximize gains in muscle strength, muscle power, and muscle size. Nevertheless, don't think of a beginner program as a simple, short-term workout. Strength training needs to be continued, progressed, and when necessary, modified in order to make continual gains in health and fitness. Otherwise, the training-induced gains from strength training begin to dissipate.

13

Beginner Programs

Pablo B. Costa and José A. Arevalo

Adults with no strength training experience and those who have not trained for several months or years should begin strength training by following a general preparation program in which the resistance is light and the main focus is on learning or relearning proper exercise technique. All too often, beginners do too much too soon. You must give your body a chance to gradually adapt to the physical stress of strength training while at the same time making fitness gains. Using the 12-week beginner program detailed in this chapter will help you gradually increase your body's ability to tolerate the stress of strength training with minimal muscle soreness. The idea is to develop healthy habits early in the training program so that strength training becomes an enjoyable, meaningful, and lifelong fitness experience. Regardless of how much weight everybody else is lifting at the local fitness center, beginners need to proceed slowly during the first few weeks of strength training as they build a foundation for more advanced training programs in the future. It is not necessary to train with a high volume or intensity early in the training program because most of the initial strength gains are due to neural adaptations rather than muscle hypertrophy.

Although all strength training programs need to be based on the fundamental principles of overload, progression, and specificity (see chapter 3), beginners respond favorably to most strength training protocols provided the exercise intensity is adequate. As you become more trained, the rate of improvement tends to slow down (figure 13.1). It is not uncommon for a beginner to increase muscular strength by about 40 percent during the first 8 to 12 weeks of strength training, whereas an advanced lifter may improve by only about 5 to 10 percent during this same time period.

The authors acknowledge the significant contributions of Avery Faigenbaum and Jay Hoffman to this chapter.

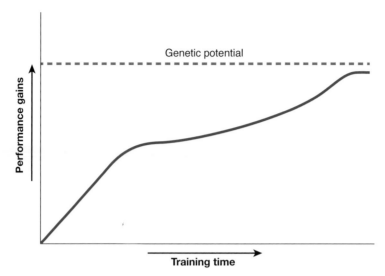

FIGURE 13.1　A theoretical training curve. Gains are made easily on the lower portion of the curve as individuals start to train and come more slowly as individuals approach their genetic potential.

Reprinted, by permission, from S. Fleck and W. Kraemer, 2014, *Designing resistance training programs*, 4th ed. (Champaign, IL: Human Kinetics), 207.

As strength training experience increases, you will get closer to your genetic potential, and it becomes increasingly difficult to make strength gains. After you have completed the beginner program successfully, you will need to modify your strength training program if you want continued gains in muscular fitness. Instead of discouraging you from continuing a strength training program, this slower rate of improvement should motivate you to put additional time and effort into your program design as your training experience increases. Of course, you need to weigh the increased time required in order to maximize gains in muscular fitness. Although small gains in strength may be the difference between winning and losing in some athletic events, as a beginner you may want only to maintain your current level of fitness. In any case, all strength training programs must be based on your needs, goals, and abilities as well as an understanding of fundamental strength training principles.

Program Design Considerations

Although men and women can benefit from strength training, the act of strength training itself does not ensure that optimal gains will be made. In other words, simply lifting light weights for a few exercises will not enhance muscular fitness. Individual effort and a systematic progression of program variables result in the most effective training outcomes. This does not mean that beginners should jump right to training with heavy weights or performing advanced exercises but rather that the program should be structured in a way that maximizes training adaptations while minimizing the risk of muscle soreness or injury. During the early phase of your training, great variations in training repetitions and sets are not needed to enhance muscle strength. Therefore, a general program design is used during the first 8 to 12 weeks of strength training. Over time, the strength training program can become more specific in order to maximize gains in muscle strength or muscle size.

Warm up before every strength training workout by performing 8 to 12 repetitions at approximately 50 percent of the intensity used for the first set (Abad et al. 2011). Not only does a warm-up reduce the risk of injury, but it also enhances muscular performance by preparing your body for the demands of strength exercise. It is a good idea to exercise with an experienced training partner who can serve as a spotter on selected exercises and can provide motivation and encouragement when needed. Be sure to review the safety precautions discussed in chapter 8 as well as in the general strength training guidelines in this chapter.

As discussed in parts I and II, several variables must be considered when setting up a strength training program, including the choice and order of exercises, the intensity, the volume, the frequency, and the progression of the training. Let's review each of these variables as they apply to a strength training program for beginners.

Choice and Order of Exercises

Beginners should perform a total-body workout that includes one or two exercises for each major muscle group. This is an effective and time-efficient method for

General Strength Training Guidelines for Beginners

- ☐ Make sure that the exercise environment is free of clutter.
- ☐ Warm up for about 5 to 10 minutes before strength training.
- ☐ A specific resistance training warm-up is preferred over a general warm-up.
- ☐ Take time to learn proper exercise technique.
- ☐ Perform exercises for larger muscles (i.e., barbell bench press) before performing exercises for smaller muscles (i.e., biceps curl), and begin with a weight you can handle for 8 to 12 repetitions.
- ☐ Begin with 1 set and progress to 2 to 4 sets on selected exercises.
- ☐ Rest about 1 to 2 minutes between sets and exercises.
- ☐ Perform all exercises throughout the full range of motion.
- ☐ Avoid jerky, uncontrolled movements while strength training.
- ☐ Strength train 2 to 3 days per week on nonconsecutive days.

improving muscular fitness. Both single-joint exercises (e.g., dumbbell biceps curl and leg extension) and multijoint exercises (e.g., barbell bench press and leg press) are effective for increasing muscular strength. Although it's important to include both exercise types in a strength training workout, over time you need to emphasize multijoint exercises in order to maximize gains. Multijoint exercises are more complex and involve more muscle mass; consequently, more weight can be lifted. In addition, multijoint exercises more closely mimic activities of daily life and sport activities. It's best to perform multijoint exercises early in a workout when the muscles are fresh and fatigue is minimal.

As a beginner, you can include exercises that use both weight machines and free weights (i.e., barbells and dumbbells) in your program. Many beginners enjoy strength training on weight machines because the exercises are relatively easy to learn and to perform correctly and because risk of injury is low. Weight machines help stabilize the body and limit movement around specific joints. However, because weight machines are expensive and take up a lot of floor space, most people do not have these machines at home. If weight machines are not available, barbells and dumbbells can be used to strengthen all the major muscle groups. Free-weight exercises require more balance and coordination than machine exercises; therefore, it may take a longer period of time to learn proper exercise technique. However, this greater demand on balance and coordination might be desirable. In any case, all beginner exercises should be performed at a controlled movement velocity during the lifting and lowering phases. This means that you should be able to stop any lifting or lowering action at will without momentum carrying the movement to completion. Uncontrolled, jerky movements are ineffective and may result in injury. In addition, make sure to maintain a normal breathing pattern and do not hold your breath at any phase of the lift.

Exercise Intensity

Because heavy weights are not required to increase the muscular strength of beginners, weights corresponding to about 60 to 70 percent of 1RM are recommended for the first month of strength training, when individuals are learning the correct exercise technique. This training zone corresponds to about 8 to 12 repetitions. Although weights that can be lifted for 15 to 20 repetitions are effective for increasing local muscular endurance, light weights typically do not result in meaningful gains in muscular strength. Because beginners usually do not perform maximal 1RM strength tests before training, the best approach is to first establish a repetition range (e.g., 8 to 12) and to determine by trial and error the maximum load that can be handled with proper technique for the prescribed training range. It may take two or three workouts to find the desired training weight on all exercises.

As you progress into the second and third months of training, you can use additional sets and slightly heavier loads (up to 80 percent of 1RM) to keep the training stimulus effective. Performing the same training program for a long period of time likely will result in training plateaus, boredom, or overtraining (characterized by a decrease in muscle performance). Thus, the best advice is to systematically vary your training program every month or so by changing one or more of the program variables. Heavier loads and multiple sets maximize gains in muscular fitness, and other tissues (e.g., bone) respond more favorably to more advanced training programs than to single-set training with a light weight.

When training within a repetition range, the magnitude of individual effort determines the outcome of the strength training program. For example, training in a zone of 8RM to 12RM (estimated at 60 to 70 percent of 1RM) means that you should be able to perform no more than 12 repetitions with proper form with a given weight. Simply performing an exercise for 8, 9, 10, 11, or 12 repetitions does not necessarily mean that training falls within the 8RM to 12RM zone. Although you never want to sacrifice proper form, the training weight should be challenging enough to result in at least a modest degree of muscle fatigue as the last few repetitions of a set are finished. If this does not occur, gains will not be maximized.

Exercise Sets and Interset Periods

Because the number of training sets is not a critical factor during the first few weeks of strength training, beginners should start with one and progress to two to four sets for each muscle group. You can progress to more sets after the first month of training, depending on the time available for training as well as individualized training goals. If you are following a multiset protocol, keep in mind that not all exercises need to be performed for the same number of sets.

Another important consideration is the rest interval between sets and exercises because fatigue associated with the previous set or exercise will limit performance on the following set or exercise. Some fatigue is to be expected—however, not so much that it significantly affects the ability to perform subsequent sets. In general, a one- to two-minute rest period between sets and exercises is recommended for beginners.

Exercise Frequency

A total-body workout should be performed on two or three alternating days per week. Because only moderate weights are used during this early period, allowing 48 hours between workouts usually is sufficient. Longer recovery periods may be needed during more advanced training programs in which heavier weights are used. Although a training frequency of once per week can be an effective maintenance frequency for individuals who have experience in strength training, a higher training frequency is needed to maximize gains in muscular fitness.

You should maintain a training frequency of two or three days per week as you progress through training. Although changes may be made to other program variables during this time, an increase in training frequency is not needed for total-body training. After successfully completing the beginner program, you may use higher training frequencies to perform more specialized training programs.

Note that if higher training frequencies are used, specific muscle groups typically are trained only twice per week.

Program Progression

For continued gains in muscular fitness, the strength training program must be progressively altered over time so that the body can be continually challenged to adapt to the new demands. This does not mean that every workout needs to be harder than the previous workout. Rather, a systematic progression of the exercise program is needed for long-term gains in muscular fitness. Although beginners will improve at a faster rate than more advanced lifters, manipulating the program variables (i.e., the number of sets and reps) during the first few weeks of training will limit training plateaus and boredom, which may lead to loss of enthusiasm for strength training.

In addition to increasing the amount of weight that is lifted, you can progress the program by performing additional repetitions with the current weight, adding more sets to the program, altering rest periods between sets, or combining modifications of these variables to provide progressive overload. For example, you can increase the demand of your training program by first performing more repetitions within a training zone and later increasing the weight lifted (by 5 to 10 percent). If you perform 1 set of 8 repetitions with 50 pounds (22.7 kg) on the chest press, you should work toward performing 12 repetitions with 50 pounds over the next few workouts. Once this is achieved, the weight can be increased to 55 pounds (24.9 kg), and the repetitions should be reduced back to 8. The strength training program can also be advanced by adding sets on selected exercises or by adding more challenging exercises to the program.

Suggested Beginner Program

Individual goals, personal preferences, and time available for training will determine the design of more advanced training programs. As a beginner, however, performing a total-body workout two or three days per week is an effective method for improving muscular fitness. The 12-week beginner program gives you time to learn proper exercise technique and develop a fitness base for more advanced training programs as your strength and confidence improve (figure 13.2).

You should be using a training log or mobile app to monitor training progress. We provide a sample training log that you can photocopy and use. Because there is no optimal combination of sets, repetitions, and exercises that will work for everyone, you should assess the effectiveness of your training program every few weeks and make modifications when necessary. In addition, be prepared to alter the recommended workout to accommodate your state on a given day. For example, if you feel tired or sore from a previous workout, you should decrease the training intensity and number of exercises. This is where the science of designing a strength training workout needs to be combined with the art of developing an exercise program.

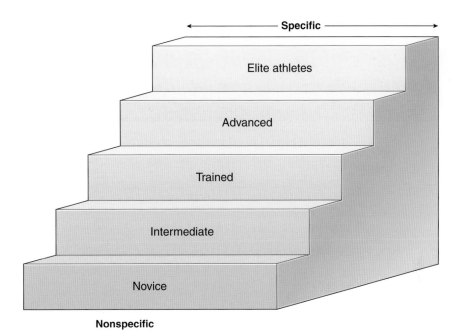

FIGURE 13.2   The design of strength training programs progresses from general programs for beginners to more specific programs for advanced lifters.

Adapted, by permission, from C. Corbin, G. Le Masurier, K. McConnell, 2014, *Fitness for life*, 6th ed. (Champaign, IL: Human Kinetics), 34.

Training Program Outline: Weeks 1 Through 4

During the first month of strength training, workouts should include 1 to 3 sets of each of the 10 to 12 different exercises with a one-minute rest between exercises (see table 13.1). Perform the exercises using a moderate weight. Beginners with a very low level of fitness may need to get in shape before participating in a strength training program that maximizes gains in muscular fitness. In other words, if you have never strength trained before, additional time for muscular adaptation is recommended. For example, instead of performing 8 to 12 exercises with a moderate weight, try performing 4 to 6 different exercises with a light weight, and perhaps perform only 1 set per exercise. This will give you an opportunity to gain confidence in your ability to strength train.

A major goal of this training phase is to learn proper form and technique on a variety of upper- and lower-body exercises while practicing training fundamentals (e.g., proper technique, controlled movements, maintaining a normal breathing pattern). Thus, an initial load of 60 to 65 percent of 1RM will allow you to be in the zone of 10 to 12 repetitions on a variety of upper- and lower-body exercises that target all the major muscle groups. Of course, you can use lighter loads when learning a new exercise or attempting to correct a flaw in exercise technique. At least one exercise for all the major muscle groups should be performed.

TRAINING LOG

Name_____

Order	Exercise	Sets	Set	Week # Day 1 1	2	3
1			Wt.			
			Reps			
2			Wt.			
			Reps			
3			Wt.			
			Reps			
4			Wt.			
			Reps			
5			Wt.			
			Reps			
6			Wt.			
			Reps			
7			Wt.			
			Reps			
8			Wt.			
			Reps			
9			Wt.			
			Reps			
10			Wt.			
			Reps			
11			Wt.			
			Reps			
Body weight						
Date						
Comments						

From National Strength Training and Conditioning Association (NSCA), 2017, *Strength training*, 2nd ed. (Champaign, IL: Human Kinetics). Reprinted from W. Westcott and T. Baechle, 1999, *Strength training for seniors: Instructor guide* (Champaign, IL: Human Kinetics), 207. By permission of W. Westcott.

							Week # _____								
	Day 2			Day 3			Day 1			Day 2			Day 3		
1	2	3	1	2	3	1	2	3	1	2	3	1	2	3	

309

TABLE 13.1   Beginner Strength Training Program: Weeks 1 Through 4*

Weight machine exercise	Page #	Free weight exercise	Page #	Sets	Reps
Leg extension	219	Back squat	210	1-3	10-12
Seated leg curl	235	Glute bridge with sliders	234	1-3	10-12
Machine chest press	174	Dumbbell bench press	182	1-3	10-12
Machine seated row	186	Dumbbell upright row	167	1-3	10-12
Machine biceps curl	201	Dumbbell biceps curl	203	1-3	10-12
Cable triceps extension	194	Lying triceps extension	199	1-3	10-12
Back extension	260	Modified Superman	266	1-3	10-12
Stability ball crunch	246	Abdominal crunch	244	1-3	10-12

* Note that progression of this workout plan is required to maximize gains in muscular fitness after the first few weeks of strength training.

Training Program Outline: Weeks 5 Through 8

During weeks 5 through 8, the workout should become more challenging as strength and coordination improve. By varying the program variables, you start to accomplish specific goals in health and fitness, and you prevent the boredom and training plateaus that eventually lead to a lack of adherence to the program or to dropping out of the program entirely. This is a good time to think about the physical and psychosocial benefits of strength training. Although positive changes in physical abilities certainly are important, so too are the qualitative changes associated with a more active lifestyle.

During this period, increase the training volume by performing 3 to 4 sets of 10 exercises at a training intensity of about 75 percent of 1RM (8-10 repetitions). Rest for about one to two minutes between sets (see table 13.2). As additional

TABLE 13.2   Beginner Strength Training Program: Weeks 5 Through 8

Weight machine exercise	Page #	Free weight exercise	Page #	Sets	Reps
Leg press	209	Back squat	210	3-4	8-10
Leg extension	219	Step-up	216	3-4	8-10
Seated leg curl	235	Glute-ham raise	230	3-4	8-10
Machine chest press	174	Dumbbell bench press	182	3-4	8-10
Machine seated row	186	Dumbbell upright row	167	3-4	8-10
Seated barbell military press	170	Dumbbell lateral raise	164	3-4	8-10
Machine biceps curl	201	Dumbbell biceps curl	203	3-4	8-10
Cable triceps extension	194	Lying triceps extension	199	3-4	8-10
Back extension	260	Modified Superman	266	3-4	8-10
Stability ball crunch	246	Abdominal crunch	244	3-4	8-10

sets are performed in the training program, continued effort will determine training outcomes. Thus, you should expect and welcome the feelings of exercise exertion. A major goal of this conditioning phase is to be confident in your abilities to overcome the continued progressive demands of strength-building exercises while maximizing training adaptations.

Training Program Outline: Weeks 9 Through 12

After the first eight weeks of strength training, improvements in muscular fitness will occur at a slower rate. Beginners who started strength training with great enthusiasm may become disappointed when gains in muscle strength become less dramatic during the third month of training. This is where you need to understand that a strength training workout that was effective during the first few weeks of training may not be effective in the long term. To make continual gains in muscular fitness and to achieve specific health and fitness goals, higher intensities and a more challenging training program are required (i.e., the principle of progressive overload). This is particularly important for people who want to maximize gains in muscle strength or muscle size.

During this phase, perform 3 to 4 sets of 8 exercises at a training intensity of 75 to 80 percent of 1RM (6-8 repetitions). Rest about two to three minutes between sets (see table 13.3). Although endless combinations of program variables can be used, continued improvement requires that you increase the training weight and reduce the repetitions to the lower end of the training zone once you have performed the desired number of repetitions on the last set. As a general recommendation, you should perform more sets on exercises for large muscle groups than on exercises for smaller muscle groups. However, research has shown that

TABLE 13.3   Beginner Strength Training Program: Weeks 9 Through 12

Weight machine exercise	Page #	Free weight exercise	Page #	Sets	Reps
Leg press	209	Front squat	212	3-4	6-8
Seated hip abduction	237	Lateral lunge with slider	221	3-4	6-8
Seated hip adduction	236	Lateral lunge with slider	221	3-4	6-8
Machine chest press	174	Barbell bench press	173	3-4	6-8
Machine chest fly	175	Lying dumbbell fly	176	3-4	6-8
Machine seated row	186	Dumbbell upright row	167	3-4	6-8
Lat pull-down	188	Medicine ball slam	289	3-4	6-8
Machine shoulder press	169	Seated barbell military press	170	3-4	6-8
Machine biceps curl	201	Dumbbell biceps curl	203	3-4	6-8
Machine seated triceps push-down	193	Lying triceps extension	199	3-4	6-8
Back extension	260	Modified Superman	266	3-4	6-8
Stability ball crunch	246	Abdominal crunch	244	3-4	6-8

beginners do not experience greater strength gains when performing more than 4 sets per exercise (Rhea 2013a). Therefore, any exercise should probably not be performed for longer than 4 sets.

Summary

Beginners can make remarkable gains in muscular fitness by following established strength training guidelines. By starting with a reasonable training weight and gradually progressing from simple to more complex exercises, novices can make strength training a safe, effective, and enjoyable activity that can be performed for a lifetime. Those who successfully complete the beginner program are more confident and prepared to move on to more advanced strength training workouts and to achieve even greater gains in muscular fitness.

Intermediate Programs

Evan E. Schick and Jared W. Coburn

During the first three months of strength training, beginners experience rapid improvements in strength. As discussed in part I, most of these improvements are related to neurological adaptations, although noticeable improvements in muscle size may also be present. However, as the duration of training progresses, the rate of strength improvement slows down. At this point, beginners need to make adjustments to their program in order to provide a new training stimulus to the exercising muscles; what may have been a sufficient stimulus for a beginner may be inadequate for an intermediate lifter (figure 14.1). This chapter discusses how to develop a training program for the intermediate lifter—someone who currently is strength training and has at least three months of regular strength training experience.

Program Design Considerations

By strength training on a regular basis for three months, a lifter has demonstrated a commitment and consistency in training that suggest the ability and desire to incorporate a more sophisticated exercise design into his or her training regimen. The workout for the beginner focuses on performing a total-body workout that involves both single-joint (e.g., machine biceps curl) and multijoint (e.g., leg press) exercises. At the intermediate level, it becomes necessary to consider increasing the frequency of training and incorporating a split routine into the training program. As you learned in chapters 3 and 7, a split routine involves separating your workouts by grouping exercises that train a certain body part. You then alternate the days that you work on each body part. This allows for the necessary recovery of the muscles while still increasing the total number of times you work out in a given week. For example, you may choose to focus on the chest, shoulders, and triceps for one workout and the legs, back, and biceps

The authors acknowledge the significant contributions of Jay Hoffman and Avery Faigenbaum to this chapter.

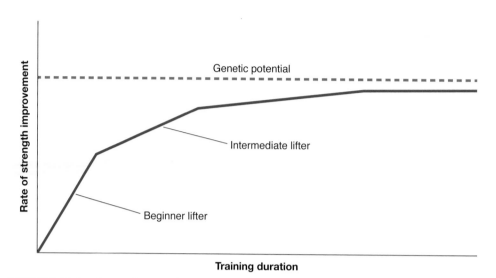

FIGURE 14.1   Rate of strength improvement relative to training duration.

Adapted, by permission, from J. Hoffman, 2014, *Physiological aspects of sports training and performance,* 2nd ed. (Champaign, IL: Human Kinetics), 97.

for the other workout. Although workouts are performed four days per week in this example, each particular muscle group is trained twice per week.

This type of split routine can also be classified as a push–pull routine. During one workout, the exercises involve primarily a pushing movement (e.g., exercises for the chest, shoulders, and triceps), whereas in the other workout the exercises involve primarily the lower body and a pulling movement (e.g., exercises for the back and biceps). Another benefit of this split routine is that the musculature being recruited for each training session is either the prime mover or a synergist for each exercise. For instance, the triceps are recruited as a synergist during the bench press and shoulder press exercises, but they are the prime movers during the triceps push-down exercise. If these exercises were performed on consecutive days, the triceps would not receive adequate rest, leading to fatigue and poor performance during the workouts. This is an important reason for splitting the routine in this fashion.

Another benefit of using a split routine is that it allows you to incorporate additional exercises per body part into the training regimen. Including assistance exercises over and above the core exercises has been shown to be especially relevant for the intermediate lifter. It generally is believed that an assistance exercise provides an added stimulus for further physiological adaptations that may lead to greater gains in muscle strength and size.

For the beginner who has been lifting consistently for several months, adding assistance exercises to the training regimen may not seem particularly important. However, in order to further your gains, you need to add these types of changes to your training program. Other changes can include increasing the number of sets performed per exercise, increasing the number of exercises performed per training session (i.e., increasing the volume of training), or using heavier loads (i.e., increasing the intensity of training).

Choice and Order of Exercises

There is no optimum number of exercises to perform per body part. The appropriate number depends on a person's experience level, training goals, available time, and ability to adequately recover between sets and workouts. As a beginner, your training program may have included only one exercise per body part, which was sufficient for providing the initial training stimulus. As an intermediate lifter, however, you need to include additional exercises per body part to effectively increase muscle strength and size.

For example, most beginner lifters use the barbell bench press or machine chest press as the core exercise for the chest—that is, the exercise that recruits the greatest amount of muscle mass for that body part. However, if your goal is to build additional muscle strength or size, then you need to add complementary exercises that move that area of the body through different angles and planes, such as the barbell incline bench press or bent-over dumbbell fly.

In general, exercises that recruit the greatest amount of muscle mass are performed before exercises that recruit a smaller muscle mass for any given body part. The primary reason for this is to prevent you from fatiguing the musculature you need to perform the core lifts. This means performing core exercises before assistance exercises. For instance, when exercising the legs, back, and biceps, the legs are the largest muscle group of the three; therefore, the legs are trained first, followed by the back and then the biceps. When training the legs, the exercise that recruits the greatest muscle mass (e.g., the back squat) is performed before the exercises that recruit a smaller muscle mass (e.g., seated leg curl, calf raise).

Exercise Intensity

As you learned in chapter 13, a strength training program for beginners generally requires a moderate training intensity of between 60 and 70 percent of 1RM. As lifters progress and focus on more specific training goals, they can adjust the intensity and vary it to help them meet those goals. For instance, individuals who are interested in maximizing strength will begin to use a higher intensity of training (i.e., >70 percent of 1RM), whereas individuals whose primary desire is to maximize muscle hypertrophy will use a relatively lower intensity of training. In addition, the rest interval between exercise sets will vary depending on the specific goals of the training program.

For example, if the exercise prescription was written as "1, 3 × 6-8RM" (the "1" indicates the initial warm-up set), you would choose a weight that you can lift at least 6 times but not more than 8 times. If you lift 100 pounds (45.4 kg) for 8 repetitions in the first set but feel that you could have easily performed a few more repetitions, then the 100-pound training weight is too light and should be increased. It may take several workouts to find the appropriate weight on all exercises, but once you find it, the progression principle necessitates strict adherence. For instance, if a workout requires the intermediate lifter to perform 3 sets of 8 repetitions (written as "3 × 8") in the squat during the first week of training, he or she may have difficulty lifting 140 pounds (63.5 kg) for 8 repetitions for all 3 sets. After several weeks of training, this lifter may have much less difficulty performing 8 repetitions for all 3 sets, and he or she may feel that it would be possible to perform 9 repetitions with proper form. At this point, the lifter needs to add weight to ensure the same relative intensity and performance gains. As muscle strength increases, the relative intensity of that particular weight decreases. This is a classic example of the way the progression principle works and how the overload principle leads to strength gains.

Exercise Sets and Interset Rest Periods

One-set training protocols may be effective for some beginners, but intermediate lifters will want to use multiple sets per exercise. This provides a better training stimulus for generating even greater gains in muscle strength and size.

The exercise prescription for the intermediate lifter should include a warm-up set followed by the number of work sets to be performed. The warm-up set usually involves a light to moderate weight that the person can lift comfortably for at least 10 repetitions. It serves to prime the muscle for the greater intensity that will be used in the next sequence of sets. It should also be mentioned that large individual variations exist in the volume and intensity of warm-ups used. It is up to each individual to select the routine that provides an adequate warm-up without inducing fatigue.

The number of sets to be performed per exercise varies. In general, three to five sets per exercise are used for the core lifts (e.g., back squat, barbell bench press), whereas two to four sets commonly are used for assistance exercises (e.g., barbell incline bench press, seated leg curl). Generally speaking, as intensity (i.e., the weight lifted) increases, the volume (i.e., sets and repetitions) decreases.

Similar to training intensity, the amount of rest allotted between sets appears to have a significant effect on desired training outcomes. Training programs of high intensity (>85 percent of 1RM for the development of strength) specify rest intervals of at least two minutes in duration. This provides sufficient time for the muscle to replenish the energy expended during the previous set, thereby maximizing recovery and providing for optimum performance in the next set.

In contrast, when muscle hypertrophy is the goal, the rest interval between sets is shorter (approximately 30-90 seconds). Fatigue associated with lower training intensities and shorter rest intervals appears to be an important factor in stimulating anabolic hormone secretions. This physiological response helps maximize muscle hypertrophy (see chapter 2). Such training programs are common for bodybuilders who want maximal muscle growth. For the lifter who has begun to focus on specific training goals, the proper combination of training intensity and rest intervals provides the opportunity to maximize those goals.

Exercise Frequency

Similar to the beginner, the intermediate lifter may still exercise two or three days per week using one exercise per body part (although, as stated previously, more exercises are recommended). This training program may be based on necessity (i.e., time constraints) or desire. The intermediate lifter may add an assistance exercise for the larger or multijoint muscle groups and maintain a single exercise for some of the smaller or single-joint muscle groups. For instance, the intermediate lifter exercising two or three days per week may want to add the barbell incline bench press to the upper-body or chest routine and add the seated leg curl to the lower-body routine.

Suggested Intermediate Programs

The remainder of this chapter provides various examples and explanations of intermediate-level strength training programs. The selection of a program that is right for you should be based on several factors. Most notably, you must decide what your goals are for training and how much time you have available to train. The programs listed offer an array of possibilities to choose from.

You'll want to limit the time you spend on any one of these programs without change for two to three months. Setting this limit will prevent you from getting too bored with the program, hitting a training plateau, or experiencing chronic fatigue. After two or three months with one program, you may choose to alter your training goal. For example, after two months of general muscular conditioning, you may proceed to a two- to three-month muscular hypertrophy program, followed by two to three months of a muscular strength program. Depending on your goals or needs, the training program can continue focusing on strength development, enter an active rest period during which you do not lift but do participate in other forms of activity, or proceed to a more advanced resistance training program.

General Muscular Conditioning

The first program (see table 14.1) is a three-days-per-week general muscular conditioning program. During each training session, the entire body is trained. The training routines for each session use different exercises for each body part in order to provide a variety that can relieve the potential monotony of performing the same exercise routine every workout. In addition, the change of exercises provides a different stimulus to the musculature. The rest period between sets should be between 30 and 90 seconds, and at least 48 hours of rest should be allowed between each workout. Note that the intensity of training is prescribed as 8 to 10RM, which requires the lifter to select a resistance with which he or she can perform at least 8 but not more than 10 repetitions.

For individuals who are interested in general conditioning but want to exercise four days per week, table 14.2 provides a sample split routine. The legs, back,

TABLE 14.1 General Muscular Conditioning Program (3 Days per Week)

Exercise	Page #	Sets × reps
Monday		
Back squat	210	3 × 8-10RM
Machine chest press	174	3 × 8-10RM
Machine shoulder press	169	3 × 8-10RM
Lat pull-down	188	3 × 8-10RM
Back extension	260	3 × 8-10RM
Seated leg curl	235	3 × 8-10RM
Machine seated triceps push-down	193	3 × 8-10RM
Dumbbell biceps curl	203	3 × 8-10RM
Abdominal crunch	244	3 × 20
Wednesday		
Suspension trainer elevated rear-foot split squat	218	3 × 8-10RM
Barbell incline bench press	180	3 × 8-10RM
Dumbbell upright row	167	3 × 8-10RM
Cable seated row	187	3 × 8-10RM
Back extension	260	3 × 8-10RM
Romanian deadlift	224	3 × 8-10RM
Lying triceps extension	199	3 × 8-10RM
EZ-bar curl	205	3 × 8-10RM
Abdominal crunch	244	3 × 20
Friday		
Step-up	216	3 × 8-10RM
Dumbbell bench press	182	3 × 8-10RM
Dumbbell lateral raise	164	3 × 8-10RM
Dumbbell single-arm row	191	3 × 8-10RM
Back extension	260	3 × 8-10RM
Seated leg curl	235	3 × 8-10RM
Close-grip bench press	197	3 × 8-10RM
Machine biceps curl	201	3 × 8-10RM
Bent-knee sit-up	243	3 × 20

and biceps are trained on days 1 (Monday) and 3 (Thursday) of the week. The chest, shoulders, and triceps are trained on days 2 (Tuesday) and 4 (Friday) of the week. In contrast to the three-days-per-week training model, this four-day split routine allows you to include additional assistance exercises in the program. Although the workouts are performed on some consecutive days, at least

TABLE 14.2   General Muscular Conditioning Program (4 Days per Week)

Monday			Tuesday		
Exercise	**Page #**	**Sets × reps**	**Exercise**	**Page #**	**Sets × reps**
Leg press	209	1, 4 × 8-10RM	Dumbbell bench press	182	1, 4 × 8-10RM
Leg extension	219	3 × 8-10RM	Dumbbell incline bench press	184	3 × 8-10RM
Seated leg curl	235	3 × 8-10RM	Machine shoulder press	169	1, 4 × 8-10RM
Calf raise	238	3 × 8-10RM	Dumbbell upright row	167	4 × 8-10RM
Lat pull-down	188	1, 4 × 8-10RM	Machine seated triceps push-down	193	4 × 8-10RM
Back extension	260	3 × 8-10RM	Lying triceps extension	199	3 × 8-10RM
Dumbbell biceps curl	203	4 × 8-10RM	Ankle touch	245	3 × 20
Abdominal crunch	244	3 × 20			

Thursday			Friday		
Exercise	**Page #**	**Sets × reps**	**Exercise**	**Page #**	**Sets × reps**
Lateral lunge	220	1, 4 × 8-10RM	Barbell bench press	178	1, 4 × 8-10RM
Step-up	216	3 × 8-10RM	Dumbbell incline bench press	184	3 × 8-10RM
Romanian deadlift	224	3 × 8-10RM	Standing military press	172	1, 4 × 8-10RM
Calf raise	238	3 × 8-10RM	Dumbbell front raise	165	4 × 8-10RM
Bent-over row	192	1, 4 × 8-10RM	Close-grip bench press	197	4 × 8-10RM
Back extension	260	3 × 8-10RM	Machine seated triceps push-down	193	3 × 8-10RM
Dumbbell hammer curl	204	4 × 8-10RM	Side plank	257	3 × 20
Jackknife	249	3 × 20			

The "1" before the number of sets and repetitions of select exercises indicates that one warm-up set should be performed before the main set.

72 hours of rest is always allotted for the specific body parts that are trained to ensure adequate recovery between workouts. The rest period between sets should be between 30 and 90 seconds.

You can perform this four-day workout with variable-resistance machines, free weights, or a combination of both. If you use free weights, you easily can substitute the back squat or lateral lunge for the leg press. Similarly, the barbell bench press and standing barbell military press can replace the machine chest press (see table 14.2) and machine shoulder press, respectively.

Determining whether to use machines or free weights is an important decision. In terms of comfort and ease of use, variable-resistance machines are often recommended. However, people who want to increase the chances of gaining carryover strength may want to include as many free-weight exercises as possible. *Carryover strength* refers to the degree of strength improvement achieved during exercise that is reflected in improved performance in another activity (i.e., activities of daily living or sporting events). For instance, if an athlete improves his or her squat performance by 20 percent, this does not necessarily translate into a 20-percent improvement in athletic performance. To ensure the greatest degree of carryover strength, the exercise chosen should simulate the activity as closely as possible. Exercises may progress from general (e.g., leg press) to more specific (e.g., back squat) to highly specific (e.g., split squat) over the course of a training program. In most sporting activities, the athlete performs in an upright position; thus, the best way to improve leg strength that will carry over to sport is to incorporate the back squat exercise into training for the lower body. Furthermore, research suggests that free-weight training can increase the activation of stabilizer muscles, thereby making training more efficient and effective.

Circuit Training

Tables 14.3 and 14.4 show circuit training programs that can be performed either two or three days per week. (Note that you should allow at least 48 hours of rest between each workout.) This program develops general muscle fitness,

TABLE 14.3 Circuit Training Program: Machines (Performed 2 or 3 Days per Week)

Exercise	Page #	Sets × reps
Leg press	209	1 × 12-15RM
Machine chest press	174	1 × 12-15RM
Seated leg curl	235	1 × 12-15RM
Machine shoulder press	169	1 × 12-15RM
Leg extension	219	1 × 12-15RM
Lat pull-down	188	1 × 12-15RM
Machine seated triceps push-down	193	1 × 12-15RM
Back extension	260	1 × 12-15RM
Machine biceps curl	201	1 × 12-15RM
Roll-out	248	1 × 12-15
Cycle ergometer	148	5 min

TABLE 14.4 Circuit Training Program:
Free Weights (Performed 2 or 3 Days per Week)

Exercise	Page #	Sets × reps
Step-up	216	1 × 12-15RM
Dumbbell bench press	182	1 × 12-15RM
Romanian deadlift	224	1 × 12-15RM
Dumbbell upright row	167	1 × 12-15RM
Lateral lunge	220	1 × 12-15RM
Dumbbell single-arm row	191	1 × 12-15RM
Lying triceps extension	199	1 × 12-15RM
Kettlebell swing	264	1 × 12-15RM
Dumbbell biceps curl	203	1 × 12-15RM
Abdominal crunch	244	1 × 12-15
Cycle ergometer	148	5 min

enhances local muscle endurance, and improves cardiovascular fitness. It is well rounded, especially for individuals who have limited time to devote to physical activity. Although it does not impart the magnitude of cardiovascular benefit that strict endurance exercise (e.g., jogging or cycling) provides, this program has been shown to improve aerobic capacity by 5 to 8 percent in some individuals, particularly those with a low initial level of conditioning.

Circuit training requires that you perform one set per exercise, alternating between an upper-body exercise and a lower-body exercise, with minimal rest (about 30 seconds or less) between exercises. Then you repeat the circuit if desired. To maximize caloric expenditure during exercise, incorporate as many multijoint exercises as possible. To maintain the rotation between upper- and lower-body exercises and ensure constant blood flow among body parts, several assistance exercises need to be included. At the end of each circuit is a cardiovascular station where you perform three to five minutes of exercise on a cycle ergometer or a treadmill.

Circuit training may be ideal for people who have limited time to exercise. This is the basis for many franchise fitness centers that cater to individuals who want to perform a quick circuit of strength exercises. Depending on their available time and level of conditioning, individuals can perform up to three circuits in one workout. This type of training will enhance the aerobic conditioning effect.

Maximal Strength Training

For people whose training goal is to maximize strength improvement, the resistance training programs outlined in tables 14.5 and 14.6 may be the best

TABLE 14.5   Strength Development Program (3 Days per Week)

Exercise	Page #	Sets × reps*
Monday		
Back squat	210	1, 3 × 4-6RM
Dumbbell bench press	182	1, 3 × 4-6RM
Machine shoulder press	169	1, 3 × 4-6RM
Lat pull-down	188	1, 3 × 4-6RM
Seated leg curl	235	3 × 6RM
Machine seated triceps push-down	193	3 × 6RM
Dumbbell biceps curl	203	3 × 6RM
Abdominal crunch	244	3 × 20
Wednesday		
Leg press	209	1, 3 × 4-6RM
Barbell incline bench press	180	1, 3 × 4-6RM
Dumbbell upright row	167	1, 3 × 4-6RM
Cable seated row	187	1, 3 × 4-6RM
Leg extension	219	3 × 6RM
Lying triceps extension	199	3 × 6RM
EZ-bar curl	205	3 × 6RM
Ankle crunch	244	3 × 20
Friday		
Split squat	214	1, 3 × 4-6RM
Dumbbell bench press	182	1, 3 × 4-6RM
Dumbbell lateral raise	164	1, 3 × 4-6RM
Dumbbell single-arm row	191	1, 3 × 4-6RM
Romanian deadlift	224	3 × 6RM
Close-grip bench press	197	3 × 6RM
Machine biceps curl	201	3 × 6RM
Stability ball crunch	246	3 × 20

*The "1" before the number of sets and repetitions of select exercises indicates that one warm-up set should be performed before the main set.

options. Table 14.5 is a three-days-per-week program that maximizes strength improvement in the intermediate lifter. Table 14.6 provides a four-days-per-week training program for strength improvement in these individuals. The three-days-per-week program allows 48 hours of rest between each training session. The four-day program is a split routine that requires at least 72 hours of rest for the body parts being worked; however, you perform the workouts for days 1 and 2 on consecutive days and the workouts for days 3 and 4 on consecutive days.

TABLE 14.6 Strength Development Program (4 Days per Week)

Monday			Tuesday		
Exercise	**Page #**	**Sets × reps***	**Exercise**	**Page #**	**Sets × reps**
Squat (front or back)	212 or 210	1, 4 × 4-6RM	Barbell bench press	178	1, 4 × 4-6RM
Leg extension	219	4 × 6RM	Barbell incline bench press	180	4 × 4-6RM
Romanian deadlift	224	4 × 6RM	Machine shoulder press	169	1, 4 × 4-6RM
Calf raise	238	4 × 6RM	Dumbbell upright row	167	4 × 4-6RM
Cable seated row	187	1, 4 × 4-6RM	Machine seated triceps push-down	193	4 × 6RM
Dumbbell biceps curl	203	4 × 6RM	Abdominal crunch	244	3 × 20
Back extension	250	4 × 6RM			
Abdominal crunch	244	3 × 20			
Thursday			Friday		
Exercise	**Page #**	**Sets × reps**	**Exercise**	**Page #**	**Sets × reps**
Leg press	209	1, 4 × 4-6RM	Dumbbell bench press	182	1, 4 × 4-6RM
Step-up	216	4 × 6RM	Dumbbell incline bench press	194	4 × 4-6RM
Deadlift	223	4 × 6RM	Standing military press	172	1, 4 × 4-6RM
Calf raise	238	4 × 6RM	Dumbbell front raise	165	4 × 4-6RM
Bent-over row	192	1, 4 × 4-6RM	Close-grip bench press	197	4 × 6RM
Back extension	260	4 × 6RM	Side plank	257	3 × 20
Dumbbell hammer curl	204	4 × 6RM			
Medicine ball overhead reach	250	3 × 20			

*The "1" before the number of sets and repetitions of select exercises indicates that one warm-up set should be performed before the main set.

Because strength development is the primary goal, you should take at least two minutes of rest between each set for either of these training programs.

As discussed earlier, maintaining the proper training intensity is critical for developing maximum strength. If the training program requires 3 sets of 4 to 6RM, you need to select a resistance that you can lift for at least 4 but not more than 6 repetitions while maintaining correct form. Once you can perform 3 sets of 6 repetitions, in order to maintain the appropriate training intensity and overload, you will need to add resistance to the exercise for the next session. Most intermediate strength programs (including both of the provided programs) focus on free-weight exercises. The primary difference between the two programs is that you can include more assistance exercises in the four-day program.

Hypertrophy Training

Table 14.7 depicts a program for people who are interested in maximizing muscle growth. This is a split routine training regimen that should be performed four days per week. To maximize muscle hypertrophy, assistance exercises must be

TABLE 14.7 Muscle Hypertrophy Program (4 Days per Week)

Monday			Tuesday		
Exercise	**Page #**	**Sets × reps***	**Exercise**	**Page #**	**Sets × reps**
Front squat	212	1, 4 × 10-12RM	Dumbbell incline bench press	194	1, 4 × 10-12RM
Lateral lunge with slider	221	4 × 10-12RM	Machine chest fly	175	4 × 10-12RM
Romanian deadlift	224	4 × 10-12RM	Bent-over dumbbell fly	166	1, 4 × 10-12RM
Calf raise	238	4 × 10-12RM	Barbell shrug	173	4 × 10-12RM
Dumbbell single-arm row	191	1, 4 × 10-12RM	Dip	196	4 × 10-12RM
Machine biceps curl	201	4 × 10-12RM	Hanging leg raise	251	3 × 20
Back extension	260	4 × 10-12RM			
Russian twist	254	3 × 20			
Thursday			**Friday**		
Exercise	**Page #**	**Sets × reps**	**Exercise**	**Page #**	**Sets × reps**
Leg press	209	1, 4 × 10-12RM	Barbell bench press	178	1, 4 × 10-12RM
Lateral lunge	220	4 × 10-12RM	Machine chest press	174	4 × 10-12RM
Seated leg curl	235	4 × 10-12RM	Seated barbell military press	170	1, 4 × 10-12RM
Calf raise	238	4 × 10-12RM	Cable lateral raise	163	4 × 10-12RM
Pull-up	190	1, 4 × 10-12RM	Machine seated triceps push-down	193	4 × 10-12RM
Back extension	260	4 × 10-12RM	Outside calf touch	255	3 × 20
EZ-bar curl	205	4 × 10-12RM			
Prone plank	256	3 × 20			

*The "1" before the number of sets and repetitions of select exercises indicates that one warm-up set should be performed before the main set.

incorporated into the training routine, hence the recommendation for a split routine program. The rest period between sets is another important factor for training programs that focus on muscle growth. For these programs, lifters generally will reduce the rest period between sets to 30 to 90 seconds to induce fatigue, which has been demonstrated to be a potent stimulator of anabolic hormone secretion.

The overload principle is still an important concept for increasing muscle growth even though the intensity of exercise is much lower than that of a strength program. The lifter who is interested in maximizing muscle growth still needs to exercise the muscle at a level that provides the required stimulus. Therefore, it is just as important for this type of lifter to increase the resistance when he or she has met a given training protocol—for example, 3 sets of 10 to 12RM—as it is for a lifter who is focusing on maximal strength development.

An important difference between muscle hypertrophy and muscle strength development is the relationship between training intensity and training volume. Training volume typically is defined as the number of sets multiplied by the number of repetitions performed per set. Those interested in maximizing muscle hypertrophy focus on high volume and low intensity—typical of a bodybuilder's resistance training program. On the other hand, those interested in maximal strength development focus on low volume and high intensity. Interestingly, a natural inverse relationship exists between training intensity and training volume. As the intensity of exercise increases, the number of repetitions that can be performed with correct form is reduced (i.e., training volume is decreased). Likewise, as the intensity of exercise is reduced, the number of repetitions is increased (i.e., training volume is increased). In addition to exercise intensity and training volume, the rest interval used between sets is important in eliciting the desired training adaptations. Table 14.8 provides a brief overview of the intensity, volume, and rest intervals used for the various training paradigms.

TABLE 14.8 Comparison of Various Training Paradigms for the Intermediate Lifter

Training paradigm	Training intensity	Training volume	Rest interval between sets
Muscular endurance	>12RM	2-3 sets	<30 s
Muscle hypertrophy	6-12RM	3-6 sets	30-90 s
Muscle strength	<6RM	2-6 sets	2-5 min

Summary

The intermediate lifter can begin to maximize gains in muscle strength and muscle size moreso than a beginner lifter. Specific training paradigms can be designed to help the intermediate lifter achieve his or her training objectives. This chapter highlights training program variables that need to be addressed when developing these specific training programs and provides examples of various exercise protocols for the intermediate lifter.

15

Advanced Programs

Kristen C. Cochrane-Snyman and Jared W. Coburn

As you become more experienced and your body becomes more accustomed to the stresses imposed on it by lifting, your ability to stimulate further physiological change is reduced. Without further modification to the training stimulus, the program becomes less effective and performance improvements begin to wane. The reduced rate of improvement may be acceptable for some intermediate lifters, but it may lead to frustration for others.

This chapter discusses the design and development of advanced resistance training programs. It describes how to further manipulate training variables in order to maximize your desired improvements in performance outcomes while peaking at the desired time, such as a competition or life event (e.g., wedding).

Chronic Program Adaptations

The strength training program for the lifter who progresses from an intermediate to a more advanced level may begin to resemble that of a competitive athlete. The fundamental difference between the training of an advanced lifter and that of a competitive athlete is that the competitive athlete has a defined period of competition. The advanced lifter who is not a competitive athlete may train toward reaching peak physical condition at a time of his or her own choosing rather than maximizing athletic potential at a predetermined period related to a competition schedule.

However, it is difficult to maintain peak physical condition for a prolonged period of time without becoming fatigued or overtrained. By systematically manipulating both training volume and intensity as well as the exercises utilized, an advanced lifter can make the necessary physiological adaptations while reaching peak condition at the appropriate time. In addition, by altering the volume and intensity of training with appropriately timed, short (one to two

The authors acknowledge the significant contributions of Jay Hoffman and Avery Faigenbaum to this chapter.

weeks) reduced-loading phases, the advanced lifter will minimize his or her risk of becoming fatigued or experiencing a plateau in performance improvements. Feelings of fatigue and the inability to perform to one's desired level are often associated with a syndrome called *overtraining,* which can occur when training intensity and volume are increased without interspersing periods of rest and recovery in the training cycle. This eventually results in a decrease in performance and, in some cases, illness and injury.

It is well known that athletes are unable to maintain a high intensity of training stimulus for a prolonged duration without suffering some sort of performance or physiological detriment. To reduce the risk of this occurring, sport scientists have developed periodized training programs that separate a training year, known as a *macrocycle,* into four different training phases (see also chapters 3 and 7 for more discussion of periodization). These phases are referred to as *mesocycles.* The duration of each mesocycle is approximately two to three months, depending on the individual lifter and his or her specific training goals.

As you'll recall from chapter 3, periodization is partially based on principles related to the general adaptation syndrome developed by Dr. Hans Selye, a Czech-trained endocrinologist who became well known for his work on the study of stress. The general adaptation syndrome principle (figure 15.1) suggests that the body experiences three distinct phases in response to the stressful demands that are placed on it. The first phase, known as the *alarm phase,* is the body's initial response to a stimulus (e.g., exercise). This phase consists of both shock and soreness in response to a new exercise stimulus, and it frequently results in a reduction in performance. The second phase is an *adaptation* to this new stimulus. During this phase, the body has adapted to the training stimulus, resulting in an observable improvement in performance. The third phase is one of *exhaustion.* During this phase, the body is unable to make any further

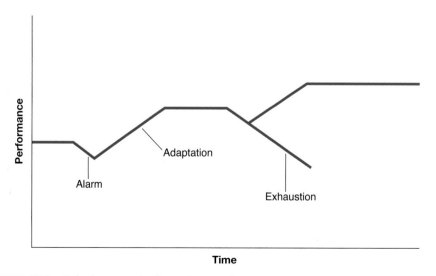

FIGURE 15.1 Selye's general adaptation syndrome.

Adapted from H. Selye, 1956, *The stress of life* (New York: McGraw-Hill Companies).

adaptation to the training stimulus. Unless this stimulus is reduced, a situation leading to prolonged fatigue (i.e., overtraining) may occur. On the other hand, if the body is allowed sufficient recovery, it can then make further adaptations, and performance may increase further. The purpose of periodization is to maintain an effective training stimulus that leads to consistent long-term improvements in performance while minimizing the risk of illness, injury, or burnout.

Periodization is based on the manipulation of both training volume and training intensity. During the first mesocycle of a linear periodization model, often referred to as the *preparatory* or *hypertrophy* phase, training volume (i.e., total number of repetitions) is high and training intensity (i.e., percentage of the individual's maximal lifting ability in a particular exercise) is low. In addition, the lifter puts little effort into choosing sport-specific exercises, or exercises with movement patterns similar to the sport for which he or she is training. For the advanced lifter, this phase of the training cycle focuses on increasing muscle mass and muscle endurance. A secondary objective is to help prepare the lifter for the more intense training cycles that will occur later in the training program. During the next two mesocycles—referred to as *strength* and *strength-power*—intensity of training is increased, whereas the volume of training is reduced. During these two mesocycles, the advanced lifter primarily is concerned with strength and power development and performs more sport-specific exercises. The final mesocycle of the training year is the *peaking* phase. This phase is geared toward the competitive athlete who wants to attain peak conditioning for a specific competition or the most important competitions of the year. During this mesocycle, training volume is again reduced, whereas training intensity is at its highest level. Table 15.1 shows the volume and intensity typically seen during the various mesocycles in a training cycle.

Although the purpose of a periodized training program is to prepare an athlete to reach peak condition for a specific event during the year, many advanced lifters participate in sports that place importance on an entire season of competition, such as American football, baseball, and basketball. For these athletes, peak strength must be achieved by the onset of the competitive year and maintained throughout the competitive season. The peaking phase for these athletes generally

TABLE 15.1 Typical Intensities and Volumes of Training for a Periodized Training Program for an Advanced Strength or Power Athlete

	Phase of training				
	Muscular endurance	Hypertrophy	Strength	Power*	
				Single effort	Multiple effort
Sets	2-3	3-6	2-6	3-5	3-5
Repetitions	>12	6-12	<6	1-2	3-5
Intensity (% 1RM)	<67	67-85	>85	80-90	75-85

*Single effort = sport event such as shot put or high jump; multiple effort = sport event such as basketball or volleyball.

occurs several weeks before the preseason period. However, once the competitive season begins, the athlete performs an additional mesocycle, known as the *maintenance* phase, to maintain the strength, power, and size gains made during the off-season strength and conditioning program. During this phase of training, exercise intensity often is reduced to the levels used during the strength mesocycle, whereas training volume is lowered by reducing the number of assistance exercises performed during each workout. It is not uncommon for the advanced lifter to use short training cycles that last between several days and two weeks, known as *microcycles*, to transition from mesocycle to mesocycle.

Periodized Programs

The basic model of periodization focuses on strategic changes in training intensity and volume between each mesocycle, but these training variables remain relatively constant within each mesocycle. This periodization model, sometimes referred to as a *linear* model, is the traditional or classical form used for designing most periodized training programs. However, nonlinear or undulating models of periodization are also becoming popular. In this type of periodization scheme, the volume and intensity of training vary from workout to workout. Table 15.2 provides an example of a nonlinear training model. The intensity of the workouts varies among light, moderate, and heavy training.

This nonlinear training model is appropriate for advanced lifters. It can also be advantageous for athletes who participate in sports that involve a varied schedule with several games or competitions in a given week, such as basketball, hockey, baseball, or soccer. Additionally, it may be effective for lifters who participate in sports with a variable game or travel schedule that does not permit a regularly scheduled strength maintenance program during the season. Some coaches and athletes may prefer to use relatively light training intensities before or on days of competition. In the undulating periodized program, the athlete can still train at a high intensity but at a more appropriate time of the week given his or her competition schedule.

General Muscular Conditioning

For the advanced lifter whose primary training goal is to improve general muscular conditioning, an undulating program design may be the most appropriate. For these individuals, the primary purpose is general fitness. They are not preparing

TABLE 15.2 Sample Nonlinear Periodized Training Program

Day	Program	Sets	Repetitions (RM)	Rest between sets (min)
1	Power	3-5	1-5	2-5
2	Strength	2-6	<6	2-5
3	Hypertrophy	3-6	6-12	.5-1.5

for a specific competition or a season of competition, so a program that has them peak for a specific time frame is irrelevant. Table 15.3 depicts an undulating program for an advanced lifter who is interested in general muscular fitness.

On careful examination of this program, it appears quite similar to the three-days-per-week general muscular fitness program for the intermediate lifter (see

TABLE 15.3 Undulating Program for General Muscular Conditioning

Exercise	Page #	Sets × reps
Monday		
Leg press	209	3 × 4-6RM
Machine chest press	174	3 × 4-6RM
Seated barbell military press	170	3 × 4-6RM
Lat pull-down	188	3 × 4-6RM
Back extension	260	3 × 4-6RM
Seated leg curl	235	3 × 4-6RM
Machine seated triceps push-down	193	3 × 4-6RM
Dumbbell biceps curl	203	3 × 4-6RM
Bent-knee sit-up	243	3 × 20
Wednesday		
Lateral lunge	220	3 × 10-12RM
Barbell incline bench press	180	3 × 10-12RM
Dumbbell upright row	167	3 × 10-12RM
Cable seated row	187	3 × 10-12RM
Back extension	260	3 × 10-12RM
Romanian deadlift	224	3 × 10-12RM
Lying triceps extension	199	3 × 10-12RM
EZ-bar curl	205	3 × 10-12RM
Jackknife	249	3 × 20
Friday		
Step-up	216	3 × 15RM
Dumbbell bench press	182	3 × 15RM
Dumbbell lateral raise	164	3 × 15RM
Dumbbell single-arm row	191	3 × 15RM
Back extension	260	3 × 15RM
Seated leg curl	235	3 × 15RM
Close-grip bench press	197	3 × 15RM
Machine biceps curl	201	3 × 15RM
Bent-knee sit-up	243	3 × 20

table 14.1). It is unlikely that a person could maintain that training program for a prolonged time period without suffering some form of decline in performance or other symptom associated with overtraining syndrome. Thus, as these individuals move on to the advanced lifting program, they need to manipulate their weekly training sessions. On Monday, the lifter focuses on basic strength. Each exercise should be performed with a resistance that can be performed for at least 4 but not more than 6 repetitions, with two to five minutes of rest between each set. On Wednesday, the workout focuses on muscle hypertrophy by requiring a lighter resistance that allows the lifter to perform a greater number of repetitions (10-12) per set, with 30 to 90 seconds of rest between sets. On Friday, the workout involves a low intensity and high volume (15RM), with 30 seconds of rest between each set. Advanced lifters should rest for approximately 48 hours between each training session for a given muscle group.

Strength and Power Training

Table 15.4 depicts a three-days-per-week undulating (nonlinear) training program for the competitive strength or power athlete. A whole-body workout is performed during each training session. The difference between each workout is the variety of exercises, the intensity and volume of the training session, and the rest period. These acute program variables correspond to the goal of the training session. The first workout of the week focuses on strength and power, whereas the second and third workouts emphasize muscle strength and hypertrophy, respectively. Rest periods between sets should be approximately two to three minutes during the first two training sessions and approximately 30 to 90 seconds during the muscle hypertrophy workout. Typically, 48 hours of rest should be included between each training session. As discussed earlier in this chapter, this training program may also be used by athletes who are involved in a season of competition.

Table 15.5 provides an example of a periodized (linear) yearly training program for advanced lifters who are interested in maximizing strength and power development. This program would be appropriate for a strength or power athlete such as a powerlifter, football player, or basketball player. It would not be the ideal training program for the recreational athlete or lifter who is not attempting to reach a peak in performance for a specific time of the year. This program uses a four-days-per-week split routine. Similar to other four-day split routines that have been described, the workouts on days 1 and 2 are performed consecutively, as are the training sessions on days 3 and 4. However, at least 72 hours of rest is allotted between workouts 1 and 3 and between workouts 2 and 4 in order to provide adequate rest for the specific muscle groups. The rest interval between sets is determined by the mesocycle in which the individual is training. During the hypertrophy (or preparatory) phase, the rest between sets is approximately 30 to 90 seconds. During the strength, strength-power, and peaking phases, the rest interval is two to five minutes between sets.

TABLE 15.4 Undulating Program for the Competitive Athlete

Exercise	Page #	Sets × reps
Monday		
Push press	281	3 × 1-2RM
High pull	273	3 × 1-2RM
Back squat	210	3 × 3-5RM
Barbell bench press	178	3 × 3-5RM
Lat pull-down	188	3 × 3-5RM
Machine seated triceps push-down	193	3 × 3-5RM
Dumbbell biceps curl	203	3 × 3-5RM
Wednesday		
Step-up	216	3 × 4-6RM
Dumbbell incline bench press	184	3 × 4-6RM
Dumbbell upright row	167	3 × 4-6RM
Cable seated row	187	3 × 4-6RM
Back extension	260	3 × 4-6RM
Romanian deadlift	224	3 × 4-6RM
Lying triceps extension	199	3 × 4-6RM
EZ-bar curl	205	3 × 4-6RM
Abdominal crunch	244	3 × 20
Friday		
Step-up	216	3 × 10-12RM
Dumbbell bench press	182	3 × 10-12RM
Dumbbell lateral raise	164	3 × 10-12RM
Dumbbell single-arm row	191	3 × 10-12RM
Kettlebell swing	265	3 × 10-12RM
Seated leg curl	235	3 × 10-12RM
Close-grip bench press	197	3 × 10-12RM
Machine biceps curl	201	3 × 10-12RM
Stability ball crunch	246	3 × 20

In the linear program, each phase of training should last from six to eight weeks, with a one-week unloading period between each phase. During unloading periods, the individual does not perform any resistance training but may be recreationally active (e.g., playing racket sports, jogging). The unloading period should consist of a reduction in training volume (i.e., fewer exercises; lower weights, sets, and reps) but not an absence of training. The peaking phase may

TABLE 15.5 Periodized Training for Strength and Power*

Phase I: preparatory or hypertrophy	Page #	Phase II: basic strength	Page #	Phase III: strength-power	Page #	Phase IV: peaking	Page #
Days 1 and 3							
Back squat (1, 4 × 8-10RM)	210	Back squat (1, 4 × 5-6RM)	210	Back squat (1, 3 × 3-5RM)	210	Back squat (1, 3 × 1-2RM)	210
Leg extension (3 × 8-10RM)	219	Deadlift (4 × 5-6RM)	222	Deadlift (3 × 3-5RM)	222	Deadlift (3 × 1-2RM)	222
Seated leg curl (3 × 8-10RM)	235	Seated leg curl (3 × 5-6RM)	235	Seated leg curl (3 × 5-6RM)	235	Seated leg curl (3 × 5-6RM)	235
Calf raise (3 × 8-10RM)	238	Calf raise (3 × 5-6RM)	238	Lat pull-down (1, 3 × 3-5RM)	188	Lat pull-down (1, 3 × 5-6RM)	188
Lat pull-down (1, 4 × 8-10RM)	188	Lat pull-down (1, 4 × 5-6RM)	188	Cable seated row (3 × 5-6RM)	187	Cable seated row (5 × 4-6RM)	187
Cable seated row (4 × 8-10RM)	187	Cable seated row (4 × 5-6RM)	187	Dumbbell biceps curl (3 × 5-6RM)	203	Dumbbell biceps curl (3 × 4-6RM)	203
Dumbbell biceps curl (3 × 8-10RM)	203	Dumbbell biceps curl (3 × 5-6RM)	203	EZ-bar curl (3 × 5-6RM)	205	Back extension (3 × 30)	260
EZ-bar curl (3 × 8-10RM)	205	EZ-bar curl (3 × 5-6RM)	205	Back extension (3 × 5-6RM)	260	Abdominal crunch (3 × 20)	244
Back extension (3 × 8-10RM)	260	Back extension (3 × 5-6RM)	260	Abdominal crunch (3 × 20)	244		
Abdominal crunch (3 × 20)	244	Abdominal crunch (3 × 20)	244				
Days 2 and 4							
Barbell bench press (1, 4 × 8-10RM)	178	High pull (1, 4 × 5-6RM)	273	High pull (1, 3 × 3-5RM)	273	Power clean (1, 3 × 1-2RM)	268
Barbell incline bench press (3 × 8-10RM)	180	Barbell bench press (1, 4 × 5-6RM)	178	Push press (1, 3 × 3-5RM)	281	Push jerk (1, 3 × 1-2RM)	285
Lying dumbbell fly (3 × 8-10RM)	176	Barbell incline bench press (3 × 5-6RM)	180	Barbell bench press (1, 3 × 3-5RM)	178	Barbell bench press (1, 3 × 1-2RM)	178
Seated barbell military press (1, 4 × 8-10RM)	170	Lying dumbbell fly (3 × 5-6RM)	176	Barbell incline bench press (3 × 3-5RM)	180	Barbell incline bench press (3 × 1-2RM)	180
Dumbbell upright row (3 × 8-10RM)	167	Seated barbell military press (3 × 5-6RM)	170	Dumbbell upright row (3 × 5-6RM)	167	Dumbbell upright row (3 × 5-6RM)	167
Dumbbell lateral raise (3 × 8-10RM)	164	Dumbbell front raise (3 × 5-6RM)	165	Lying triceps extension (3 × 5-6RM)	199	Lying triceps extension (3 × 5-6RM)	199

Phase I: preparatory or hypertrophy	Page #	Phase II: basic strength	Page #	Phase III: strength-power	Page #	Phase IV: peaking	Page #
Machine seated triceps push-down (3 × 8-10RM)	193	Lying triceps extension (3 × 5-6RM)	195	Assisted dip (3 × 5-6RM)	195	Assisted dip (3 × 5-6RM)	195
Lying triceps extension (3 × 8-10RM)	199	Machine seated triceps push-down (3 × 5-6RM)	193	Abdominal crunch (3 × 20)	244	Abdominal crunch (3 × 20)	244
Abdominal crunch (3 × 20)	244	Medicine ball overhead reach (3 × 20)	250				

*The "1" before the number of sets and repetitions of select exercises indicates that one warm-up set should be performed before the main set.

be shorter in duration, lasting approximately four to six weeks. Some advanced lifters may repeat these cycles to provide greater variability in their yearly training program. For instance, football players may perform these cycles before spring football and then repeat the same training paradigm after spring football and leading into preseason training camp.

Hypertrophy Training

For the advanced lifter who is interested in maximizing muscle growth, the primary change from the intermediate-level hypertrophy program is the number and type of exercises. Because lifters who are interested in maximizing muscle hypertrophy generally use high volume, low intensity, and short rest (30-90 seconds between sets) in their training programs, the variations you can introduce in these acute program variables are limited. Although some individuals who train in this manner may incorporate several higher-intensity exercise routines, for the most part these training protocols are often similar in regard to volume, intensity, and rest.

What the advanced lifter may do is vary the selection and order of exercises in the program. For instance, some bodybuilders will change the order of exercise so that instead of performing the exercises that recruit the larger muscle mass first, they first perform the assistance exercises to prefatigue the muscle. Although this may seem to contradict what was said in earlier chapters, the focus for these lifters is not to maximize strength gains but rather to maximize muscle growth. By prefatiguing the muscle fibers, these lifters are trying to achieve a greater anabolic effect on the muscle. Exercise order can also be manipulated through super setting and compound setting. You'll recall from chapter 3 that super setting involves alternating exercises for agonist and antagonist muscle groups (e.g., machine biceps curl and machine seated triceps push-down) with little or no rest between exercises. Compound setting involves performing different exercises for the same muscle group (e.g., barbell incline bench press and bent-over dumbbell fly) in an alternating fashion with little or no rest between exercises.

Many advanced lifters interested in body sculpting may employ a four- or six-days-per-week split routine. Tables 15.6 and 15.7 provide examples of both of these options.

The primary reason why some advanced lifters prefer a six-days-per-week training program is that it provides greater opportunity to focus on a single muscle group per workout session. In addition, it can provide adequate time in a program to add assistance exercises for the selected group or groups. Another feature of the six-day training program is the increased number of compound

TABLE 15.6 Advanced Program for Muscle Hypertrophy (4 Days per Week)*

Monday			Tuesday		
Exercise	Page #	Sets × reps	Exercise	Page #	Sets × reps
Back squat	210	1, 4 × 8-10RM	Barbell bench press	178	1, 4 × 8-10RM
Leg press	209	3 × 8-10RM	Dumbbell incline bench press	184	3 × 8-10RM
Superset: Leg extension Seated leg curl	219 235	3 × 8-10RM	Lying dumbbell fly	176	3 × 8-10RM
Calf raise	238	3 × 8-10RM	Seated barbell military press	170	4 × 8-10RM
Lat pull-down	188	1, 4 × 8-10RM	**Compound set:** Dumbbell upright row Dumbbell lateral raise	167 164	3 × 8-10RM
Cable seated row	187	4 × 8-10RM	Barbell shrug	173	3 × 8-10RM
Back extension	260	4 × 8-10RM	Machine seated triceps push-down	193	4 × 8-10RM
EZ-bar curl	205	4 × 8-10RM	Lying triceps extension	199	4 × 8-10RM
Dumbbell biceps curl	203	4 × 8-10RM	Alternate-touch crunch	253	4 × 20
Abdominal crunch	244	4 × 20			

and super sets that can be incorporated, allowing for greater fatigue to occur during each training session. However, it is difficult for most individuals—even advanced lifters—to maintain a six-days-per-week training program for more than a month. Such training protocols often pose problems when it comes to providing adequate recovery.

Similar to other split routine training programs, both sample programs in tables 15.6 and 15.7 include at least 72 hours of rest between workouts of the same body part. For the six-day program, workouts on days 1, 2, and 3 can be performed on consecutive days, so there is one day of complete rest before day 4. Although not necessary, you may consider interchanging different exercises for those listed in the training program to help reduce potential monotony.

Thursday			Friday		
Exercise	Page #	Sets × reps	Exercise	Page #	Sets × reps
Front squat	212	1, 4 × 8-10RM	Dumbbell bench press	182	1, 4 × 8-10RM
Lateral lunge with slider	221	3 × 8-10RM	Dumbbell incline bench press	184	3 × 8-10RM
Step-up	216	3 × 8-10RM	Machine chest press	174	3 × 8-10RM
Romanian deadlift	224	3 × 8-10RM	Standing military press	172	1, 4 × 8-10RM
Calf raise	238	3 × 8-10RM	**Compound set:** Dumbbell front raise Bent-over dumbbell fly	165 166	3 × 8-10RM
Bent-over row	192	1, 4 × 8-10RM	Close-grip bench press	197	4 × 8-10RM
Machine seated row	186	4 × 8-10RM	Machine seated triceps push-down	193	4 × 8-10RM
Dumbbell hammer curl	204	4 × 8-10RM	Outside calf touch	255	4 × 20
Machine biceps curl	201	4 × 8-10RM	Side plank	257	4 × 20
Side bend	258	4 × 20			

*The "1" before the number of sets and repetitions of select exercises indicates that one warm-up set should be performed before the main set.

TABLE 15.7 Advanced Program for Muscle Hypertrophy (6 Days per Week)

Day 1			Day 4		
Chest and triceps					
Exercise	**Page #**	**Sets × reps**	**Exercise**	**Page #**	**Sets × reps**
Barbell bench press	178	4 × 6-12RM	Dumbbell bench press	192	4 × 6-12RM
Dumbbell incline bench press	184	4 × 6-12RM	Barbell incline bench press	180	4 × 6-12RM
Machine chest press	174	4 × 6-12RM	Machine chest fly	175	4 × 6-12RM
Dip	196	4 × 6-12RM	Assisted dip	195	4 × 6-12RM
Lying triceps extension	199	4 × 6-12RM	Close-grip bench press	197	4 × 6-12RM
Machine seated triceps push-down	193	4 × 6-12RM	Machine seated triceps push-down	193	4 × 6-12RM
Abdominal crunch	244	3 × 20	Prone plank	256	3 × 20
Day 2			**Day 5**		
Back and shoulders					
Exercise	**Page #**	**Sets × reps**	**Exercise**	**Page #**	**Sets × reps**
Machine shoulder press	169	4 × 6-12RM	Seated barbell military press	170	4 × 6-12RM
Dumbbell upright row	167	4 × 6-12RM	Bent-over dumbbell fly	166	4 × 6-12RM
Compound set: Dumbbell front raise Dumbbell lateral raise	 165 164	3 × 6-12RM	Cable lateral raise	163	4 × 6-12RM
Assisted pull-up	189	4 × 6-12RM	Dumbbell single-arm row	191	4 × 6-12RM
Lat pull-down	188	4 × 6-12RM	Cable seated row	187	4 × 6-12RM
Bent-over row	192	4 × 6-12RM	Machine seated row	186	4 × 6-12RM
Modified Superman	266	4 × 6-12RM	Kettlebell swing	264	4 × 6-12RM
Day 3			**Day 6**		
Legs and biceps					
Exercise	**Page #**	**Sets × reps**	**Exercise**	**Page #**	**Sets × reps**
Back squat	210	4 × 6-12RM	Leg Press	209	4 × 6-12RM
Step-up	216	4 × 6-12RM	Front squat	212	4 × 6-12RM
Superset: Leg extension Seated leg curl	 219 235	3 × 6-12RM	**Superset:** Seated leg curl Leg extension	 235 219	3 × 6-12RM
Calf raise	238	3 × 6-12RM	Calf raise	238	3 × 6-12RM
Compound set: Dumbbell biceps curl EZ-bar curl	 203 205	3 × 6-12RM	**Compound set:** Dumbbell hammer curl Machine biceps curl	 204 201	3 × 6-12RM

Summary

The advanced lifting programs are geared toward individuals who have remained committed to resistance training for a prolonged period. Although the goals described in the chapter on intermediate lifting are still relevant, they are addressed and maintained by the advanced lifter via the manipulation of acute program variables over the course of a yearly training program. The systematic manipulation of these acute program variables to develop the yearly training protocol is known as *periodization*.

A periodized training program for a recreational athlete or lifter whose goal is to reach peak performance at a specific time period may resemble that of a competitive athlete. An experienced recreational lifter who is primarily interested in general muscular fitness, on the other hand, may put together a different periodized program or may decide that the move from an intermediate-level program to an advanced program is not necessary. This chapter focused on how the acute training program variables can be manipulated during a training year to meet the individual goals of experienced lifters.

16

Youth Programs

Pablo B. Costa and David H. Fukuda

Children and adolescents traditionally have been encouraged to participate regularly in aerobic activities such as swimming and bicycling to enhance and maintain their cardiovascular fitness. However, a compelling body of evidence indicates that strength training can also be a safe, effective, and fun method of exercise for boys and girls as young as seven years of age provided that appropriate training guidelines are followed. Over the past decade, strength training has become a popular conditioning tool with proven benefits for children and adolescents who want to improve their health, fitness, and sport performance. Today, boys and girls are strength training as part of a general fitness program in physical education classes, in after-school programs, at recreation centers, and at sport camps. In support, 10 major professional sports medicine, exercise science, and pediatric organizations combined to endorse the *Position Statement on Youth Resistance Training: The 2014 International Consensus* (Lloyd et al. 2014a), which outlines the benefits of strength training and provides general guidelines for implementation in this population. In conjunction, in 2016 the National Strength and Conditioning Association released a *Position Statement on Long-Term Athletic Development*, which incorporates these benefits and guidelines for strength training within a long-term approach to physical activity and exercise participation. The same Position Statement clarifies that the terms *youth* and *young athletes* represent both children (up to approximately age 11 years in girls and 13 years in boys) and adolescents (typically including girls aged 12-18 years and boys aged 14-18 years).

Despite the previously held belief that strength training was inappropriate or unsafe for children, the acceptance of youth strength training by professional organizations has become universal. In fact, *Physical Activity Guidelines for Americans* (Physical Activity Guidelines Advisory Committee 2008) recommends that

The authors acknowledge the significant contributions of Jay Hoffman and Avery Faigenbaum to this chapter.

341

children and adolescents engage in moderate to vigorous activity that includes resistance exercise and bone-loading activities at least three days per week, and *Global Recommendations on Physical Activity for Health* (World Health Organization 2010) includes resistance training as part of its guidelines for children. Indeed, a strong musculoskeletal system is recognized as an important component of health-related physical fitness (along with aerobic fitness, flexibility, balance, and appropriate body composition). Unfortunately, less than half of all children and adolescents meet these guidelines. Like riding a bike and playing basketball, participation in a youth strength training program provides boys and girls with yet another opportunity to improve their health, fitness, and quality of life.

Although a growing number of boys and girls participate in strength training programs in schools, camps, YMCAs, and fitness centers, some parents and coaches have lingering concerns about the safety of youth strength training. Others are unsure whether the potential benefits of youth strength training outweigh the risks.

Benefits of Strength Training for Youths

When appropriately designed and competently supervised, youth strength training programs can offer observable health and fitness benefits to boys and girls, including the following:

- Increases in muscle strength and power
- Increases in local muscle endurance
- Increases in bone mineral density
- Improvements in blood lipid profile
- Improvements in body composition
- Increases in motor skill performance (balance, jumping, throwing, and sprinting)
- Improvements in athletic ability
- Increases in resistance to sport-related injuries
- Improvements in body image and self-confidence
- A more positive attitude toward lifetime physical activity

In addition to increasing muscular strength and power, strength training has the potential to positively influence local muscular endurance (i.e., the ability to perform more repetitions at a given weight), body composition, bone mineral density, and motor performance skills such as sprinting, jumping, and throwing. Furthermore, aspiring young athletes who participate in a preseason conditioning program that includes strength training tend to suffer fewer sport-related injuries during practice and competition compared with children and adolescents who do not strength train.

In the United States, approximately 70 percent of children and adolescents in 3rd through 12th grades participate in team or organized sports (Sabo and

■■■■ Dispelling the Myths

Many myths surrounding youth strength training persist today. The most prevalent myths and the facts that refute them include the following:

Myth: Strength training stunts the growth of children.

Fact: No scientific evidence supports the belief that strength training stunts the growth of children. Despite concerns associated with this type of training, properly performed strength training exercises do not put too much pressure on the developing growth plates of young athletes. In addition, lateral impact on the bone is not typical in strength training, unlike what is seen in contact sports commonly played by youths. Physical activity is essential for normal growth and development. Therefore, regular participation in strength training activities will likely have a favorable influence on growth during childhood and adolescence because it provides longitudinal weight-bearing stimulus to the bone. Additional concerns associated with this myth are discussed later in this chapter.

Myth: Children cannot increase muscle strength because they do not have enough testosterone.

Fact: Testosterone is not essential for achieving strength gains, as evidenced by women who experience impressive gains in strength even though they have little testosterone. In addition, strength gains without increases in muscle mass are possible due to neurological adaptations. On a relative or percentage basis, training-induced strength gains during childhood are comparable with those made during adulthood.

Myth: Strength training is unsafe for children.

Fact: The risks associated with strength training are not greater than those associated with other physical activities in which children regularly participate. The key is to provide qualified supervision, age-specific instruction and programming, and a safe training environment. However, as with all types of physical activity, accidents can happen if coaches, parents, or children do not follow established training guidelines and adhere to safety rules.

Myth: Strength training is for fit young athletes only.

Fact: Regular participation in a youth strength training program can be a safe, effective, and worthwhile experience for boys and girls of all abilities. Strength training certainly can make young athletes faster and stronger, but it may also spark an interest in physical activity in sedentary or overweight youths who tend to dislike prolonged periods of continuous aerobic exercise.

Myth: Strength training will make kids "muscle bound" and inflexible.

Fact: Performing strength-building exercises throughout the full range of motion will not result in a loss of flexibility. In fact, strength training combined with stretching exercises may actually improve flexibility in children and adolescents.

Veliz 2008). Unfortunately, along with this remarkable interest in youth sport, an accompanying increase has occurred in the number of sport-related injuries, possibly due to poorly prepared or improperly trained young athletes. Although factors such as improper footwear and hard playing surfaces have been implicated as risk factors for overuse injuries (e.g., stress fractures and tendinitis), we must also consider the current physical activity level of boys and girls who want to play a competitive sport. Generally, today's youths spend less time being physically active and more time with sedentary pursuits such as using the computer or playing video games. Parents need to recognize that participation in physical activity should not begin with competitive sport; rather, it should evolve out of preparatory conditioning that includes playing, daily physical activity, and strength training. To obtain the specific benefits from strength training, boys and girls need to participate regularly in a strength training program.

Accordingly, if children and adolescents spend more time developing fundamental physical abilities (e.g., muscular fitness) before participating in sport, their musculoskeletal system will be better prepared for the demands of practice and competition. Although the total elimination of sport-related injuries is an unrealistic goal, strength training may help decrease the incidence of injuries in youth sport by strengthening the supporting structures (ligaments, tendons, and bones), enhancing muscle fitness, and developing muscle balance around a joint. Aspiring young athletes should be advised to participate in at least six weeks of preparatory conditioning (including strength, aerobic, and flexibility training) before competitive sport participation (see figure 16.1). This type of conditioning will better prepare boys and girls for the demands of practice and

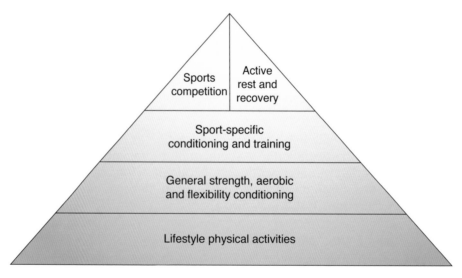

FIGURE 16.1   Physical activity pyramid.

Reprinted, by permission, from A. Faigenbaum, 2001, "Progression conditioning for high school athletes," *Strength and Conditioning* 23(1): 70-72.

competition and may decrease the likelihood that some will drop out of a sport because of frustration, embarrassment, failure, or injury.

In addition to helping young athletes, strength training can be beneficial from a health perspective. Although aerobic exercise typically is prescribed for decreasing body fat, it appears that regular participation in a strength training program can have a favorable influence on the body composition of overweight youths. In addition, youngsters who are not accustomed to physical activity tend to enjoy strength training because it is not aerobically taxing, and the easily adaptable nature of strength training gives all participants a chance to experience success and feel good about their performance regardless of body size and fitness ability. Along with support from family and friends, regular participation in a physical activity program that includes strength training may be part of the solution for long-term fat loss and weight management in overweight boys and girls. However, youth strength training programs need to be properly designed to be effective and safe.

Risks and Concerns

In general, the risk of injury associated with strength training is similar for children and adults. However, one of the unique concerns associated with youth strength training involves the potential for injury to the epiphyses, or growth plates, of the long bones (e.g., the radius in the arms and the femur in the legs). The growth of the long bones in a child is initiated from a section of cartilage, known as an *epiphyseal plate* (growth plate), at the end of each long bone (see figure 16.2). This area is the weak link in the developing skeleton because growth cartilage is not as strong as bone. Although children and adolescents are susceptible to growth plate fractures, this type of injury has not been reported in any research study of youth strength training involving programs that were properly designed and supervised by qualified adults. It appears that the risk of a growth plate fracture is minimal if boys and girls are taught how to strength train properly and use appropriate training loads. In fact, sideways impacts that are common in sports such as soccer, football, and basketball are more likely to cause injuries to the growth plates.

The greatest concern for children and adolescents

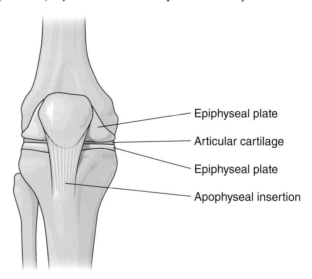

FIGURE 16.2   Growth plate cartilage in the knee.

Epiphyseal plate

Articular cartilage

Epiphyseal plate

Apophyseal insertion

who engage in strength training is the risk of repetitive or overuse injuries to the soft tissue of the muscles, tendons, and ligaments. Although the incidence of this type of injury is difficult to determine because it does not always result in a visit to a physician, limited evidence suggests that the risk of developing this kind of injury is worth mentioning. In studies involving teenage athletes, about half of the reported injuries from strength training occurred in the lower back region. Although these young athletes presumably trained with very heavy weights and/or improper exercise techniques, similar injuries could occur in boys and girls who participate in school-based or recreational programs. These findings highlight the importance of following safety standards (e.g., adult supervision, spotters, safe equipment) and using proper exercise technique, appropriate weights, and program design. Thus, youth strength training programs need to be carefully designed and appropriately progressed because serious accidents can happen if safety guidelines are not followed.

No justifiable safety reasons exist to preclude children and adolescents from participating in strength-building activities. In addition, some youths spend too much time training their "mirror muscles" (e.g., chest and biceps) and not enough time—or no time at all—strengthening their abdominal and lower-back muscles. Hence, additional guidance often is needed to help youths develop a balanced strength training program. In fact, because of the potential for lower-back injuries noted previously and the high prevalence of low-back pain among the general population, it would be reasonable for all boys and girls (as well as adults) to include abdominal and lower-back strengthening exercises in their general fitness program. Finally, because children generally do not dissipate as much heat as adults, particular attention should be paid to hydration status. Because children are not likely to stop exercising when having fun, water breaks can be implemented in order to ensure adequate fluid intake.

Program Design Considerations

There is no widely accepted minimum age requirement for participating in a youth strength training program. However, all children who participate should have the emotional maturity to accept and follow directions and should understand the benefits and risks associated with this type of training. In general, if a child is ready for participation in sport, then he or she may be ready for some type of strength training. Although children as young as age seven or eight have participated in supervised youth strength training programs, cautionary measures need to be taken when youths of any age want to participate in strength training. In addition, strength training should be just one part of a total physical activity program for children and adolescents that also includes free play and recreational physical activities.

Because no major difference exists in relative strength between prepubescent boys and girls (generally under age 13), strength training programs for both sexes can be similar in design. In only a short period of time (about 8-12 weeks), untrained boys and girls can increase their strength by up to about 40 percent. Although most of this increase is attributable to neuromuscular adaptations, this relative gain is similar to the relative gains made by adolescents and adults. Even though boys and girls will get stronger on their own simply because of normal growth, a well-designed strength training program helps optimize training-induced strength gains in youths beyond those obtained through the development and maturation process.

No matter how big or strong a child is, adult training philosophies (e.g., "no pain, no gain") should not be imposed on boys and girls who are physically and psychologically less mature. When designing strength training programs for youths, it is always better to underestimate their physical abilities and gradually increase the intensity or weight than to overestimate their abilities and risk an injury. Some beginners may want to see how much weight they can lift on the first day of the program. If this occurs, try to redirect their enthusiasm and interest in lifting heavy weights toward the development of proper form and technique on a variety of strength-building exercises using lighter loads. In any case, youths

Youth Strength Training Guidelines

- ☐ Provide qualified adult supervision and instruction.
- ☐ Ensure that the exercise environment is safe and free of hazards.
- ☐ Begin each session with a 5- to 10-minute general warm-up period.
- ☐ Conduct specific warm-up sets for each exercise (approximately half of the starting weight).
- ☐ Start with 1 or 2 sets of 1 to 3 repetitions (<60 percent of 1RM) on a variety of exercises in order to emphasize technical competencies.
- ☐ Progress to 2 to 4 sets of 6 to 12 repetitions (60-80 percent of 1RM) depending on individual needs and goals.
- ☐ Perform a total of 6 to 10 exercises for the upper body, lower body, and midsection.
- ☐ Increase the resistance gradually (e.g., 5-10 percent) as strength improves, and consider fewer repetitions.
- ☐ Focus on the correct exercise technique instead of the amount of weight lifted.
- ☐ Strength train two or three times per week on nonconsecutive days.
- ☐ Use individualized workout logs to monitor progress.
- ☐ Provide proper spotting when necessary to actively assist in the event of a failed repetition.
- ☐ Keep the program fresh and challenging by systematically varying the training program.

should always learn proper form and technique with a light weight (or even a wooden dowel) before adding weight to the bar.

Tangible outcome measures such as increasing muscle strength are important, but they are not the only benefits associated with a youth strength training program. When instructing children, focus on intrinsic rewards such as skill improvement, personal success, and having fun. Throughout the program, teach children and adolescents about proper lifting techniques and safe training procedures (e.g., controlled movements and proper breathing). In addition, do not overlook the importance of youths developing a more positive attitude toward strength training and other types of physical activity. Rather than competing against each other in the weight room, with appropriate guidance and supervision boys and girls can learn to embrace self-improvement and feel good about their own accomplishments. Using individualized workout cards can help focus each child or adolescent on his or her own performance. Other issues to address in designing an effective strength training program for children and adolescents include the quality of instruction, mode of training, choice and order of exercises, and rate of progression as well as those provided under the Youth Strength Training Guidelines.

Quality of Instruction

Children and adolescents should strength train only when under the watchful eye of a qualified adult. Although the efforts of inexperienced adults are appreciated, it is unlikely that they will be able to provide the quality of instruction that is needed for safe and effective training. Parents, youth coaches, and fitness trainers should have a thorough understanding of youth strength training guidelines and safety procedures. Accordingly, adults supervising youth strength training should be aware of proper spotting procedures, speak to children and adolescents at a level they understand, and model appropriate behavior. They should also keep the program fun and challenging while recognizing the importance of adhering to safe training procedures. All exercises must be clearly explained and properly demonstrated to all participants. Easy-to-follow explanations and verbal learning cues (e.g., "back erect," "eyes forward") can facilitate the learning of a desired skill or movement.

Unsafe behavior in the strength training area should not be tolerated under any circumstances. We do not recommend strength training at home for youths unless a competent adult is willing to provide supervision and instruction to ensure that proper training guidelines and exercise technique are always followed. Some home exercise equipment, such as that used for the bench press, can cause serious injury if used inappropriately without a spotter or if an accident occurs. With competent instruction and quality practice time, children and adolescents can learn the skills needed for successful and enjoyable participation in a youth strength training program. The first step is to get boys and girls interested in strength training so it becomes a regular part of their weekly routine.

When introducing young people to strength training, keep in mind that they are active in different ways than adults are and for different reasons. Attempting to sell strength training to kids by explaining that it will enhance their quality of life is a losing proposition. Thus, an understanding of their motivations for engaging in strength training and an explanation of appropriate goal setting are essential. Boys and girls should be aware of the potential health- and fitness-related benefits associated with regular strength training, but enthusiastic leadership, positive reinforcement, and effective teaching are more likely to get youths energized about participating in a strength training program. Provide an environment in which children and adolescents can have fun, socialize with friends, and interact with adults who are positive and can provide age-appropriate training tips. It may be fitting for adults to tell youths why they strength train and how they stay healthy, fit, and strong as part of the modeling process. The following list provides additional tips for teaching youths.

- Listen to each of their concerns and answer any questions they have.
- Speak to them using words they understand.
- Demonstrate proper form on each exercise.
- Provide constructive feedback when appropriate or necessary.
- Focus on proper exercise technique, not the amount of weight lifted.
- Highlight personal successes and value the importance of having fun.
- Remind them that it takes time to learn a new exercise and to get in shape.
- Offer a variety of activities and avoid regimentation.
- Playing music while strength training may be acceptable, but give consideration to both volume (in order to minimize distraction) and tempo (in order to align with the goals of the training session).

Mode of Training

Different modes of training can be effective in youth strength training programs, including performing exercises using body weight as resistance and using rubber tubing, medicine balls, free weights, and child-size weight machines. When evaluating strength training equipment for boys and girls, consider factors such as the cost, quality of instruction, adjustability, proper fit, and weight stack increments. Sometimes the initial minimal weight or the weight increments on exercise equipment designed for adults might be too much for children. In addition, adjustments for children's sizes may not be possible.

Most children are too small to use adult-size weight machines, but many adolescents can fit into these machines if extra pads are used. Note that a common problem with adult weight machines is that the increments on the weight stacks are often too large—10 to 20 pounds (4.5-9.1 kg)—for most youths, who typically increase the weight by increments of 2 to 5 pounds (0.9-2.3 kg). Specific child-size weight machines are a viable alternative and have proven to be safe and effective for youths, but the cost is relatively expensive compared with most other modes of training. Free weights, rubber tubing, and medicine balls are relatively inexpensive and can be used with youths of all ages and abilities.

If equipment is not available, you can also develop a circuit of bodyweight exercises. However, this type of training may be too challenging for sedentary or overweight boys and girls, who may not have the muscular strength and local muscular endurance to perform exercises such as the push-up or pull-up. If available, weight-assisted machines that reduce body weight by using a counterweight system can be used to perform the pull-up and dip.

The best training results are likely to occur when children and adolescents have an opportunity to participate in different strength training programs and develop proper form and technique on a variety of exercises. However, young people also need to warm up properly and begin strength training with appropriate weights and exercises that are consistent with each individual's needs and abilities. The idea is for youths to understand the concept of a fitness workout while enhancing their strength and gaining confidence in their abilities to perform strength exercise.

Choice and Order of Exercises

Single-joint (e.g., machine biceps curl), multijoint (e.g., back squat), or power-oriented (e.g., power clean) exercises can be incorporated into a youth strength training program (Sadres et al. 2001). Single-joint exercises are relatively easy to perform and are appropriate for beginners when the activation of a specific muscle group is desired, whereas multijoint and power-oriented exercises require the coordinated action of many muscle groups. When preparing young athletes for sport participation, you should include multijoint and power-oriented exercises in the workout program because they are more specific to sporting activities. This type of exercise also requires more balance and stabilization and promotes the coordinated use of multijoint movements that an athlete will perform in his or her sport. In addition, the variety of exercises in a program should focus on the upper body, lower body, and midsection.

The sequence of exercises in a training session can be arranged in many ways. Traditionally, experts recommend performing exercises for large muscle groups before those for smaller muscle groups and performing multijoint exercises before single-joint exercises. Following this exercise order allows heavier weights to be used on the multijoint or power-oriented exercises because the muscles are not fatigued by previous exercises. It is also helpful to perform more challenging exercises earlier in the workout when the neuromuscular system is less fatigued. Following the same exercise order every workout is not necessary. Sometimes it might be reasonable to strengthen weaker muscle groups early in the workout, when they are less fatigued. This method of training is referred to as the *priority system.*

Training Intensity

Most experts recommend that youths perform somewhere between 6 and 12 repetitions on each exercise. However, when introducing boys and girls to strength training, have them begin with a light to moderate weight (<60 percent of 1RM) that they can lift for 10 to 15 repetitions. Even though the child may be able to lift the selected weight 10 to 15 times, the repetition range utilized should be lower. This allows for positive changes in muscular performance and provides an opportunity for youths to focus on technique and feel good about their performance. The best approach may be to first establish the repetition training range (e.g., 6-12) and then by conservative trial and error determine the appropriate load that can be handled for that repetition range.

When learning a multijoint exercise such as the back squat or a power-oriented exercise such as the power clean, it is a good idea for young weightlifters to start with a long wooden dowel instead of a loaded barbell. In addition, the number of repetitions (1-3) may be decreased in order for the strength training professional to provide appropriate feedback. This is safer and helps youths learn how to perform an exercise correctly first, which is easier than trying to break bad habits later on. After gaining technical competence in a particular exercise, adolescents may then utilize greater intensities (approximately 80 percent of 1RM; Faigenbaum et al. 2012; Harries et al. 2016).

Another issue to note is training speed. Although various speeds of movement can be effective for strength development, fast lifting speeds are not recommended for general strength training in youths. Controlled lifting speeds with a consistent application of force are recommended for children and adolescents.

Training Sets and Rest

Youths should perform one to three sets on a variety of exercises. However, they do not need to perform all exercises for the same number of sets. A good strategy is to begin strength training with a single set on each exercise and then add additional sets on selected exercises depending on the individual's needs, goals, and time available for training.

In general, youths should rest about one minute between sets and exercises. Although longer rest periods (about two to three minutes) may be appropriate for some young athletes who are following an advanced strength training program, youths have shorter attention spans than adults and likely will get bored if they have to "stand around" and wait for an extended period before doing the next exercise. Nonetheless, rest periods should be of sufficient duration to ensure that correct lifting technique is maintained.

Training Session Frequency

A strength training frequency of two or three nonconsecutive days per week is recommended for boys and girls who are participating in an introductory strength training program. This allows for adequate recovery between workouts, which is essential for maximizing training adaptations. Adolescents who perform more advanced strength training programs may increase the training session frequency, but specific muscle groups should be trained only two or three times per week.

Rate of Progression

A fundamental principle of strength training is that as the muscle adapts to the strength training stimulus, the demands placed on the muscle need to become more challenging in order to maintain the same relative training intensity. As you learned in previous chapters, this does not mean that every strength training session needs to be more intense than the previous session. However, over a period of weeks, the training stimulus needs to be advanced by gradually increasing the resistance or the number of sets. On average, a 5- to 10-percent increase in training load is appropriate for increasing the intensity of most exercises. Remember that young lifters should always develop proper form and technique before the weight is increased.

Youths should start with a basic workout using relatively light weights for the first four weeks, with an emphasis on learning proper technique. This important introductory period gives muscles, tendons, and ligaments time to adapt to the demands of strength exercise. A common mistake is for youths to begin strength training with a relatively heavy weight instead of mastering correct exercise technique. This misguided approach to strength training can result in injury and burnout. In addition, poor technique can be difficult to modify later on in the exercise program.

Once adolescents develop proper form and technique on a variety of exercises and understand the concept of progression, they can advance to more challenging workouts. This may include heavier weights, extra sets, or the addition of advanced exercises to the workout plan. As long as qualified instruction is available and age-appropriate weights are used, youths who successfully complete a beginner program can progress to more advanced programs discussed in this book that are adapted to suit their skill sets. However, because of individual differences in the ability of youths to tolerate advanced strength training workouts, each child and adolescent must be treated as an individual and be carefully observed for signs of burnout or overtraining that would require modification in the frequency, intensity, or volume of training.

Additional Considerations

Because strength training should be only one part of a child or adolescent's weekly physical activity routine, a total-body conditioning workout performed two or three nonconsecutive days per week is recommended for boys and girls who have no experience strength training. Children and adolescents who have experience strength training may perform the more advanced training programs outlined in this book (Sadres et al. 2001); however, they should first learn proper form and technique on a variety of movement patterns and upper- and lower-body exercises before progressing to more complex training programs. In addition, youths need to genuinely appreciate the potential benefits and concerns associated with strength training if this type of exercise is to become a lifelong physical activity.

Keep in mind that no matter how big or strong a child is, that child is still growing and may be experiencing a game or activity for the first time. When introducing boys and girls to strength-building exercises, you must respect their feelings and appreciate the fact that their thinking is different from yours. Remember that the primary reason children engage in physical activity is to have fun and feel successful. If boys and girls have a positive experience while strength training, they likely will become adults who regularly strength train.

Despite outdated concerns and misconceptions associated with youth strength training, qualified and respected professional organizations now recommend strength training for boys and girls provided that specific training guidelines are followed. With qualified supervision and an appropriate progression of the training program, boys and girls of all abilities—from the inactive child to the adolescent athlete—can benefit from regular participation in a strength training program. Along with other types of physical activity, strength training provides boys and girls with yet another opportunity to enhance their health, fitness, and quality of life.

Age- and Skill-Appropriate Programming

Due to the variable nature of the onset of puberty and its subsequent effects on muscular strength development, age is a major consideration for programming in youths. However, chronological age should be differentiated from biological age, which considers a child's maturity status (Lloyd et al. 2014a, b). Thus, recommendations for strength training should differ throughout the various developmental processes that occur throughout childhood and adolescence. Several approaches regarding this concept exist, including the long-term athlete development and youth physical development models (Lloyd et al. 2012, 2015).

Generally, younger children (males: 6-9 years; females: 6-8 years) should focus on fundamental movement skills with unstructured programming before progressing to learning the strength training exercise movement patterns (males: 9-12 years; females: 8-11 years). Typically, light-weight (<60 percent of 1RM) or bodyweight exercises should be utilized in order to ensure safety and allow for technical development as children in this age group benefit from increased brain maturation. Table 16.1 shows a sample workout for children in this age range.

Before and after the onset of puberty (males: 12-16 years; females: 11-15 years), which coincides with the maximal rates of growth in height and weight, reinforcement of technical proficiency should be paramount in order to cultivate appropriate lifting habits and to combat adolescent awkwardness. Performance can become an additional aim of training programs. Table 16.2 shows a sample workout for this age group. Finally, as growth rates begin to decrease (males:

16+ years; females: 15+ years), highly structured programs intended to maximize performance through increased intensities and utilization of greater movement speeds can be considered (see chapter 15 for advanced programs).

TABLE 16.1   Child Workout*

Exercise	Page #	Sets	Repetitions	Intensity
Hollow position or modified Superman	263 or 266	1	10	BW
Back squat	210	1	10	<60% 1RM/BW
Medicine ball slam	289	2	8	1-2 kg, approximately 10 in. (25 cm) in diameter
Countermovement squat jump or split jump	293 or 294	2	8	BW
Dumbbell bench press	182	1	10	<60% 1RM/BW
Dumbbell single-arm row	191	1	10 each side	<60% 1RM
Split squat	214	2	8 each side	BW
Medicine ball rotational throw	291	2	8 each side	1-2 kg, approximately 10 in. (25 cm) in diameter
Glute-ham raise	230	2	10	BW

*Male < 12 years; female < 11 years. BW = body weight; RM = repetitions maximum.

TABLE 16.2   Adolescent Workout*

Exercise	Page #	Sets	Repetitions	Intensity
Hollow position or modified Superman	263 or 266	1	10	BW
Back squat or front squat	210 or 212	2	6	<80% 1RM
Dumbbell bench press	182	2	6	<80% 1RM
Countermovement squat jump or split jump	293 or 294	3	6	BW+
Seated barbell military press	170	2	6	<80% 1RM
Russian twist	254	3	6	BW+
Pull-up or high pull	190 or 273	3	6	BW+<80% 1RM
Hip thrust	232	3	8 each side	BW

*Male > 12 years; female > 11 years. BW = body weight; RM = repetitions maximum.

Summary

Although chronological age and biological age are apparent in these guidelines, another point of emphasis should be training age, which quantifies the amount of time a child or adolescent has been engaged in a particular activity (Myer et al. 2013). Regardless of a child's chronological age or maturity status, experience with strength training should be determined, and programming should be adjusted accordingly.

17

Senior Programs

Pablo B. Costa and Ryan T. McManus

Americans now live nearly twice as long as they did only 100 years ago. Older adults can be defined as those aged 65 years and older (Nelson et al. 2007). The number of men and women over age 65 continues to increase, and by the year 2050 the number of Americans over age 65 likely will reach 84 million (Ortman 2014). The aging of our population has resulted in the development of interventions to optimize health and reduce health care costs.

Although aerobic exercise such as walking and swimming has long been recognized as an important recommendation for older adults, recent research studies and clinical observations indicate that strength training can also offer numerous health and fitness benefits for this segment of our population. Strength training can reverse or arrest much of the body's deterioration, especially in regards to muscle strength, functional capacity, functional independence, and overall quality of life. These benefits can offset the natural declines in musculoskeletal health that occur with aging. Hence, for many, this equates to a reduction in the rate of decline that occurs naturally with aging.

Because physical inactivity can lead to deterioration in general health and the ability to perform activities of daily life (e.g., climbing stairs and carrying groceries), it is not surprising that regular strength training can help maintain and enhance musculoskeletal health. Of particular importance to older adults is the observation that regular participation in a well-designed strength training program can reduce the risk of falls and hip fractures. Per 100,000 older adults, approximately 369 to 1,051 have hip fractures, depending on age and sex (Brauer et al. 2009). In addition, roughly 30 percent of older adults suffering from a hip fracture die in the subsequent year (Brauer et al. 2009). Given the potential long-term loss of function or even death associated with hip fractures, this reduced risk is an important benefit.

Concerns that strength training is unnecessary, ineffective, or unsafe for older adults are outdated. Current research clearly indicates that older adults have

The authors acknowledge the significant contributions of Avery Faigenbaum and Jay Hoffman to this chapter.

a significant ability to benefit from strength-building exercises. In fact, even individuals over age 90 can enhance their muscular fitness by strength training. Major health and fitness organizations, including the National Strength and Conditioning Association, recommend strength training for older adults to help maintain and enhance musculoskeletal health, fitness, and well-being. When incorporated into a comprehensive exercise program that includes aerobic exercise and stretching, strength training can help offset the age-related declines in bone density, muscle mass, and strength that often make activities of daily life more difficult.

Benefits of Strength Training for Older Adults

It is well established that aerobic exercise such as walking and swimming is effective for burning calories and improving cardiovascular fitness. However, the benefits of strength exercise are equally impressive, especially for older men and women. Strength training is well known for enhancing sport-specific fitness, but it can also have profound effects on an individual's health and functional capacity. In addition to enhancing strength and preserving muscle mass, regular participation in a strength training program can reduce body fat, increase metabolic rate, decrease resting blood pressure, lower cholesterol, improve glucose tolerance and insulin resistance, improve sleep quality, reduce lower-back pain, and reduce the risk of developing osteoporosis and colon cancer. Collectively, these benefits can help individuals maintain long-term independence and enhance self-confidence as muscle strength and function improve. As such, these potential benefits are important incentives for older adults to initiate an exercise program that includes safe and proper strength training.

Advancing age is associated with a number of changes that are detrimental to health and performance. The age-related progressive loss of muscle mass and strength in older adults is referred to as *sarcopenia*. Sarcopenia results in weakness, reduced physical activity, and an increased risk of falls or injury. Research studies indicate that muscle strength declines by about 15 percent per decade in the sixth and seventh decades of life and by about 30 percent thereafter. Decreased muscular strength and mass make activities such as walking and standing up from a chair more difficult and can result in physical disability and loss of independence. Moreover, the loss of muscle that occurs with aging is accompanied by a decline in resting metabolic rate, which can lead to unwanted fat gain if declining caloric needs are not matched with an appropriate decline in caloric intake.

Strength training is a powerful stimulus that decreases the effects of sarcopenia in older adults. Because muscle is metabolically active and therefore burns calories, regular participation in muscle-building activities can increase resting metabolic rate. This in turn assists in maintaining a desirable body weight and composition. These potential benefits are particularly important for older adults because advancing age typically is associated with a loss of muscle and a gain of fat (see figure 17.1).

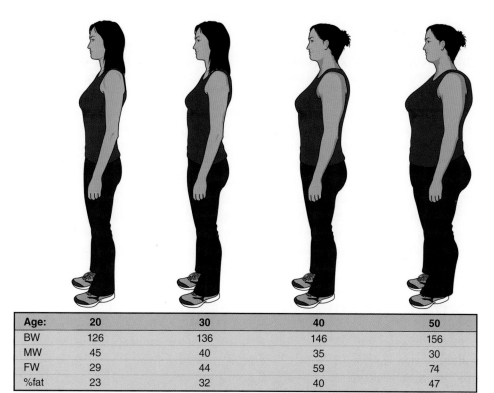

Age:	20	30	40	50
BW	126	136	146	156
MW	45	40	35	30
FW	29	44	59	74
%fat	23	32	40	47

Abbreviations: BW, body weight; MW, muscle weight; FW, fat weight; %fat, percent fat.

FIGURE 17.1 Examples of body weight and body composition changes over four decades.

Reprinted, by permission, from W. Westcott, 2003, *Building strength and stamina*, 2nd ed. (Champaign, IL: Human Kinetics), 9.

Is it possible to rebuild muscles that have already atrophied from lack of physical activity and regular strength training? Yes—and the rate of muscle development is quite impressive in older adults. Research studies have shown that the rate of age-related declines in muscle structure and function is not an inevitable consequence of aging but rather mostly a result of a sedentary lifestyle and improper nutrition (in particular, protein and caloric imbalance). Older adults can respond favorably to a strength training program that is appropriately designed and properly progressed. Therefore, strength-building exercises may be warranted to enhance muscle strength, mass, and performance in older adults. In fact, because muscle weakness is a problem for many older adults, those who increase their muscle strength may also be more likely to participate in aerobic activities such as swimming and tennis.

Another major issue related to musculoskeletal health is the progressive loss of bone mass (osteopenia), which eventually can lead to a state of low bone strength and density (osteoporosis). The prevalence of osteoporosis increases with aging, and osteoporosis is associated with fractures in the hip, back, and forearm. For older adults, fractures are a serious medical concern and could be potentially life threatening. Because bone mass and strength decrease with age, the enhancement or even maintenance of bone strength is a desirable result of regular strength training for older adults. Bone tissue is a living system and is constantly being reabsorbed and formed. Hence, strength training can offer an important stimulus to this bone remodeling process at any age by providing stresses and strains, which strengthen the bone. Although any type of weight-bearing physical activity can have a favorable effect on bone strength, a total-body strength training workout involving high-impact cyclical loading can enhance or maintain bone strength in the upper body, lower body, and midsection. Low-impact activity can have, at most, a modest favorable effect on bone remodeling, whereas higher-impact exercises, such as the back squat, are likely to have more significant effects. Hence, strength training should be considered an essential component of a well-rounded exercise program for older adults—including those with osteoporosis—who want to enhance their musculoskeletal health and quality of life.

Program Design Considerations

To maximize the benefits of strength training for older adults, the fundamental principles of overload, progression, and specificity must be followed, and the program variables must be manipulated over time to keep the program effective. In addition, training-induced improvements in health and performance will depend on the program design as well as an individual's training status or level of fitness. For example, a previously untrained older adult will make remarkable gains in muscle strength and performance during the first eight weeks of strength training, whereas a senior who has been strength training for several months or even years will show a much slower rate of improvement. These differences highlight the importance of proper program design, sensible progression, and realistic expectations. In some cases, older adults who have attained a certain level of fitness may wish to train for maintenance rather than progression. In addition, older adults might benefit from multijoint exercises because multijoint exercises promote improvements in balance and stability and decrease the risk of falls. The next section details recommendations to consider when designing strength training programs for older adults.

Safety Considerations

Safety should be the primary concern in any exercise program, and this is especially true for older adults. Some older adults have physical or mental conditions that make it difficult for them to participate in a traditional strength training program. Thus, the first step is to obtain clearance specifically for resistance exercise—as well as recommendations and training modifications, if needed—from a physician or health care provider. Older adults must be especially observant if they have any pre-existing medical condition (e.g., heart disease, high blood

◀ ■■ ■■ Strength Training Guidelines for Older Adults

- ☐ Undergo a health screening by a physician or health care provider before participating.
- ☐ Perform a preprogram evaluation to document baseline measurements. This will allow for the assessment of responses to specific exercise modalities.
- ☐ Use a 5- to 10-minute specific warm-up period before each strength training workout.
- ☐ Begin with 1 set of 10 to 15 repetitions for 8 to 10 separate exercises.
- ☐ Strength train two or three days per week on nonconsecutive days. Perform each repetition through a pain-free range of motion.
- ☐ Focus on proper breathing patterns while strength training.
- ☐ Seek guidance from a qualified fitness professional if needed.

pressure, or diabetes) that may require close supervision or some type of modification in their exercise program. Any undesirable responses to exercise, such as lightheadedness, chest pain, or joint discomfort, should result in immediate cessation of exercise and should be addressed with a medical professional as soon as possible.

To ensure a safe and productive strength training experience, older adults should also adhere to the following safety recommendations:

- Make sure the exercise area is well lit, adequately ventilated, and spacious, with plenty of room between equipment and machines.
- Avoid exercising in areas with a cluttered floor, which increases the risk of tripping and falling.
- Wear comfortable, lightweight clothing that allows for freedom of movement.
- Wear athletic shoes that provide adequate support and good traction to prevent slipping.

Above all, use common sense when strength training, and always respect your body. For example, be sure the correct load is selected on a weight machine, and have a spotter nearby to assist if performing a free-weight exercise such as the barbell bench press. If you are feeling tired or if your muscles are still sore from your last exercise session, modify the training session by using lighter weights, train different muscle groups, or simply skip the workout altogether.

Because advancing age is associated with increased muscle stiffness and reduced elasticity of the supporting structures, older adults must perform a proper warm-up before each strength training session. This can reduce the risk of injury and may even enhance performance. A 5- to 10-minute warm-up consisting of low-intensity aerobic exercise such as walking (at a level where you can maintain a conversation), calisthenics, or a specific strength training warm-up is often sufficient, but increase or modify accordingly if a longer warm-up is needed. Be sure to cool down after each strength training session as well. End your workout with several minutes of slow walking and static stretching. Because the body will have warmed up from the workout, postexercise stretching will be easier because your muscles, tendons, and ligaments will be more compliant.

Training Technique

The key to safe and successful strength training is to perform each exercise with proper form and technique. In addition to the technical guidelines discussed in part III, older adults need to pay particular attention to their movement speed, movement range, and exercise breathing.

Strength training exercises should be performed at a controlled speed of about two seconds for the lifting phase and two to three seconds for the lowering phase. Although different movement speeds may be acceptable, older adults should perform each repetition under control. An exception to this would be when older adults are engaging in specific strength training for developing power.

Furthermore, the goal is to perform each repetition through a pain-free range of motion. Older adults should attempt to perform each repetition through the full range of joint motion whenever possible, but some older adults may be limited by arthritis, joint pain, or other physical conditions. Therefore, older adults should perform strength exercises throughout a range of motion that does not exceed normal joint limits or result in pain. Avoid hyperextending or locking joints, and do not exercise if the joint is in pain or inflamed. For example, if you cannot perform a back squat exercise through the full range of motion, modify the exercise by bending your knees and hips to a lesser extent. As you continue to perform the modified squat exercise and your strength and flexibility improve, you may be able to gradually increase the range of motion. Alternatively, partial exercises can be used to train the range of motion that is free of pain. Nevertheless, older adults should discontinue any exercise that causes pain.

Older adults must also avoid the Valsalva maneuver (i.e., holding the breath during exertion). Practicing proper breathing during each repetition is important for older adults because holding the breath may result in elevated blood pressure and heart rate responses that can be harmful for this population. Common practice is to exhale when you lift the weight and inhale when you lower the weight.

Choice and Order of Exercises

Older adults can use different types of exercise equipment, including weight machines, free weights (barbells and dumbbells), and simple devices such as ankle bags filled with sand or household objects such as plastic milk jugs filled with water. Whatever the type of equipment used, the training program should address all the major muscle groups that are used in everyday activities, paying particular attention to developing muscle balance. For example, if you perform an exercise for the chest muscles, you should also perform an exercise using the back muscles. If you do not give equal attention to opposing muscle groups on your upper body, midsection, and lower body, you may develop poor posture and muscle imbalances and increase your risk of developing an injury.

You can incorporate both single-joint (e.g., dumbbell biceps curl) and multijoint (e.g., back squat) exercises into the training program. Bear in mind that on some weight machines the lightest weight may be too heavy or the increments—for example, 10 pounds (4.5 kg)—may be too large. Furthermore, linear movements on weight machines may not address some common daily movement patterns that require balance and coordination. Nevertheless, if you have access to weight machines, you may want to start strength training with them and gradually progress to free-weight exercises that require more balance, skill, and coordination.

As with younger adults, it is preferable for older adults to exercise large muscle groups first and then progress to smaller muscle groups. This exercise order allows you to work with heavy weights early in the workout, when these muscles are fresh. After training the legs, you can perform exercises for the chest, back, shoulders, and arms. Near the end of your workout, train the abdominal and lower-back muscles around the midsection. However, you do not have to follow the same exercise order in every workout. Sometimes it makes sense to strengthen the weaker muscle groups early in the workout, when you are less fatigued. (This is called using the priority method.) Keep in mind that altering the exercise order may change the weight you can lift and the number of repetitions you can perform. If a workout consists of both strength and aerobic exercise, you might want to begin with strength training and then progress to the aerobic activity.

Training Intensity

A variety of strength training programs have proven to be effective for older adults. The key is to start with a weight that allows you to lift the prescribed number of repetitions using proper form and then gradually increase the demands placed on the exercising muscles. In short, the goal of the exercise program should be to challenge your muscles so they adapt to the training program and become stronger.

Older adults should begin strength training with 10 to 15 repetitions per set of 8 to 10 exercises that use all the major muscle groups (American College of Sports Medicine 2009). It is always prudent to err on the side of safety when starting a strength training program, and the higher repetition range represents relatively lower exercise resistance (approximately 40-50 percent of 1RM).

However, as strength increases, you should progress to higher exercise resistance and fewer repetitions per set because the intensity of the strength training workout determines the magnitude of the gains in strength and, to a certain extent, muscle size. An acceptable resistance range may extend from 60 to 85 percent of 1RM, with a corresponding range of 8 to 12 repetitions. If the intensity of the exercise is too low (i.e., the weight can be lifted for more than 20 repetitions), gains in local muscular endurance are likely, but gains in muscle strength or muscle mass will be limited.

As a general guideline, beginning older adults may train with 40 to 50 percent of maximum resistance (10-15 repetitions). Older adults with several months of strength training experience may train with 75 to 90 percent of maximum resistance (6 repetitions or fewer) on selected exercises for large muscle groups in order to enhance strength development. Training variety enhances strength development and reduces the risk of overtraining. Therefore, the best approach for advanced older adults may be to periodically vary the training intensity by performing fewer repetitions with a relatively heavier weight and more repetitions with a relatively lighter weight. Heavier weights typically are used on leg exercises compared with arm exercises because the legs have more muscle mass.

Training Sets and Rest

Older adults should begin strength training with a single set on each exercise. This is an efficient and effective way to enhance muscle strength during the first six to eight weeks of training. However, as you become more advanced, you may want to perform a second or third set on selected exercises in order to keep the training program effective by applying progressive overload. If multiple sets are performed, be sure to include one to three minutes of rest between sets and maintain a balanced training program. For example, if you perform two sets of a chest exercise, you should also perform two sets of a back exercise. In addition, allow ample time to adjust to postural changes and balance during the transition between exercises.

Keep in mind that not all exercises need to be performed for the same number of sets. If time permits, you may want to progress to two or three sets on exercises for large muscle groups and stay with only one set on exercises for smaller muscle groups. If you perform multiple sets, you can use the same weight or you can change the weight and the repetitions on the second and third sets. For example, advanced older adults could perform a set of 10 repetitions on the leg press with 100 pounds (45.4 kg), a second set of 8 repetitions with 120 pounds (54.4 kg), and a third set of 6 repetitions with 140 pounds (63.5 kg). If you perform multiple sets with a heavier weight, you should rest about two minutes between each set to allow yourself time to recover.

Training Frequency

For best results, older adults should strength train two or three nonconsecutive days per week using a full-body workout (most major muscle groups) in each exercise session. Another alternative is to use split routines, or work different body parts on consecutive days. This approach is especially beneficial for older adults who enjoy training more frequently. Regardless of choice, after each strength training session, the targeted muscles need about 48 to 72 hours to recover and rebuild in order to adapt and get stronger. Therefore, strength training the same muscle group on two consecutive days can be counterproductive. For older adults, strength training every other day is a reasonable recommendation that will result in larger, stronger muscles. This training frequency also increases the likelihood of training consistency, which is essential for long-term gains. Short-term programs may increase muscle strength; however, long-term (lifetime) training is necessary to ensure lasting improvements in muscle strength and other physical factors that reduce the risk of various diseases and physical ailments associated with aging.

Programs for Older Adults

Regular participation in strength training workouts is essential for enhancing and maintaining muscular fitness so that older adults can live a physically independent lifestyle. The training overload must be adequate, and the program must be progressive. In addition, older adults need to learn how to properly strength train right from the start. Poor exercise technique and haphazard programming increase the risk of injury and undermine the purpose of strength training. We also recommend that you keep careful records of your strength training workouts. This information provides you with important material for future program design and can serve as a powerful motivational tool. It is always better to develop good habits right from the start than to try to break bad habits later on.

Older adults can start with the program outlined in tables 17.1, 17.2, or 17.3 or the beginner program discussed in chapter 13. The goal should be to develop proper exercise technique on a variety of exercises that use all the major muscle groups. Beginning with 1 set of 8 to 12 repetitions, older adults should first increase the number of repetitions (up to 15) and then gradually increase the weight as strength improves. Very deconditioned or frail older adults can begin with a lower resistance (40-50 percent of 1RM). As older adults progress from one exercise to the next, they may need a little extra time to adjust to postural changes such as moving from a supine lying or seated position to standing. With these considerations in mind, older adults may find it worthwhile to learn proper exercise technique from a qualified fitness trainer who understands their individual needs, goals, and medical history.

A growing number of recreation centers and fitness facilities offer supervised strength training workouts for older adults. In these settings, certified strength and conditioning specialists and fitness trainers can provide positive reinforcement for correct technique and specific suggestions for improved performance. Strength training with a fitness trainer or a friend makes the workout more enjoyable and increases safety and the likelihood that you will stick with the exercise program.

Strength training with friends and family members is a perfect opportunity to stay healthy and strong while having fun. An advantage strength training has over other types of exercise is that older adults can talk to their friends between sets.

TABLE 17.1 Older Adult: General Muscular Conditioning

Exercise	Page #	Sets	Repetitions	Intensity
Leg press	209	1-2	8-12	65-80%
Seated leg curl	235	1-2	8-12	65-80%
Leg extension	219	1-2	8-12	65-80%
Machine chest press	174	1-2	8-12	65-80%
Machine seated row	180	1-2	8-12	65-80%
Ankle touch	245	1-2	10	BW
Back extension	260	1-2	10	BW
Side plank	257	2	8 s each side	BW
Prone plank	256	2	15-30 s	BW

BW = body weight.

TABLE 17.2 Older Adult: Strength Training

Exercise	Page #	Sets	Repetitions	Intensity
Step-up	216	1-3	2-5	85-95%
Dumbbell bench press	182	1-3	2-5	85-95%
Dumbbell upright row	167	1-3	2-5	85-95%
Dumbbell biceps curl	203	1-3	2-5	85-95%
Cable triceps extension	194	1-3	2-5	85-95%
Abdominal crunch	244	1-3	10	BW
Prone plank	256	1-3	15-30 s	BW

BW = body weight.

TABLE 17.3 Older Adult: Power Training

Exercise	Page #	Sets	Repetitions	Intensity
High pull	273	1-3	2-5	BW
Push press	281	1-3	2-5	30-60%
Medicine ball put	290	1-3	2-5	30-60%
Medicine ball slam	289	1-3	2-5	30-60%
Leg press (for power)	209	1-3	2-5	30-60%

BW = body weight.

Summary

It is clear that men and women of all ages retain the capacity to adapt to strength training. Because muscle and bone weakness is a common characteristic of advancing age, older adults can benefit from physical activity programs that preserve or enhance muscular fitness and bone strength. Regular strength training can improve muscle function, increase bone strength, improve balance and coordination, and have a meaningful effect on the ability of older adults to maintain a high-quality lifestyle. Although the principles of strength training are similar for individuals of all ages and abilities, unique factors specific to older adults must be considered when designing strength training programs. Perhaps the best recommendation for older adults who want to optimize their current and future health is to begin a sensible strength training program that is consistent with their current needs, abilities, and medical history.

References

Abad, C.C., M.L. Prado, C. Ugrinowitsch, V. Tricoli, and R. Barroso. 2011. Combination of general and specific warm-ups improves leg-press one repetition maximum compared with specific warm-up in trained individuals. *J. Strength Cond. Res.* 25:2242-2245.

Ahtiainen, J.P., A. Pakarinen, W.J. Kraemer, and K. Häkkinen. 2004. Acute hormonal responses to heavy resistance exercise in strength athletes versus nonathletes. *Can. J. Appl. Physiol.* 29(5):527-543.

Alway, S.E., W.H. Grumbt, W.J. Gonyea, and J. Stray-Gundersen. 1989. Contrasts in muscle and myofibers of elite male and female bodybuilders. *J. Appl. Physiol.* 67(1):24-31.

American College of Sports Medicine. 2009. American College of Sports Medicine position stand. Progression models in resistance training for healthy adults. *Med. Sci. Sports Exerc.* 41(3):687-708.

Atkins, S.J., I. Bentley, D.B. Brooks, M.P. Burrows, H.T. Hurst, and J.K. Sinclair. 2015. Electromyographic response of global abdominal stabilizers in response to stable- and unstable-base isometric exercise. *J. Strength Cond. Res.* 29(6):1609-1615.

Blaauw, B., and C. Reggiani. 2014. The role of satellite cells in muscle hypertrophy. *J. Muscle Res. Cell Motil.* 35(1):3-10.

Brauer, C.A., M. Coca-Perraillon, D.M. Cutler, and A.B. Rosen. 2009. Incidence and mortality of hip fractures in the United States. *J. Amer. Med. Assoc.* 302(14):1573-1579.

Brown, L.E., and J.P. Weir. 2001. ASEP procedures recommendation I: Accurate assessment of muscular strength and power. *JEPonline* 4(3):1-21.

Bruusgaard, J.C., I.B. Johansen, I.M. Egner, Z.A. Rana, and K. Gundersen. 2010. Myonuclei acquired by overload exercise precede hypertrophy and are not lost on detraining. *Proc. Nat. Acad. Sci. USA* 107(34):15111-15116.

Camera, D.M., D.W. West, N.A. Burd, S.M. Phillips, A.P. Garnham, J.A. Hawley, and V.G. Coffey. 2012. Low muscle glycogen concentration does not suppress the anabolic response to resistance exercise. *J. Appl. Physiol.* 113(2):206-214.

Campos, G.E., T.J. Luecke, H.K. Wendeln, K. Toma, F.C. Hagerman, T.F. Murray, K.E. Ragg, N.A. Ratamess, W.J. Kraemer, and R.S. Staron. 2002. Muscular adaptations in response to three different resistance-training regimens: Specificity of repetition maximum training zones. *Eur. J. Appl. Physiol.* 88(1-2):50-60.

Cramer, J.T., T.J. Housh, G.O. Johnson, J.M. Miller, J.W. Coburn, T.W. Beck. 2004. Acute effects of static stretching on peak torque in women. *J Strength Cond Res.* 18(2):236-41.

Damas, F., S. Phillips, F.C. Vechin, and C. Ugrinowitsch. 2015. A review of resistance training-induced changes in skeletal muscle protein synthesis and their contribution to hypertrophy. *Sports Med.* 45(6):801-807.

Dudley, G.A., P.A. Tesch, B.J. Miller, and P. Buchanan. 1991. Importance of eccentric actions in performance adaptations to resistance training. *Aviation Space Environ. Med.* 62:543-550.

Faigenbaum, A.D., J.E. McFarland, R.E. Herman, F. Naclerio, N.A. Ratamess, J. Kang, and G.D. Myer. 2012. Reliability of the one-repetition-maximum power clean test in adolescent athletes. *J. Strength Cond. Res.* 26(2):432-437.

Fleck, S.J., and W.J. Kraemer. 2014. *Designing resistance training programs.* 4th ed. Champaign, IL: Human Kinetics.

Fragala, M.S., W.J. Kraemer, C.R. Denegar, C.M. Maresh, A.M. Mastro, and J.S. Volek. 2011. Neuro-endocrine-immune interactions and responses to exercise. *Sports Med.* 41(8):621-639.

Haff, G., and N.T. Triplett, eds. 2016. *Essentials of strength training and conditioning.* 4th ed. Champaign, IL: Human Kinetics.

Hansen, S., T. Kvornign, M. Kajaer, and G. Sjogaard. 2001. The effect of short-term strength training on human skeletal muscle: The importance of physiologically elevated hormone levels. *Scand. J. Med. Sci. Sports* 11:347-354.

Harman, E.A., M.T. Rosenstein, P.N. Frykman, R.M. Rosenstein, and W.J. Kraemer. 1991. Estimation of human power output from vertical jump. *J. Appl. Sports Sci. Res.* 5:116-120.

Harries, S.K., D.R. Lubans, and R. Callister. 2016. Comparison of resistance training progression models on maximal strength in sub-elite adolescent rugby union players. *J. Sci. Med. Sport* 19(2):163-169.

Hatfield, D.L., W.J. Kraemer, B.A. Spiering, K. Häkkinen, J.S. Volek, T. Shimano, L.P. Spreuwenberg, R. Silvestre, J.L. Vingren, M.S. Fragala, A.L. Gómez, S.J. Fleck, R.U. Newton, and C.M. Maresh. 2006. The impact of velocity of movement on performance factors in resistance exercise. *J. Strength Cond. Res.* 20(4):760-766.

Hather, B.M., P.A. Tesch, P. Buchanan, and G.A. Dudley. 1991. Influence of eccentric actions on skeletal muscle adaptations to resistance training. *Acta Physiol. Scand.* 143:177-185.

Hawke, T.J. 2005. Muscle stem cells and exercise training. *Exerc. Sport Sci. Rev.* 33:63-68.

Hoeger, W.W.K., S.L. Barette, D.F. Hale, and D.R. Hopkins. 1990. Relationship between repetitions and selected percentages of one repetition maximum. *J. Appl. Sport Sci. Res.* 4(2):47-54.

Hoffman, J. 2006. *Norms for fitness, performance, and health.* Champaign, IL: Human Kinetics.

Huxley, H.E. 2004. Fifty years of muscle and the sliding filament hypothesis. *Eur J Biochem* 271(8):1403-15. Johnson, D.L., and R. Bahamonde. 1996. Power output estimates in university athletes. *J. Strength Cond. Res.* 10(3):161-166.

Kadi, F., and L.E. Thornell. 2000. Concomitant increases in myonuclear and satellite cell content in female trapezius muscle following strength training. *Histochem. Cell Biol.* 113:99-103.

Kalamen, J.L. 1968. Measurement of maximum muscular power in man. PhD diss., Ohio State Univ., Columbus.

Knuttgen, H.G., and W.J. Kraemer. 1987. Terminology and measurement in exercise performance. *J. Strength Cond. Res.* 1(1):1-10.

Kraemer, W.J., C. Dunn-Lewis, B.A. Comstock, G.A. Thomas, J.E. Clark, and B.C. Nindl. 2010. Growth hormone, exercise, and athletic performance: A continued evolution of complexity. *Curr. Sports Med. Rep.* 9(4):242-252.

Kraemer, W.J., and S.J. Fleck. 2007. *Optimizing strength training.* Champaign, IL: Human Kinetics.

Kraemer, W.J., S.J. Fleck, and M.R. Deschenes. 2016. *Exercise physiology: Integrating theory and applications.* 2nd ed. Philadelphia: Kluwer/Lippincott, Williams & Wilkins.

Kraemer, W.J., S.E. Gordon, S.J. Fleck, L.J. Marchitelli, R. Mello, J.E. Dziados, K. Friedl, E. Harman, C. Maresh, and A.C. Fry. 1991. Endogenous anabolic hormonal and growth factor responses to heavy resistance exercise in males and females. *Int. J. Sports Med.* 12:228-235.

Kraemer, W.J., L. Marchitelli, S.E. Gordon, E. Harman, J.E. Dziados, R. Mello, P. Frykman, D. McCurry, and S.J. Fleck. 1990. Hormonal and growth factor responses to heavy resistance exercise protocols. *J. Appl. Physiol.* 69:1442-1450.

Kraemer, W.J., and N.A. Ratamess. 2005. Hormonal responses and adaptations to resistance exercise and training. *Sports Med.* 35:336-361.

Kvorning, T., M. Andersen, K. Brixen, and K. Madsen. 2006a. Suppression of endogenous testosterone production attenuates the response to strength training: A randomized, placebo-controlled, and blinded intervention study. *Am. J. Physiol. Endocrinol. Metab.* 291(6):E1325-E1332.

Kvorning, T., M. Bagger, P. Caserotti, and K. Madsen. 2006b. Effects of vibration and resistance training on neuromuscular and hormonal measures. *Eur. J. Appl. Physiol.* 96(5):615-625.

Kvorning, T., M. Andersen, K. Brixen, P. Schjerling, C. Suetta, K. Madsen. 2007. Suppression of testosterone does not blunt mRNA expression of myoD, myogenin, IGF, myostatin or androgen receptor post strength training in humans. *Physiol.* Jan 15; 578 (Pt 2): 579-93.

Lake, J.P., and M.A. Lauder. 2012. Kettlebell swing training improves maximal and explosive strength. *J. Strength Cond. Res.* 26(8):2228-2233.

Lewis, P.B., D. Ruby, and C.A. Bush-Joseph. 2012. Muscle soreness and delayed-onset muscle soreness. *Sports Med.* 31(2):255-262.

Lloyd, R.S., A.D. Faigenbaum, M.H. Stone, J.L. Oliver, I. Jeffreys, J.A. Moody, C. Brewer, K. Pierce, T.M. McCambridge, R. Howard, L. Herrington, B. Hainline, L.J. Micheli, R. Jaques, W.J. Kraemer, M.G. McBride, T.M. Best, D.A. Chu, B.A. Alvar, and G.D. Myer. 2014a. Position statement on youth resistance training: The 2014 International consensus. *Br. J. Sports Med.* 48(7):498-505.

Lloyd, R.S., J.L. Oliver, A.D. Faigenbaum, R. Howard, M.B.D.S. Croix, C.A. Williams, T.M. Best, B.A. Alvar, L.J. Micheli, D.P. Thomas, D.L. Hatfield, J.B. Cronin, and G.D. Myer. 2015. Long-term athletic development-Part 1: A pathway for all youth. *J. Strength Cond. Res.* 29(5):1439-1450.

Lloyd, R.S., J.L. Oliver, A.D. Faigenbaum, G.D. Myer, and M.B.D.S. Croix. 2014b. Chronological age vs. biological maturation: Implications for exercise programming in youth. *J. Strength Cond. Res.* 28(5):1454-1464.

Lloyd, R.S., J.L. Oliver, R.W. Meyers, J.A. Moody, and M.H. Stone. 2012. Long-term athletic development and its application to youth weightlifting. *Strength Cond. J.* 34(4):55-66.

Ma, S., G.R. Neto, P.B. Costa, T.M. Gomes, C.M. Bentes, A.F. Brown, and J.S. Novaes. 2015. Acute effects of different stretching techniques on the number of repetitions in a single lower body resistance training session. *J. Hum. Kinet.* 45:177-185.

MacDougall, J.D., D.G. Sale, S.E. Alway, and J.R. Sutton. 1984. Muscle fiber number in biceps brachii in bodybuilders and control subjects. *J. Appl. Physiol. Respir. Environ. Exerc. Physiol.* 57(5):1399-1403.

Malliaropoulos, N., S. Papalexandris, A. Papalada, and E. Papacostas. 2004. The role of stretching in rehabilitation of hamstring injuries: 80 athletes follow-up. *Med. Sci. Sports Exerc.* 36(5):756-759.

Manocchia, P., D.K. Spierer, A.S. Lufkin, J. Minichiello, and J. Castro. 2013. Transference of kettlebell training to strength, power, and endurance. *J. Strength Cond. Res.* 27(2):477-484.

Margaria, R., P. Aghemo, and E. Rovelli. 1966. Measurement of muscular power (anaerobic) in man. *J. Appl. Physiol.* 21(5):1662-1664.

Matheny, R.W., Jr., B.C. Nindl, and M.L. Adamo. 2010. Mechano-growth factor: A putative product of IGF-I gene expression involved in tissue repair and regeneration. *Endocrinology* 151(3):865-875.

McBride, J.M., T. Triplett-McBride, A. Davie, and R.U. Newton. 2002. The effect of heavy- vs. lightload jump squats on the development of strength, power, and speed. *J. Strength Cond. Res.* 16(1):75–82.

McCall, G.E., W.C. Byrnes, A. Dickinson, P.M. Pattany, and S.J. Fleck. 1996. Muscle fiber hypertrophy, hyperplasia, and capillary density in college men after resistance training. *J. Appl. Physiol.* 81(5):2004-2012.

Miranda, F., R. Simão, M. Rhea, D. Bunker, J. Prestes, R.D. Leite, H. Miranda, B.F. de Salles, and J. Novaes. 2011. Effects of linear vs. daily undulatory periodized resistance training on maximal and submaximal strength gains. *J. Strength Cond. Res.* 25(7):1824-1830.

Moritani, T., and H.A. deVries. 1979. Neural factors versus hypertrophy in the time course of muscle strength gain. *Am. J. Phys. Med.* 58:115–130.

Myer, G.D., R.S. Lloyd, J.L. Brent, and A.D. Faigenbaum. 2013. How young is "too young" to start training? *ACSM Health Fitness J.* 17(5):14-23.

Nelson, M.E., W.J. Rejeski, S.N. Blair, P.W. Duncan, J.O. Judge, A.C. King, C.A. Macera, and C. Castaneda-Sceppa. 2007. Physical activity and public health in older adults: Recommendation from the American College of Sports Medicine and the American Heart Association. *Med. Sci. Sports Exerc.* 39(8):1435-1445.

Nindl, B.C., W.J. Kraemer, J.O. Marx, A.P. Tuckow, and W.C. Hymer. 2003. Growth hormone molecular heterogeneity and exercise. *Exerc. Sport Sci. Rev.* 31(4):161-166.

Nindl, B.C., and J.R. Pierce. 2010. Insulin-like growth factor I as a biomarker of health, fitness, and training status. *Med. Sci. Sports Exerc.* 42(1):39-49.

Noakes, T., J.S. Volek, and S.D. Phinney. 2014. Low-carbohydrate diets for athletes: What evidence? *Br. J. Sports Med.* 48(14):1077-1078.

Ortman, J.M., V.A. Velkoff, and H. Hogan. 2014. *An aging nation: The older population in the United States.* Washington, DC: U.S. Census Bureau.

Paoli, A., A. Rubini, J.S. Volek, and K.A. Grimaldi. 2013. Beyond weight loss: A review of the therapeutic uses of very-low-carbohydrate (ketogenic) diets. *Eur. J. Clin. Nutr.* 67(8):789-796.

Peterson, M.D., M.R. Rhea, and B.A. Alvar. 2004. Maximizing strength development in athletes: A meta-analysis to determine the dose-response relationship. *J. Strength Cond. Res.* 18(2):377-382.

Peterson, M.D., M.R. Rhea, and B.A. Alvar. 2005. Applications of the dose-response for muscular strength development: A review of meta-analytic efficacy and reliability for designing training prescription. *J. Strength Cond. Res.* 19(4):950-958.

Peterson, M.D., M.R. Rhea, A. Sen, and P.M. Gordon. 2010. Resistance exercise for muscular strength in older adults: A meta-analysis. *Ageing Res. Rev.* 9(3):226-237.

Physical Activity Guidelines Advisory Committee. 2008. *Physical activity guidelines for Americans.* Washington, DC: U.S. Department of Health and Human Services.

Plisk, S.S., and M.H. Stone. 2003. Periodization strategies. *Strength Cond. J.* 25(6):19-37.

Ratamess, N.A., B.A. Alvar, T.K. Evetoch, T.J. Housh, W.B. Kibler, W.J. Kraemer, and N.T. Triplett. 2009. Progression models in resistance in healthy adults. American College of Sports Medicine position stand. *Med. Sci. Sports Exerc.* 41(3):687-708.

Reed, J.L., J.L. Bowell, B.R. Hill, B.A. Williams, M.J. De Souza, and N.I. Williams. 2011. Exercising women with menstrual disturbances consume low energy dense foods and beverages. *Appl. Physiol. Nutr. Metab.* 36(3):382-394.

Rhea, M.R., B.A. Alvar, and L.N. Burkett. 2002. Single versus multiple sets for strength: A meta-analysis to address the controversy. *Res. Q. Exerc. Sport* 73(4):485-488.

Rhea, M.R., B.A. Alvar, L.N. Burkett, and S.D. Ball. 2003a. A meta-analysis to determine the dose response for strength development. *Med. Sci. Sports Exerc.* 35:456-464.

Rhea, M.R., W.T. Phillips, L.N. Burkett, W.J. Stone, S.D. Ball, B.A. Alvar, and A.B. Thomas. 2003b. A comparison of linear and daily undulating periodized programs with equated volume and intensity for local muscular endurance. *J. Strength Cond. Res.* 17(1):82-87.

Robergs, R.A., F. Ghiasvand, and D. Parker. 2004. Biochemistry of exercise-induced metabolic acidosis. *Am. J. Physiol. Regul. Integr. Comp. Physiol.* 287(3):R502-R516.

Rønnestad, B.R., H. Nygaard, and T. Raastad. 2011. Physiological elevation of endogenous hormones results in superior strength training adaptation. *Eur. J. Appl. Physiol.* 111(9):2249-2259.

Sabo, D., and P. Veliz. 2008. *Go out and play: Youth sports in America.* New York: Women's Sports Foundation.

Sadres, E., A. Eliakim, N. Constantini, R. Lidor, and B. Falk. 2001. The effect of long-term resistance training on anthropometric measures, muscle strength, and self concept in pre-pubertal boys. *Pediatr. Exerc. Sci.* 13:357-372.

Schoenfeld, B.J. 2012. Does exercise-induced muscle damage play a role in skeletal muscle hypertrophy? *J. Strength Cond. Res.* 26(5):1441-1453.

Schuenke, M.D., J. Herman, and R.S. Staron. 2013. Preponderance of evidence proves "big" weights optimize hypertrophic and strength adaptations. *Eur. J. Appl. Physiol.* 113(1):269-271.

Selye, H. 1956. *The stress of life*. New York: McGraw-Hill Companies.

Selye, H. 1976. *The stress of life*. Rev. ed. New York: McGraw-Hill Companies.

Selye, H. 1950. Stress and the general adaptation syndrome. *Br Med J.* Jun 17;1(4667):1383-92.

Shimano, T., W.J. Kraemer, B.A. Spiering, J.S. Volek, D.L. Hatfield, R. Silvestre, J.L. Vingren, M.S. Fragala, C.M. Maresh, S.J. Fleck, R.U. Newton, L.P. Spreuwenberg, and K. Häkkinen. 2006. Relationship between the number of repetitions and selected percentages of one repetition maximum in free weight exercises in trained and untrained men. *J. Strength Cond. Res.* 20(4):819-823.

Snijders, T., L.B. Verdijk, M. Beelen, B.R. McKay, G. Parise, F. Kadi, and L.J. van Loon. 2012. A single bout of exercise activates skeletal muscle satellite cells during subsequent overnight recovery. *Exp. Physiol.* 97(6):762-773.

Spiering, B.A., W.J. Kraemer, J.M. Anderson, L.E. Armstrong, B.C. Nindl, J.S. Volek, D.A. Judelson, M. Joseph, J.L. Vingren, D.L. Hatfield, M.S. Fragala, J.Y. Ho, and C.M. Maresh. 2008a. Effects of elevated circulating hormones on resistance exercise-induced Akt signaling. *Med. Sci. Sports Exerc.* 40(6):1039-1048.

Spiering, B.A., W.J. Kraemer, J.M. Anderson, L.E. Armstrong, B.C. Nindl, J.S. Volek, and C.M. Maresh. 2008b. Resistance exercise biology: Manipulation of resistance exercise programme variables determines the responses of cellular and molecular signalling pathways. *Sports Med.* 38(7):527-540.

Staron, R.S., D.L. Karapondo, W.J. Kraemer, A.C. Fry, S.E. Gordon, J.E. Falkel, F.C. Hagerman, and R.S. Hikida. 1994. Skeletal muscle adaptations during early phase of heavy resistance training in men and women. *J. Appl. Physiol.* 76:1247-1255.

Szivak, T.K., D.R. Hooper, C. Dunn-Lewis, B.A. Comstock, B.R. Kupchak, J.M. Apicella, C. Saenz, C.M. Maresh, C.R. Denegar, and W.J. Kraemer. 2013. Adrenal cortical responses to high-intensity, short rest, resistance exercise in men and women. *J. Strength Cond. Res.* 27(3):748-760.

Tan, B. 1999. Manipulating resistance training program variables to optimize maximum strength in men: a review. *J. Strength Cond. Res.* 13(3), 289–304.

Tharion, W.J., T.M. Rausch, E.A. Harman, and W.J. Kraemer. 1991. Effects of different resistance exercise protocols on mood states. *J. Appl. Sport Sci. Res.* 5(2):60-65.

Thomas, J.F., K.L. Larson, D.B. Hollander, and R.R. Kraemer. 2014. Comparison of two-handed kettlebell exercise and graded treadmill walking: Effectiveness as a stimulus for cardiorespiratory fitness. *J. Strength Cond. Res.* 28(4):998-1006.

Todd, J.S., J.P. Shurley, T.C. Todd, and L. Thomas. 2012. DeLorme and the science of progressive resistance exercise. *J. Strength Cond. Res.* 26(11):2913-2923.

Vingren, J.L., W.J. Kraemer, D.L. Hatfield, J.S. Volek, N.A. Ratamess, J.M. Anderson, K. Häkkinen, J. Ahtiainen, M.S. Fragala, G.A. Thomas, J.Y. Ho, and C.M. Maresh. 2009. Effect of resistance exercise on muscle steroid receptor protein content in strength-trained men and women. *Steroids* 74(13-14):1033-1039.

Vingren, J.L., W.J. Kraemer, N.A. Ratamess, J.M. Anderson, J.S. Volek, and C.M. Maresh. 2010. Testosterone physiology in resistance exercise and training: The up-stream regulatory elements. *Sports Med.* 40(12):1037-1053.

Volek, J.S., C.E. Forsythe, and W.J. Kraemer. 2006. Nutritional aspects of women strength athletes. *Br. J. Sports Med.* 40(9):742-748.

Volek J.S., D.J. Freidenreich, C. Saenz, L.J. Kunces, B.C. Creighton, J.M. Bartley, P.M. Davitt, C.X. Munoz, J.M. Anderson, C.M. Maresh, E.C. Lee, M.D. Schuenke, G. Aerni, W.J. Kraemer, S.D. Phinney. 2016. Metabolic characteristics of keto-adapted ultra-endurance runners. *Metabolism* 65(3): 100-10.

Volek, J.S., K. Houseknecht, and W.J. Kraemer. 1997. Nutritional strategies to enhance performance of high-intensity exercise. *Strength Cond. J.* 19(1):11-17.

Volek, J.S., T. Noakes, and S.D. Phinney. 2015. Rethinking fat as a fuel for endurance exercise. *Eur. J. Sport Sci.* 15(1):13-20.

Volk, B.M., L.J. Kunces, D.J. Freidenreich, B.R. Kupchak, C. Saenz, J.C. Artistizabal, M.L. Fernandez, R.S. Bruno, C.M. Maresh, W.J. Kraemer, S.D. Phinney, and J.S. Volek. 2014. Effects of step-wise increases in dietary carbohydrate on circulating saturated fatty acids and palmitoleic acid in adults with metabolic syndrome. *PLoS One* 9(11):e113605.

Wolfe, A.E., L.E. Brown, J.W. Coburn, R.D. Kersey, and M. Bottaro. 2011. Time course of the effects of static stretching on cycling economy. *J. Strength Cond. Res.* 25(11):2980-2984.

World Health Organization. 2010. *Global recommendations on physical activity for health.* Geneva: World Health Organization Press.

Index

Note: The italicized *f* and *t* following page numbers refer to figures and tables, respectively.

About the NSCA

The **National Strength and Conditioning Association (NSCA)** is the world's leading organization in the field of sport conditioning. Drawing on the resources and expertise of the most recognized professionals in strength training and conditioning, sport science, performance research, education, and sports medicine, the NSCA is the world's trusted source of knowledge and training guidelines for coaches and athletes. The NSCA provides the crucial link between the lab and the field.

About the Editor

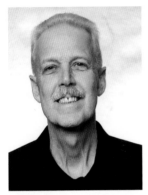

Photo courtesy of California State University, Fullerton.

Lee E. Brown, EdD, CSCS,*D, FNSCA, FACSM, is a former president of the National Strength and Conditioning Association (NSCA) Board of Directors. In 2014 he received the NSCA's Lifetime Achievement Award for his work with the association. Brown holds a master's degree in exercise science and a doctorate in educational leadership from Florida Atlantic University. Formerly a high school physical education teacher and coach of numerous sports, he is now a professor of strength and conditioning in the department of kinesiology at California State University, Fullerton. He and his wife, Theresa, reside in Buena Park, California.

About the Contributors

José A. Arevalo, MS, was born in Guatemala and grew up in East Los Angeles. He received his master of science degree in kinesiology from the California State University at Fullerton. His thesis research involved determining a relationship between leg dominance and muscle fiber type composition. Working under Dr. Andy Galpin, José was also the director of the Biochemistry and Molecular Exercise Physiology laboratory. At Fullerton, he also taught both lecture and laboratory portions of the human anatomy and physiology course. He is a graduate of the University of California at Berkeley; he decided to return to his scientific interest of exercise and muscle physiology, which he aspires to continue through a doctoral program.

James R. Bagley, PhD, is an assistant professor (tenure-track) of kinesiology, director of the Muscle Physiology Laboratory, and codirector of the Exercise Physiology Laboratory at San Francisco State University. He holds a PhD in human bioenergetics from Ball State University in Muncie, Indiana, and MS and BS degrees in kinesiology from California State University at Fullerton and California Polytechnic State University at San Luis Obispo, respectively. Before his faculty positon at SF State, Dr. Bagley spent one year as a visiting scholar in the Biochemistry and Molecular Exercise Physiology Laboratory at CSUF. His research interests include muscle physiology (hypertrophy and atrophy mechanisms), cellular imaging, and sport performance. Dr. Bagley is an active member of the American College of Sports Medicine, American Physiological Society, and National Strength and Conditioning Association.

J. Albert Bartolini, MS, is an instructor in the kinesiology department at California State University at Fullerton where he earned his bachelor of arts degree in psychology and his master of science degree in kinesiology. His affiliation with CSUF's Center for Sport Performance has afforded him the opportunity to collect preseason data on NHL teams as well as do research for national apparel companies. Albert has worked as a track and field coach, primarily the sprint events. He has also worked with team sports including baseball, football, basketball, and soccer. He has worked with levels ranging from youth to elite. Albert has presented at several American College of Sports Medicine and National Strength and Conditioning Association conferences. His research interest is training for sport performance.

Katherine E. Bathgate, MS, CSCS, earned a master's degree in kinesiology from California State University at Fullerton and a bachelor's degree (summa cum laude) in kinesiology from the same institution. As an undergraduate, Katie competed on CSUF's NCAA DI track and cross-country teams in the 5,000-meter and 3,000-meter steeplechase. In addition to her graduate studies, Katie worked as a teaching associate for the kinesiology department, assistant coach for the CSUF cross-country team, and strength and conditioning coach for the 15-time national champion CSUF dance team. Her research interests include muscle physiology and training for sport performance. Katie is an active member of the American College of Sports Medicine and National Strength and Conditioning Association.

Jared W. Coburn, PhD, CSCS*D, FNSCA, is a professor of kinesiology at California State University at Fullerton, where he teaches courses in strength and conditioning, exercise physiology, and research methods. He earned his PhD in exercise physiology from the University of Nebraska at Lincoln in 2005. His primary research interest is the underlying physiology behind strength and power performance using electromyography and mechanomyography. In addition to writing textbook chapters, Dr. Coburn has published extensively in peer-reviewed journals, including the *Journal of Strength and Conditioning Research (JSCR)*. He coedited the second edition of *NSCA's Essentials of Personal Training* textbook. He is also a senior editor for *JSCR* and has served on numerous committees in the NSCA.

Kristen C. Cochrane-Snyman, PhD, CSCS*D, is an assistant professor of exercise physiology at California State Polytechnic University at Pomona. She received her PhD from the University of Nebraska at Lincoln with an emphasis in exercise physiology and is an active certified member of the National Strength and Conditioning Association as well as an active member of the American College of Sports Medicine. Her research interests include fatigue mechanisms associated with aerobic and anaerobic exercise, neuromuscular adaptations, and perception of effort during exercise.

Pablo B. Costa, PhD, CSCS, is an associate professor in the department of kinesiology at California State University at Fullerton. Dr. Costa has a master's degree in exercise physiology from Florida Atlantic University and a doctorate in exercise physiology from the University of Oklahoma. His primary research interests involve the noninvasive assessment of neuromuscular function and the physiological effects of exercise on health, fitness, and performance. Areas of research include resistance training, sport nutrition, balance, body composition, injury risk, acceleration, and rate of force development. Dr. Costa has authored and coauthored more than 150 research publications, book chapters, conference presentations, and abstracts. In addition, he is a member of the National Strength and Conditioning Association (NSCA) as well as the American College of Sports Medicine and serves as a reviewer for more than 30 journals.

Dustin D. Dunnick, MS, is a doctoral student at the University of Nevada at Las Vegas (UNLV). Before attending UNLV, Dustin earned his master's degree in kinesiology from California State University at Fullerton and his bachelor's degree in health and exercise science from the University of Oklahoma. During his time at CSUF, Dustin served as the assistant director of the Human Performance Laboratory under the supervision of Dr. Lee E. Brown. His research interests include sports performance and electromyography.

Steven J. Fleck, PhD, CSCS, FNSCA, FACSM, is the executive director of the Andrews Research and Education Foundation in Gulf Breeze, Florida. Before this position he was the chair of the sport science and kinesiology departments at several universities. Dr. Fleck's research interests are physiological adaptations to resistance training and the application of research to optimize resistance training program design. He has authored several books and numerous research and lay articles on resistance training. He is a fellow of both the National Strength and Conditioning Association and the American College of Sports Medicine. Dr. Fleck is a past president of the National Strength and Conditioning Association and has been honored with both the National Strength and Conditioning Association's Sports Scientist of the Year Award and the Lifetime Achievement Award.

Maren S. Fragala, PhD, CSCS*D, is a sport scientist and certified strength and conditioning specialist with distinction through the National Strength and Conditioning Association. She is currently the director of athlete health and performance for Quest Diagnostics, a Fortune 500 company. She joined Quest Diagnostics from academia, where her research focused on the science of sport performance. Having held positions at the Harvard School of Public Health and University of Central Florida, publishing more than 100 scientific manuscripts, and serving on the Biomarkers Consortium of the Foundations of the National Institutes of Health, she is a leading researcher and practitioner in strength training, sport nutrition, skeletal muscle adaptations, and biomarkers. Fragala holds a master's degree in exercise science from the University of Massachusetts and a doctorate in kinesiology from the University of Connecticut. She also completed additional postdoctoral research in muscle physiology at UConn Health Center. With a background in gymnastics and dance, she is a lifelong athlete with a passion for power yoga and strength training.

David H. Fukuda, PhD, CSCS*D, is an assistant professor in the sport and exercise science program at the University of Central Florida. His undergraduate training in production and operations management at Boise State University offered a systems-based approach to problem solving, which provides him with a unique perspective to both teaching and scientific inquiry in the field of exercise science. While completing his doctoral program at the University of Oklahoma in exercise physiology, he devised a noninvasive approach to the classification of body composition phenotypes in older adults. Dr. Fukuda's research interests include the development of performance-based testing methodologies, analysis of physiological profiles, and assessment of adaptations to exercise training and nutrition interventions in various populations, including youth and combat sport athletes. In these areas, he has coauthored more than 100 peer-reviewed publications.

Andrew J. Galpin, CSCS*D, NSCA-CPT*D, is an associate professor of strength and conditioning in the Center for Sport Performance at California State University at Fullerton. Dr. Galpin is also the director of the Biochemistry and Molecular Exercise Physiology Laboratory. Before his position at CSUF, he attained a master's degree in human movement sciences and a PhD in human bioenergetics. His research is focused on human performance and uses the muscle biopsy procedure to examine acute responses and chronic adaptations to high-power exercise from the whole body, all the way down to the gene. As an educator, he disseminates information in graduate and undergraduate courses, podcasts, YouTube videos, media interviews, and his personal website. Dr. Galpin is also a practitioner, having competed for a national championship in two sports and serving as a coach and consultant for numerous professional athletes and organizations and technology, supplement, and industry companies. He is an active member in the American College of Sports Medicine and National Strength and Conditioning Association.

Kylie K. Harmon, MS, CSCS, is a researcher and certified strength and conditioning specialist with a master's degree in kinesiology from California State University at Fullerton. While at CSU Fullerton, Kylie instructed resistance training courses and served as director of the Human Performance Laboratory under the supervision of Dr. Lee E. Brown. Before pursuing her master's degree, she received her bachelor's degree from Binghamton University, where she began a career in kinesiology via strength coaching. She has coached in both the collegiate and the private sector, from youth to professional athletes. Her greatest area of interest, however, is human performance research, and she hopes to pursue a PhD in the near future.

Disa L. Hatfield, PhD, MA, CSCS*D, is an associate professor at the University of Rhode Island in the department of kinesiology. Dr. Hatfield earned her first master's degree in psychology at Antioch University in Santa Barbara and her second in kinesiology from the University of Connecticut and PhD from the University of Connecticut. Dr. Hatfield's research interests include the hormonal responses to resistance exercise, the role of supplementation in resistance exercise, and physical activity in young children. Her current research focuses on enhancing athletic performance through various training modalities and athletic development in children.

William J. Kraemer, PhD, CSCS, is a full professor in the department of human sciences at Ohio State University. Dr Kraemer is a fellow of the American College of Sports Medicine, the National Strength and Conditioning Association, and the American College of Nutrition. He earned the NSCA's Lifetime Achievement Award among many of his professional achievements. He is the editor in chief of the NSCA's *Journal of Strength and Conditioning Research,* an editor of the *European Journal of Applied Physiology,* and an associate editor of the *Journal of the American College of Nutrition.* He holds many other editorial board positions in the field. Dr. Kraemer has published more than 450 peer-reviewed papers in the scientific literature and published 10 books. With a total of almost 40,000 citations on Harzing's Publish or Perish lists, his scholarly impact has been impressive.

Ryan T. McManus, MS, CSCS, is a master's student at California State University at Fullerton, where he also earned his bachelor's degree. His primary research interests involve muscle physiology and how it adapts to exercise and sport performance. Areas of research include resistance exercise, body composition, stretching, and molecular muscle physiology. He is also a member of the National Strength and Conditioning Association.

Vanessa M. Rojo, MS, earned her master's degree in kinesiology from California State University at Fullerton in 2015, where she studied the effects of music as a diverting activity during exercise performance. She is an academic advisor and major exploration coordinator at CSUF. Her research interests include muscle fatigue, diverting activity, and neurophysiology.

Rob W. Salatto, MS, CSCS, received his bachelor's degree in kinesiology with cum laude honors from California State University at Fullerton in 2014. He earned his master's degree in kinesiology from CSUF in 2016. Currently, he works as a teaching associate, instructing anatomy labs for the kinesiology department.

Evan E. Schick, PhD, CSCS, is an assistant professor of exercise physiology at California State University at Long Beach and codirector of the Physiology of Exercise and Sport Laboratory. He holds a master's degree in strength conditioning from California State University at Fullerton and a doctorate degree in exercise science from the University of Toledo and is certified through the National Strength and

Conditioning Association as a certified strength and conditioning specialist. Dr. Schick teaches a range of courses related to exercise biochemistry and strength and conditioning and spent 10 years training a variety of athletes. His research interests center on the impact of resistance training on whole-body and cellular metabolism and hormonal regulation.

Kavin K.W. Tsang, PhD, ATC, is an associate professor in the athletic training program at California State University at Fullerton; he serves as the chair of the department of kinesiology. He is a certified athletic trainer by the Board of Certification, Inc., and an active member of the National Athletic Trainers' Association (NATA). He serves on the Board of Directors of the NATA Research and Education Foundation (NATA REF) and has been involved with Free Communications and Convention Program Committees at both the national and district levels. Dr. Tsang is a past chair of the Far West Athletic Trainers' Association Research and Grants Committee. His clinical experiences encompass physical therapy clinics, high school athletics, collegiate intramural programs, and intercollegiate athletics. He has more than 15 years of teaching experience in athletic training education curricula. His research interests include therapeutic modalities and interventions in the treatment of soft-tissue injuries.

Jakob L. Vingren, PhD, CSCS*D, FACSM, is an associate professor of exercise physiology at the University of North Texas and codirector of the Applied Physiology Laboratory. His major research interests are in exercise endocrinology and resistance training physiology related to muscle adaptations and signaling and how these are affected by alcohol. He is an active member of the National Strength and Conditioning Association and the American College of Sports Medicine and has been appointed as a fellow of the ACSM. He has authored or coauthored more than 70 peer-reviewed scientific publications, 8 book chapters, and more than 100 conference presentations in exercise physiology.

Jeff S. Volek, PhD, RD, is a registered dietitian and professor in the department of human sciences at Ohio State University. For the last two decades, he has performed cutting-edge research elucidating how humans adapt to diets restricted in carbohydrate with a dual focus on clinical and performance applications. He has also performed seminal research on a range of dietary supplements (e.g., creatine, chromium, whey protein, caffeine, carnitine, and HMB) that can augment performance and recovery. His scholarly work includes more than 300 peer-reviewed scientific manuscripts and five books, including a *New York Times* best seller.

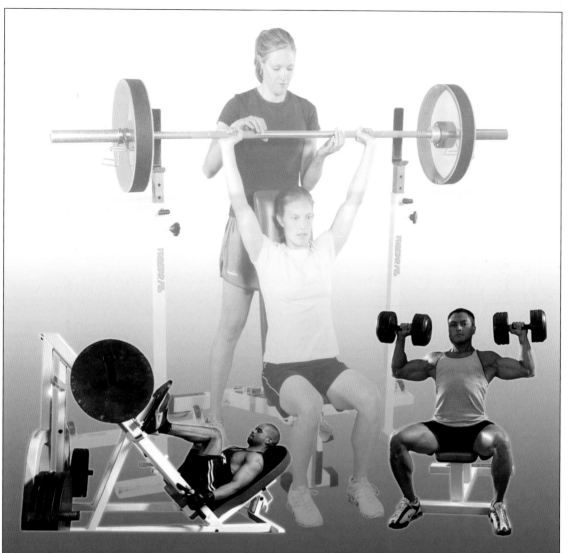

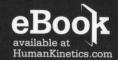